Handbook of
Neuroanesthesia

*Clinical and
Physiologic
Essentials*

Handbook of Neuroanesthesia

*Clinical and
Physiologic
Essentials*

Edited by
Philippa Newfield, M.D.
*Assistant Clinical Professor of Anesthesia and
Neurosurgery, University of California, San Francisco,
School of Medicine; Attending Anesthetist,
Children's Hospital of San Francisco*

James E. Cottrell, M.D.
*Professor and Chairman, Department of
Anesthesiology, State University of New York,
Downstate Medical Center College of Medicine;
Director, Department of Anesthesiology, Kings County
Hospital Center, Brooklyn*

Foreword by Charles B. Wilson, M.D.
*Professor and Chairman, Department of Neurological
Surgery, University of California, San Francisco,
School of Medicine; Attending Neurosurgeon,
University of California Medical Center, San Francisco*

Little, Brown and Company
Boston/Toronto

To Maurice Albin, M.D.,
*whose unfailing adherence to a single standard
of clinical and scientific excellence has been
an inspiration to anesthesiologists and
neurosurgeons the world over*

Contents

Foreword

That a handbook such as this has been conceived by two neuroanesthesiologists comes as no surprise. As neurosurgery emerged as a surgical specialty in the 1900s, the unique anesthetic and monitoring problems presented by neurosurgical procedures caught the attention of a few inquisitive minds. These perceptive individuals became the first neuroanesthesiologists. Neuroanesthesia has since earned its place as a defined specialty, very much as neurosurgery separated from surgery when the demands of the new discipline required a physician's full-time commitment.

I distinguish a legitimate specialty from an area of special interest. Whereas a special interest is the study of a facet of a larger field, a specialty, such as neuroanesthesia, is a discipline requiring focus, preparation, special competency, and depth and scope of practice. At the risk of offending members of other anesthesia specialties, I offer my conviction that among surgeons, no group has greater respect for, or greater dependence on, its counterparts in anesthesia than neurosurgeons. I am permitted to make this observation as a neurosurgeon who has witnessed firsthand the significant contributions specialists in neuroanesthesia have made to the excellence of patient care in neurosurgical procedures.

Why a multiauthored handbook? Quite simply, no single person today can obtain the breadth of knowledge necessary to speak with authority on the many component parts of this specialty. The length of time required for one or two authors to research and adequately represent all areas of professional interest to neuroanesthesiologists would make it virtually impossible for them to report the latest developments in this art. The editors' approach to this volume assures the reader of a current, comprehensive view.

This is an excellent handbook, representing the best efforts of many contributors—among them, some of my colleagues in neurosurgery. The reader of this book, whether a neuroanesthesiologist or a neurosurgeon, can expect a superb educational experience.

Charles B. Wilson

Preface

The expansion of the scientific basis and clinical practice of neuroanesthesia is responsible in great part for the increasing sophistication and success of neurosurgical procedures. Because of our better understanding of how pharmacologic and mechanical maneuvers influence intracranial dynamics, neurosurgeons can now perform more intricate operations on more seriously compromised patients with improved results.

This book was written for both anesthetists and neurosurgeons and is a compendium of the many facets of clinical neuroanesthesia and the scientific foundations on which they are based. The information is presented in a form conducive to ready reference and convenient use through division of the chapters into three areas: general considerations, intensive care, and anesthetic management. Discussions of cerebral physiology, the effect of anesthetics on cerebral blood flow and metabolism, electrophysiologic monitoring of the brain and spinal cord, and barbiturates and cerebral protection are included in the general considerations. The section on intensive care covers respiratory and cardiovascular treatment as well as the management of fluid and electrolyte balance in the neurosurgical patient.

Both neurosurgeons and anesthetists contributed to the section on anesthetic management of neurosurgical problems such as intracranial aneurysms, ischemic cerebrovascular disease, neurovascular lesions in the pregnant patient, vascular disorders and tumors of the posterior fossa, tumors of the pituitary, trauma to the head and spinal cord, and neurogenic airway and swallowing disorders. There is a separate chapter on pediatric neurosurgery because children, despite their smaller size, require the same kind of care as that given to adults; their monitoring needs and the interaction between anesthetics and cerebral pathophysiology merit consideration equal to that in adult cases. The discussion of anesthesia for neuroradiologic procedures is included because neurosurgical diagnosis relies so heavily on neuroradiologic studies. Both general and standby anesthesia is frequently needed here because the patient population includes many children and neurologically compromised adults. The same anesthetic judgment and precautions that are exercised in the operating room must be observed in other locations as well. The selection of anesthetic drugs for neurodiagnostic procedures is based on their effect on intracranial dynamics, just as it is for the definitive operation.

That neurosurgeons as well as anesthetists have contributed to this book reflects a factor of paramount importance: consultation and collaboration between the two specialties have improved the perioperative care of patients who have complicated neurosurgical problems. This spirit of mutual cooperation and regard is equally important in the management of secondary neurological injuries and the postoperative effects of intraoperative care.

Sophisticated monitoring for all neurosurgical patients is essential to identify problematic trends at an early stage, to facilitate rapid intervention, and to avert catastrophe. Because of the complexity of many neurosurgical operations, the information generated by direct measurement of arterial, central venous, pulmonary artery, pulmonary capillary wedge, and intracranial pressures has become integral to perioperative management. In addition to a discussion of the indications for the use of these techniques, the principles and methods of monitoring evoked potentials, electroencephalogram, and cerebral blood flow, as described in this manual, can also provide invaluable data affecting intraoperative care. As these modalities are developed for widespread clinical use, both anesthetic and neurosurgical care will improve.

None of these advances would have been possible, however, without the intellectual curiosity and uncompromising resolve to deliver the best possible care on the part of the specialists involved in the treatment of neurosurgical patients. We wish to acknowledge—through the authors who have so generously contributed to this manual—those neuroanesthetists who have worked to disseminate the principles of the safe and enlightened practice of neuroanesthesia. We also would like to express our appreciation to the neurosurgeons, neuroradiologists, neuropathologists, and neuroophthalmologists for their cooperation and support. The willingness of the specialists in each of these disciplines to share knowledge, information, and responsibility accounts for the concerned and informed care that neurosurgical patients enjoy.

Finally, we wish to thank Betty L. Grundy, M.D., and artist Jon Coulter for the design and execution of the evoked potential motif of the cover illustration.

P. N.
J. E. C.

Contributing Authors

Robert F. Bedford, M.D. *Associate Professor, Departments of Anesthesiology and Neurological Surgery, University of Virginia School of Medicine; Attending Anesthesiologist, University of Virginia Medical Center, Charlottesville*

Derek A. Bruce, M.B., Ch.B. *Associate Professor of Neurosurgery and Pediatrics, Department of Neurosurgery, The University of Pennsylvania School of Medicine; Associate Neurosurgeon, Children's Hospital of Philadelphia*

Neal H. Cohen, M.D., M.P.H. *Assistant Professor of Anesthesia and Epidemiology, University of California, San Francisco, School of Medicine; Associate Director, Intensive Care Unit, University of California Medical Center, San Francisco*

Peter S. Colley, M.D. *Associate Professor of Anesthesiology, University of Washington School of Medicine; Chief, Neurosurgical Anesthesia, University Hospital, Seattle*

James E. Cottrell, M.D. *Professor and Chairman, Department of Anesthesiology, State University of New York, Downstate Medical Center College of Medicine; Director, Department of Anesthesiology, Kings County Hospital Center, Brooklyn*

Khurshed J. Dastur, M.D. *Attending Neuroradiologist, Department of Radiology, Mercy Hospital, Pittsburgh*

Judith Donegan, M.D. Ph.D. *Associate Professor of Anesthesiology, The Medical College of Wisconsin; Attending Anesthesiologist, Froedtert Memorial Lutheran Hospital, Milwaukee*

Elizabeth A. M. Frost, M.B., Ch.B. *Professor of Anesthesiology, Albert Einstein College of Medicine of Yeshiva University; Attending Anesthesiologist, Bronx Municipal Hospital Center, New York*

Adrian W. Gelb, M.D., F.R.C.P.(C) *Assistant Professor, Department of Anaesthesia, The University of Western Ontario Faculty of Medicine; Co-Coordinator, Intensive Care Unit, University Hospital, London, Ontario*

Joseph P. Giffin, M.D. *Assistant Professor of Anesthesia, State University of New York, Downstate Medical Center College of Medicine; Clinical Director of Anesthesia, Kings County Hospital Center, Brooklyn*

Betty L. Grundy, M.D. *Professor and Chairman, Department of Anesthesiology, Oral Roberts University School of Medicine; Director of Anesthesia Services, City of Faith Medical and Research Center, Tulsa, Oklahoma*

William D. Hetrick, M.D. *Clinical Assistant Professor of Anesthesiology, University of Pittsburgh School of Medicine; Staff Anesthesiologist, Mercy Hospital, Pittsburgh*

Robert L. Iverson, Jr., M.D. *Co-Director, Department of Critical Care, Methodist Hospital Graduate Medical Center, Indianapolis*

Jane Matjasko, M.D. *Associate Professor of Anesthesiology, University of Maryland School of Medicine; Staff Anesthesiologist, University of Maryland Hospital, Baltimore*

Robert D. McKay, M.D. *Associate Professor of Anesthesiology, The University of Alabama School of Medicine; Director of Neurosurgical Anesthesia, Department of Anesthesiology, University of Alabama Hospitals, Birmingham*

Frederick G. Mihm, M.D. *Assistant Professor of Anesthesia, Stanford University School of Medicine; Associate Medical Director, Intensive Care Units, Stanford University Hospital, Stanford, California*

Philippa Newfield, M.D. *Assistant Clinical Professor of Anesthesia and Neurosurgery, University of California, San Francisco, School of Medicine; Attending Anesthetist, Children's Hospital of San Francisco*

S. J. Peerless, M.D., F.R.C.S.(C) *Professor of Neurosurgery, The University of Western Ontario Faculty of Medicine; Chairman, Division of Neurosurgery, University Hospital, London, Ontario*

Kalmon D. Post, M.D. *Associate Professor and Vice-Chairman, Department of Neurological Surgery, Columbia University College of Physicians and Surgeons; Attending Neurosurgeon, Neurological Institute, Columbia-Presbyterian Medical Center, New York*

J. G. Reves, M.D. *Professor of Anesthesiology and Director of Anesthesia Research, University of Alabama School of Medicine; Attending Anesthesiologist, University of Alabama Hospitals, Birmingham*

Mark A. Rockoff, M.D. *Assistant Professor of Anaesthesia (Pediatrics), Harvard Medical School; Associate Director, Multidisciplinary Intensive Care Unit, Children's Hospital Medical Center, Boston*

Mark A. Rosen, M.D. *Assistant Professor in Residence, Department of Anesthesia, University of California, San Francisco, School of Medicine; Attending Anesthetist, University of California Medical Center, San Francisco*

Lee D. Rowe, M.D. *Assistant Clinical Professor of Otolaryngology, The University of Pennsylvania School of Medicine; Attending Surgeon, Pennsylvania and Northeastern Hospitals, Philadelphia*

Barbara Shwiry, C.R.N.A. *Clinical and Didactic Instructor in Neuroanesthesia, School of Anesthesia for Nurses, Kings County Hospital Center, Brooklyn*

Bernard Wolfson, M.B., Ch.B., F.F.A.R.C.S. *Clinical Professor of Anesthesiology, University of Pittsburgh School of Medicine; Staff Anesthesiologist, Mercy Hospital, Pittsburgh*

Notice

The indications and dosages of all drugs in this book have been recommended in the medical literature and conform to the practices of the general medical community. The medications described do not necessarily have specific approval by the Food and Drug Administration for use in the diseases and dosages for which they are recommended. The package insert for each drug should be consulted for use and dosage as approved by the FDA. Because standards for usage change, it is advisable to keep abreast of revised recommendations, particularly those concerning new drugs.

Neurosurgeons and Anesthesia: A Historical View

Adrian W. Gelb

Although trephining of the skull has been practiced for thousands of years, neurosurgery as we know it—the manipulation and excision of brain tissue—had to wait for three major advancements during the second half of the nineteenth century to come of age. The most important of these advances was the accumulation of knowledge about the functional anatomy of the central nervous system. This knowledge not only enabled surgeons to locate the site of neurologic disease, but also gave them the ability to remove parts of the brain without leaving the patient neurologically devastated. The second major development was the increase in the understanding of the role of microorganisms in postoperative mortality. In 1867, Joseph Lister published his article on antisepsis, which resulted in a dramatic reduction in the incidence of postoperative infections. Nineteen years later, Ernst von Bergmann, one of the first advocates of antisepsis in the management of craniocerebral wounds, introduced steam sterilization of surgical instruments, which further reduced the incidence of postoperative infection. The third major advance occurred in 1846 with the first public demonstration of anesthesia. Anesthesia allowed surgery to be performed painlessly, so that the speed of surgery became less important than the care and accuracy with which it was done.

The management of the airway during neurosurgical procedures was a great challenge to the early anesthesiologist. Not only were he and his anesthetic apparatus frequently in the surgeon's way, but the patients were often in unusual operative positions, such as sitting or prone, which required the anesthesiologist to be a contortionist to ensure both an adequate airway and satisfactory operating conditions. Before the introduction of the pharyngeal airway in 1908, one method of keeping the airway clear was for the anesthesiologist to secure the tongue in a forward position with a large clip or suture. A suitable alternative, endotracheal intubation, was suggested by Sir William Macewen in 1880 but did not become widely used until 30 years later.

Macewen, regarded by Harvey Cushing as "the chief pioneer in craniocerebral surgery," was a Scot who studied with Lister and later followed him as Professor of Surgery at the University of Glasgow. He was one of the first to use the methods of neurologic diagnosis in the localization of a surgical lesion. Although Rickman Godlee, a British surgeon and Lister's nephew, is often credited with having initiated the modern period of neurosurgery by successfully removing a glioma from a patient (Pearce, 1982), Macewen had removed a meningioma and a subdural hematoma five years earlier. In 1880, Macewen published an article entitled "Clinical Observations on the Introduction of Tracheal Tubes by the Mouth Instead of Performing Tracheostomy or Laryngotomy," in which he described four cases, two of glottic edema and two of upper airway surgery, in which oral intubations were used successfully. The first patient had a tumor removed from the pharynx and the base of the tongue, and the principles followed in that operation are still used today: the trachea was intubated while the patient was awake, the anesthetic was administered through the tube, a throat pack was placed around the tube, and the trachea was extubated when the patient regained consciousness. Despite the final statement in Macewen's 1880 paper, "such tubes may be introduced . . . for the purpose of administering the anesthetic," this technique did not come into use until the development of intratracheal insufflation anesthesia in 1909.

One of the major transatlantic debates during the latter half of the nineteenth century was whether ether or chloroform should be the preferred agent for intracranial operations. Despite chloroform's poor safety record (it was associated with an intraoperative death three months after its introduction and continued to be a factor in intraoperative mortality thereafter), the British preferred it to ether because it produced a slight decrease in blood pressure and thus less bleeding to obscure the operative field. In addition, it was less likely than ether to cause excitement, bronchorrhea, or postoperative headache. Ether, however, was the drug of choice in the United States because it was thought to be safer, and the mild hypertension it produced was not viewed as a disadvantage. It is difficult to determine to what extent geographic chauvinism was a factor in the predilection of each country for "its" agent. Some anesthesiologists believe that the relative safety of ether made surgeons quite content to have nurses administer the drug, and that this is in part responsible for the development of the subspecialty of nurse-anesthesia in the United States today. The greater risks associated with chloroform necessitated the presence of a physician at all times, hence the absence of this nursing specialty in Britain and the Commonwealth countries.

Sir Victor Horsley, one of the founders of neurosurgery as a separate specialty in Britain, was a great proponent of chloroform, despite the associated mortality. He based his support for chloroform not only on his clinical impressions and the animal experiments he performed, but also on his personal response to being anesthetized with nitrous oxide, ether, and chloroform.

Over the years, vaporizers were developed to dispense chloroform more safely, but most did not gain popular acceptance because anesthesiologists regarded their practice as a subtle art that should not be encumbered by scientific apparatus. In 1901, at the suggestion of A. D. Waller, a British physiologist who had demonstrated the neurotoxicity of chloroform, Horsley was instrumental in establishing the British Medical Association Special Chloroform Committee. The committee concluded that 2% was the maximum safe dose, and Vernon Harcourt, a physical chemist on the committee, designed a vaporizer to fulfill this requirement, which enjoyed widespread acceptance. This was due, in part, to the quality of the vaporizer, but probably more importantly, to the growing realization that if lives were to be saved, there would have to be a dramatic change in the way in which chloroform was used.

Horsley insisted on the use of this vaporizer during his cases, and he had strong views on what percentage was needed for each stage of the operation: 2% for skin, 1% for bone, 1.5% for dura, and 0.5% or less thereafter (Horsley,

1906). Although the surgeon was well satisfied with his anesthetic protocol, Zebulon Mennell, the anesthetist with whom Horsley worked for many years, wrote that "it was customary at the National Hospital for a male nurse to be allotted for restraining the patient's movements, not only when the sensitive skin was being dealt with at the beginning and end of the operation, but often throughout its whole duration, and it was common for the patients to complain of 'dreams' after the operation" (Mennell, 1924). Surgeons and anesthesiologists always seem to have differed on what constitutes good anesthesia.

Although Horsley and others may have charted the amount of anesthetic administered and the patient's response to it, the anesthetic chart as we know it today was developed by Harvey Cushing. Cushing stands out as one of the giants of neurosurgery. Not only was he the first physician to devote his time exclusively to neurosurgery, but he also contributed greatly to the development of surgical technique and apparatus (including the Bovie cautery), the classification and pathologic description of tumors, and the elucidation of neurophysiology. While a student at Harvard Medical School, Cushing, like most of his colleagues, received no formal instruction in anesthesia but often administered ether for operations. On one such occasion, the patient died during the procedure. The distraught Cushing and his friend and fellow student Amory Codman began to look for ways of safeguarding the patient. At the suggestion of F. B. Harrington, one of their teachers, they developed an anesthetic chart that was first used in 1894. The following year, Cushing modified the chart to emphasize the importance of monitoring the pulse, respiration, and temperature. These charts were the first formal anesthetic records.

In 1901, Cushing visited Italy, where he was presented with one of Dr. Scipione Riva-Rocci's sphygmomanometers. Cushing introduced the use of this device at the Johns Hopkins Hospital and insisted on the routine monitoring and recording of blood pressure throughout his operations. In addition to using a precordial stethoscope for continuous heart monitoring, he thought that intraoperative pulse and blood pressure should always be related to the patient's normal values as obtained under normal ward conditions. In keeping with his concerns about patient safety, he believed that an apparatus for artificial respiration should be immediately available during surgery. On the subject of anesthesia for neurosurgery, Cushing wrote, "Regardless of the drug to be employed, it is essential that it be administered by an expert—preferably by one who makes this his specialty" (Cushing, 1908).

Despite Cushing's use of a tourniquet around the head to reduce scalp bleeding and Horsley's development of bone wax, obscuring of the surgical field by bleeding remained a problem. Surgeons had long noted that when a patient had partially exsanguinated, the operation became easier because the field was not hidden. James Gardner, an American neurosurgeon, attempted to take therapeutic advantage of this phenomenon by purposely inducing hypotension. In 1946, he published data on the successful use of arteriotomy for the preoperative removal, and then postoperative retransfusion, of a patient's own blood for excision of a meningioma (Gardner, 1946). Griffiths and Gillies, anesthetists in Edinburgh, preferred a pharmacologic approach and used spinal anesthesia to induce hypotension (Griffiths and Gillies, 1948). These two papers introduced the use of deliberate and controlled hypotension in surgery. They also further illustrate the useful interchange that can occur between surgeons and anesthesiologists.

References

1. Cushing, H.   Technical methods of performing certain cranial operations. *Surg. Gynecol. Obstet.* 6:227, 1908.
2. Gardner, W. J.   The control of bleeding during operation by induced hypotension. *J.A.M.A.* 132:572, 1946.
3. Griffiths, H. W. C., and Gillies, M. C.   Thoraco-lumbar splanchnicectomy and sympathectomy anaesthetic procedure. *Anaesthesia* 3:134, 1948.
4. Horsley, V.   On the technique of operations on the central nervous system. *Br. Med. J.* 2:411, 1906.
5. Keys, T. E.   *The History of Surgical Anesthesia.* New York: Dover, 1963.
6. Macewen, W.   Clinical observations on the introduction of tracheal tubes by the mouth instead of performing tracheostomy or laryngotomy. *Br. Med. J.* 2:122, 1880.
7. Mennell, Z.   Anesthesia in intracranial surgery. *Am. J. Surg.* 38:44, 1924.
8. Pearce, J. M. S.   The First Attempts at Removal of Brain Tumors. In F. C. Rose and W. F. Bynum (eds.), *Historical Aspects of the Neurosciences.* New York: Raven, 1982.
9. Thomas, K. B.   *The Development of Anaesthetic Apparatus.* Oxford: Blackwell, 1975.
10. Walker, A. E.   *A History of Neurological Surgery.* New York: Hafner, 1967.

I. General Considerations

1. Physiology and Metabolism of the Brain and Spinal Cord

Judith Donegan

I. Blood flow

A. Normal values

1. **Cerebral blood flow.** Total cerebral blood flow (CBF) in humans is about 50 ml/100 gm/min. However, flow is nonuniform; it varies both with histologic tissue type (gray or white matter) and with anatomic area. Of the two tissue types, gray matter has the higher flow at about 80 ml/100 gm/min. For white matter, the value is closer to 20 ml/100 gm/min. Overall flow normally decreases with age, the major change being in the gray matter. CBF in the various anatomic regions of the brain differs widely. An important determinant of regional CBF (rCBF) is regional metabolic activity; thus, rCBF may vary from minute to minute. When total CBF is decreased to 20 to 24 ml/100 gm/min, slowing is seen on the electroencephalogram (EEG). At CBF of 15 to 19 ml/100 gm/min, the EEG becomes flat, and when CBF is below 10 ml/100 gm/min, irreversible tissue damage occurs at normal body temperature (Lassen, 1976).

2. **Spinal cord blood flow.** The flow in the white matter of the cord, similar to that of the cerebral white matter, is 15 to 20 ml/100 gm/min. Gray matter flow in the spinal cord is about 60 ml/100 gm/min.

B. Methods of measurement.

Some methods of measuring cerebral and spinal cord blood flow are applicable only to animal studies because they require extensive surgical manipulation or tissue sampling. These techniques include the use of radioactive microspheres, classic autoradiography, and venous outflow. The following methods are available for use in awake and anesthetized humans:

1. **Inhalation of inert gas.** This method, as originally developed by Kety and Schmidt in 1945, used nitrous oxide (N_2O) as the tracer gas. It determines the mean transit time for N_2O molecules through the brain by measurement of the gas in arterial and jugular venous blood samples collected during a 10- to 15-minute period of gas inhalation. Other inert gases that have been used include argon, krypton-85 ([85]Kr), and xenon-133 (^{133}Xe), the most commonly used today.

   Regional as well as total flows can be obtained with the use of multiple collimated scintillation detectors placed in various positions over the skull. These detect photons (ionizing radiation), and the rate of photons received by a detector is directly related to the concentration of the photon-emitting radionuclide (^{133}Xe) in the volume of tissue seen by the detector.

3

2. **Intra-arterial injection of inert gas.** This method, described by Lassen and Ingvar in 1961, also measures the mean transit time of a freely diffusible tracer molecule. Although ^{85}Kr was originally used as the tracer, ^{133}Xe is now most commonly employed. The gas is dissolved in saline solution and injected as a bolus into the internal carotid or the vertebral artery. Scintillation detectors are used to measure the radionuclide, as in the inhalation method. Neither of the inert gas methods is useful for obtaining spinal cord blood flow owing to the difficulty of selective recording from the cord.

3. **Intra-arterial injection of radioactive oxygen (^{15}O).** Oxygen-15-labeled water injected into the internal carotid artery can be followed with scintillation detectors, and the same equations as are used with ^{133}Xe can be used to determine CBF. In addition, with this technique, it is possible to obtain regional oxygen consumption. The disadvantage of this method is that the half life of ^{15}O is 2.05 minutes. Thus, it can only be undertaken where a cyclotron is immediately available.

4. **Positron emission tomography (PET)** uses radionuclides that emit positrons (^{11}C, ^{15}O, ^{13}N, ^{18}F). The radionuclide is administered through inhalation or intravenous injection. PET has proven useful for determining cerebral blood volume and metabolism. A satisfactory method of measuring regional CBF employing this technique is under development. A cyclotron is required to generate the positron-emitting radionuclides.

C. **Regulation of cerebral and spinal cord blood flow**

1. **Autoregulation.** In the normal person, CBF remains almost constant, despite wide variation in the mean arterial blood pressure (MAP) (Fig. 1-1). This phenomenon, termed *autoregulation,* occurs not only in the cerebral vasculature but in the vessels of many other organs, including the heart and the kidneys, as well. The cerebral perfusion pressure (CPP) of the brain is determined by the difference between the MAP and the intracranial pressure (ICP): CPP = MAP − ICP. The normal value for CPP is about 100 mmHg. A decrease of perfusion pressure to 50 mmHg is associated with slowing of the EEG. At pressures of 25 to 40 mmHg, the EEG becomes flat; and when CPP falls below 20 mmHg, irreversible tissue damage takes place if body temperature is normal. Since, in the normal person, the ICP does not vary markedly, MAP is the major factor affecting CPP.

Autoregulation is an active vascular response; during increases in MAP, the cerebral vessels constrict (i.e., cerebrovascular resistance increases), and during decreases in arterial pres-

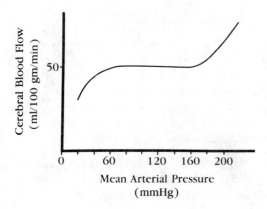

Fig. 1-1. Normal autoregulatory curve of the cerebral vasculature.

sure, the cerebral vessels dilate (i.e., cerebrovascular resistance decreases). The lower limit of autoregulation is about 50 to 60 mmHg and the upper limit is about 150 mmHg. When MAP falls below 50 to 60 mmHg, CBF decreases. When MAP exceeds 150 mmHg, "autoregulatory breakthrough" occurs. This breakthrough is associated with an increase in CBF, disruption of the blood-brain barrier at many sites, and formation of cerebral edema.

a. The time required for autoregulation to compensate for abrupt changes in systemic arterial blood pressure is 30 to 120 seconds.

b. The mechanism of cerebrosvascular autoregulation is not completely understood and may vary from organ to organ. The two major theories involve myogenic and metabolic control.

(1) Myogenic. This hypothesis states that autoregulation is an intrinsic response of the smooth muscle of the arterial wall. When the smooth muscle is stretched by increasing pressure, it contracts, producing vasoconstriction. The response of the smooth muscle to a reduction in systemic arterial tension is relaxation, thus producing vasodilatation.

(2) Metabolic. According to the metabolic hypothesis, blood flow is regulated by the metabolic activity of the tissue. Therefore, anything that interferes with oxygen delivery to the tissue (e. g., hypotension) results in the liberation of acid metabolites, which then produce local vasodilatation and increased blood flow.

c. Causes of loss of autoregulation include

(1) Hypoxia

(2) Ischemia

(3) Hypercapnia

(4) Trauma

(5) Some anesthetic agents

d. In persons who are hypertensive, the autoregulatory curve is of normal shape but is shifted to the right. Thus, the lower and upper limits of autoregulation are higher than in normotensive patients.

e. There is evidence that blood flow in the white matter of the spinal cord is autoregulated over the same range of blood pressures as is CBF. Because of the technical difficulties of measurement in a small tissue mass, comparable studies are not available for spinal cord gray matter flow.

f. CBF remains constant despite increases in ICP to approximately 30 mmHg. If ICP increases further, CBF declines. The mechanism for this differs from the mechanism for autoregulation during changes in MAP. When ICP increases, it produces brainstem ischemia, which causes an increase in systemic blood pressure through the Cushing reflex. This increase in MAP helps to preserve CPP in the presence of a higher ICP.

2. Arterial blood gases and pH

a. Arterial blood carbon dioxide tension ($PaCO_2$). Variations in $PaCO_2$ profoundly affect CBF. Cerebral blood flow varies linearly with $PaCO_2$ from 20 to 80 mmHg in normocapnic persons (Fig. 1-2).

(1) The time course of the response is approximately 30 seconds.

(2) The exact mechanism by which CO_2 exerts its effect on cerebral vessels is not completely understood. The prevailing theory is that changes in CO_2 produce alterations in the pH of the CSF surrounding the vessels and in the walls of the arterioles. This alteration occurs because CO_2 crosses the blood-brain barrier freely whereas bicarbonate crosses more slowly. Thus, increases in $PaCO_2$ decrease pH in the CSF and arteriolar walls. Because bicarbonate ions do cross the blood-brain barrier,

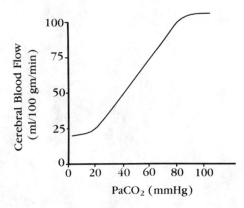

Fig. 1-2. Relationship between cerebral blood flow (CBF) and arterial carbon dioxide tension ($PaCO_2$) in the normocapnic individual.

changes in CSF pH and CBF resulting from alterations in $PaCO_2$ last only 24 to 36 hours. After this time, CBF returns to normal despite continuing hypocapnia or hypercapnia.

(3) Spinal cord blood flow reacts to CO_2 in a manner similar to CBF.

b. Arterial blood oxygen tension (PaO_2). Measurable increases in CBF do not occur until the PaO_2 is reduced below 50 mmHg (Fig. 1-3). The mechanism for the increase in flow with hypoxia is not clear. Hyperoxia, produced by the inhala-

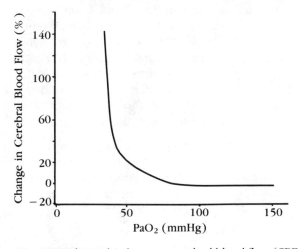

Fig. 1-3. Relationship between cerebral blood flow (CBF) and arterial oxygen tension (PaO_2).

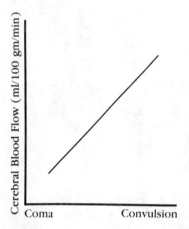

Fig. 1-4. Relationship between cerebral blood flow (CBF) and cerebral metabolism.

tion of 80% to 100% oxygen in the normal person, is associated with a 10% to 12% decrease in CBF.

c. pH. Changes in pH from respiratory variation have been discussed in section **2.a.(2).** Metabolic alterations also affect CBF, although not as profoundly as do changes in $PaCO_2$. Acidemia causes a slight increase in CBF, whereas alkalemia reduces CBF.

3. **Cerebral metabolism**

   a. Total CBF and regional CBF (rCBF). Total CBF generally parallels overall cerebral metabolism. Metabolism, and consequently CBF, are closely correlated with brain activity. When the level of activity is lowest, as in coma, metabolism and CBF are lowest. When overall brain activity is high, as in a grand mal convulsion, metabolism and CBF are high (Fig. 1-4). The same is true of activity, metabolism, and CBF at the regional level. For example, when stereognostic test objects are placed in a subject's hand, there is an increase in rCBF of the hand area of the contralateral postcentral gyrus.

   b. Sleep. Changes in CBF occurring during sleep and unrelated to variations in either $PaCO_2$ or MAP appear to reflect alterations in cerebral metabolism. CBF is reduced approximately 10% during slow-wave sleep and is increased about 10% during rapid eye movement (REM) sleep.

4. **Neurogenic factors.** The physiologic importance of the sympathetic and parasympathetic innervation of the cerebral vascula-

ture has been extensively debated and is still a matter of some controversy (Gross, 1979). Although neurogenic influences appear to be less important for overall cerebrovascular regulation than the factors just discussed, they may be operative at the upper and lower limits of autoregulation.

5. **Hematocrit.** The hematocrit affects CBF primarily by altering blood viscosity. A rise in hematocrit increases viscosity and thus reduces CBF. Decreased hematocrit has the opposite effect. Measureable changes in CBF are not seen with hematocrits between 30 and 50%.

6. **Body temperature.** A decrease in body temperature lowers cerebral metabolism, resulting in a decrease in CBF. The depression in metabolism is about 5% per degree centigrade reduction in body temperature. Similarly, raising body temperature increases CBF.

II. Cerebral metabolism

A. Cerebral metabolic rate for oxygen (CMRO$_2$)

1. **Normal values.** About 20% of resting oxygen uptake is consumed by the brain, which uses oxygen at a rate of 1.3 to 1.6 μmol/gm/min (3.0–3.5 ml/100 gm/min). As is true for CBF, CMRO$_2$ is higher in children than in adults.

2. **Regional differences.** Regional differences in CMRO$_2$ exist. The metabolic rate of the cerebral cortex is the highest in most species studied.

3. **Processes that require oxygen**

   a. The most important oxygen-consuming process in the brain is the **reduction of molecular oxygen** by the electron transport system. This process produces high-energy phosphate compounds and water.

   b. **The mixed function oxidase systems** and the **oxygen transferase systems,** two other processes that require oxygen, are involved in synthesis and detoxification. These systems contribute little to the overall oxygen consumption of the brain.

4. **Oxygen stores.** Oxygen stores in the brain are almost nonexistent. Consciousness is lost when PaO$_2$ declines to approximately 30 mmHg. If delivery of oxygen to the brain ceases, loss of consciousness occurs within 5 to 11 seconds.

B. **Cerebral metabolic rate for glucose (CMRgl)**

1. **Normal values.** Glucose is consumed by the brain at a rate of about 0.27 μmol/gm/min (5 mg/100 gm/min). More than 90% of glucose consumption is aerobic. A small amount of "anaerobic" metabolism occurs normally, producing lactic acid. The anaerobic metabolism does not signify a lack of oxygen, since the normal oxygen tensions in the brain do not limit cellular respiration. The production of lactic acid has to do, rather, with lactate concentration gradients, since if lactate levels in the brain rise, lactate production stops and, in fact, the brain can take up and metabolize lactate.

2. **Relationship between CMRO$_2$ and CMRgl.** Because most of the glucose metabolism requires oxygen, under normal steady-state conditions there is a fixed relationship between CMRO$_2$ and CMRgl. The general equation for the reaction is

   Glucose $+ \ 6 \ O_2 \rightarrow 6 \ CO_2 \ + \ 6 \ H_2O$

   Thus, the ratio of oxygen to glucose is normally six. Under certain conditions, including hypoxia (which activates glycolysis), hypercapnia (which inhibits glycolysis), and hypoglycemia (when ketone bodies are produced), the relationship does not hold. In these instances, CMRgl is not synonymous with cerebral metabolic rate.

3. **Metabolism of alternative substrates.** During starvation, the brain can metabolize acetoacetate and beta-hydroxybutyrate. These compounds appear to be the only substrates that can support cerebral energy production in the absence of glucose. Amino acids are not important in the absence of glucose, and fatty acids are not used by the brain.

C. **Production of high-energy phosphate compounds.** The aerobic metabolism of glucose produces adenosine triphosphate (ATP) according to the equation:

Glucose $+ \ 6 \ O_2 \ + \ 38 \ ADP \ + \ 38 \ P_i \rightarrow 6 \ CO_2 \ + \ 44 \ H_2O \ + \ 38 \ ATP$

The hydrolysis of ATP into adenosine diphosphate (ADP) and inorganic phosphate (P_i) is accompanied by a release of energy. Thus, the oxidation of glucose provides energy for the various synthetic and transport processes of the brain. The level of ATP is not an accurate indicator of the energy level of the brain, however, as the storage form of ATP is phosphocreatine (PCr). In addition, ATP can be produced from ADP by the adenylate kinase reaction.

$$ADP + ADP \leftrightharpoons ATP + AMP$$

Phosphocreatine can provide ATP according to the equation

$$PCr + ADP + H^+ \leftrightharpoons ATP + Cr$$

During periods of hypoxia, ATP levels are preserved, at the expense of PCr and ADP, until the hypoxic stress becomes severe.

III. Cerebrospinal fluid

A. Secretion and circulation of cerebrospinal fluid

1. **Normal values.** Cerebrospinal fluid (CSF) normally is formed at a rate of about 0.35 ml/min. The total amount of CSF circulating in the cerebrospinal subarachnoid space is 130 to 150 ml.

2. **Sites of formation.** Most CSF is formed in the choroid plexus and the ependymal lining of the cerebral ventricles. Some CSF is formed extrachoroidally by the cerebral capillary endothelium, and some may be derived from the water of oxidative metabolism.

3. **Composition.** CSF is not an ultrafiltrate of plasma, but is actively secreted by the choroid plexus and other sites. The sodium concentration of CSF is approximately 7% higher than the sodium concentration of plasma. Potassium, calcium, bicarbonate, and glucose levels are lower in CSF than in plasma, whereas chloride and magnesium levels are higher. Protein concentration in the CSF is extremely low. The pH of CSF, 7.3, is more acidic than that of plasma, and PCO_2 is higher in CSF (51 mmHg). CSF is isotonic to plasma.

4. **Factors affecting secretion**

   a. **Physiologic parameters.** The following factors reduce the rate of CSF secretion:

      (1) Decreased choroidal blood flow and choroidal capillary hydrostatic pressure

      (2) Decreased body temperature

      (3) Increased serum osmolality

      (4) Increased intraventricular hydrostatic pressure

   b. **Drugs.** Drugs that have been shown to inhibit CSF formation in mammals include acetazolamide, ouabain, corticosteroids, spironolactone, furosemide, and vasopressin. Ouabain and corticosteroids produce their effect by inhibiting Na^+, K^+-

ATPase. The mechanism of action of the other drugs is less clear; it may be related to their effects on sodium transport, or, in the case of acetazolamide, the effect on bicarbonate formation.

5. **Circulation of CSF.** CSF flows from its sources within the ventricles through the medial (foramen of Magendie) and lateral (foramina of Luschka) foramina of the fourth ventricle into the cerebellomedullary cistern (cisterna magna). From the cisterna magna, the fluid circulates in the subarachnoid spaces surrounding the brain and spinal cord. The flow in the spinal subarachnoid space is extremely sluggish compared to the flow in the cranial subarachnoid space.

B. Absorption of cerebrospinal fluid

1. **Sites of absorption.** The major sites of absorption of CSF are the arachnoid villi that protrude into the cerebral venous sinuses. Ten to fifteen percent of the absorption occurs in the spinal subarachnoid space, while the ependyma and meningeal lymphatics take up small amounts of CSF as well. From these sites, CSF is returned to the venous system.

2. **The mechanism of absorption.** The mechanism of CSF absorption is not completely understood. At one time it was thought that the arachnoid villi had valves that prevented backflow of CSF from the cerebral sinuses to the subarachnoid space. Another theory was that the arachnoid villi consisted of a number of tubes that provided direct communication between the subarachnoid space and the venous sinuses and permitted CSF to move into the sinuses by bulk flow. There is no histologic evidence, however, for either valves or open channels in the arachnoid villi.

   More recently, giant vacuoles in the lining cells of the arachnoid villi have been described. These appear to develop from invaginations of the basal cell surface and open onto the apical cell surface, thus forming in essence a dynamic system of channels through the cells. These channels allow bulk flow of CSF to occur through the cells of the arachnoid villi.

3. **Factors affecting absorption.** The absorption of CSF is governed by a hydrostatic force. The pressure in the cerebral ventricles and the subarachnoid space is normally higher than the pressure in the venous sinuses, and the process of formation of transcellular channels is hydrostatic pressure–sensitive. Thus, factors that alter the hydrostatic pressure gradient between CSF and sinuses affect absorption. Increases in CSF pressure, such as the increases that occur with meningitis and subarachnoid

hemorrhage, cause linear increases in CSF absorption, whereas increases in venous pressure result in decreased absorption. Some causes of decreased absorption include coughing, straining, positive end-expiratory pressure, and congestive heart failure. Dural sinus thrombosis also inhibits absorption because it obstructs the venous outflow tract.

IV. Intracranial pressure

A. General principles

1. The term **intracranial pressure (ICP)** as currently used means *supratentorial CSF pressure;* that is, the pressure in a lateral ventricle or in the subarachnoid space over the convexity of the cerebral cortex. This definition is a simplification of the concept of CSF pressure, as this pressure may be markedly different in different areas of the cranium, and as CSF pressure in the cranial subarachnoid space may differ from pressure in the spinal subarachnoid space. In a normal person in the recumbent position, the CSF pressure measured at the lumbar cistern accurately reflects ICP. However, many factors, including the assumption of the upright position, can alter the relationship between cranial and spinal CSF pressure. In addition, in the presence of intracranial mass lesions, infratentorial CSF pressure (as measured in the cisterna magna or lumbar cistern) often falls while supratentorial pressure rises. Therefore, the measurement of supratentorial CSF pressure is a useful clinical concept.

2. **Volume of cranial contents.** Because the cranial vault is a rigid structure, ICP is affected by the volume of the various components found within the cranium.

   a. **Brain volume.**

   b. **Blood volume.** The intracranial blood volume occupies approximately 4% of the total intracranial volume.

   c. **CSF volume.** The CSF occupies 10% of the total intracranial volume.

3. The **normal value** for intracranial pressure is about 10 mmHg.

B. Intracranial compliance

1. **Pressure-volume curve** (Fig. 1-5). Intracranial compliance can be illustrated diagrammatically by the pressure-volume curve obtained in rhesus monkeys by Langfitt et al. (1965). They plotted supratentorial CSF pressure as a function of the volume of an expanding epidural balloon.

   a. Sullivan et al. (1978) showed that the concept of a single

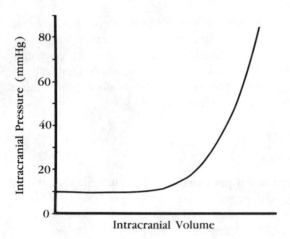

Fig. 1-5. Idealized intracranial pressure–volume curve.

pressure-volume curve is invalid, since equal volume changes in different intracranial compartments produce different effects on ICP. In addition, the shape of the curve varies from person to person and is dependent on factors such as blood pressure and $PaCO_2$. Nevertheless, the analysis of the phases of an idealized curve can be used as an aid to understanding intracranial compliance.

b. The various phases of the pressure-volume curve may be described as a flat horizontal portion (representing high compliance), a steep terminal portion (representing low compliance), and an intermediate portion (representing a transition stage). During the phase of high compliance, a considerable increase in total intracranial volume may take place before ICP increases. This initial stability occurs because there is a certain degree of elasticity in the craniospinal system; in addition, an increase in the volume of one of the intracranial contents can be partially compensated for by a decrease in the volume of the remaining contents. For example, during development of a mass lesion or of edema of the brain, some compensation is achieved by displacement of cranial CSF into the spinal subarachnoid space, by an increase in the rate of CSF absorption, by a decrease in the rate of CSF production, and by a decrease in cerebral blood volume that occurs as a result of venous compression by the mass.

2. Testing intracranial compliance. A patient may have normal or nearly normal ICP and yet be at the limit of compensatory mechanisms. Further perturbations, such as those which can occur during the induction of anesthesia, may therefore be associated with large increases in ICP and a worsening of neurologic status. A method for determining which patients are in this category would be clinically useful. Miller et al. (1973) devised a method for testing intracranial compliance in patients whose ICP is being monitored continuously by an intraventricular catheter. The ICP response to the injection of one milliliter of fluid through the catheter is assessed. An increase of greater than 4 mmHg is almost always associated with a significant mass lesion and is an indication of poor compliance.

References

1. Fitch, W., Ferguson, G. G., Sengupta, D., et al.   Autoregulation of cerebral blood flow during controlled hypotension in baboons. *J. Neurol. Neurosurg. Psychiatry* 39:1014, 1976.
2. Gross, P. M., Heistad, D. D., Strait, M. R., et al.   Cerebral vascular responses to physiological stimulation of sympathetic pathways in cats. *Circ. Res.* 44:288, 1979.
3. Kety, S. S., and Schmidt, C. F.   The determination of cerebral blood flow in man by the use of nitrous oxide in low concentrations. *Am. J. Physiol.* 143:53, 1945.
4. Kontos, H. A., Raper, A. J., and Patterson, J. L., Jr.   Analysis of vasoactivity of local pH, PCO_2 and bicarbonate on pial vessels. *Stroke* 8:358, 1977.
5. Langfitt, T. W., Weinstein, J. D., and Kassell, N. F.   Cerebral vasomotor paralysis produced by intracranial hypertension. *Neurology* 15:622, 1965.
6. Lassen, N. A., and Christensen, M. S.   Physiology of cerebral blood flow. *Br. J. Anaesth.* 48:719, 1976.
6a. Lassen, N. A., and Ingvar, D. H.   The blood flow of the cerebral cortex determined by radioactive Krypton-85. *Experientia* 17:42, 1961.
7. McDowall, D. G.   Monitoring the brain. *Anesthesiology* 45:117, 1976.
8. Mchedlishvili, G.   Physiological mechanisms controlling cerebral blood flow. *Stroke* 11:240, 1980.
9. Miller, J. D., Garibi, J., and Pickard, J. D.   Induced changes of cerebrospinal fluid volume. Effects during continuous monitoring of ventricular fluid pressure. *Arch. Neurol.* 28:265, 1973.
10. Olesen, J.   Methods for measurement of the cerebral blood flow. *Acta Neurol. Scand.* 50:Suppl. 57:2, 1974.
11. Raichle, M. E.   Quantitative in vivo autoradiography with positron emission tomography. *Brain Res.* 180:47, 1979.
12. Raichle, M. E., Grubb, R. L., Jr., Gado, M. H., et al.   Correlation between regional cerebral blood flow and oxidative metabolism. In vivo studies in man. *Arch. Neurol.* 33:523, 1976.
13. Siesjö, B. K.   Brain Energy Metabolism. Chichester, N. Y.: Wiley, 1978.
14. Sokoloff, L., Reivich, M., Kennedy, C., et al.   The (^{14}C) deoxyglucose method for the measurement of local cerebral glucose utilization: Theory, procedure, and normal values in the conscious and anesthetized albino rat. *J. Neurochem.* 28:897, 1977.
15. Strandgaard, S., Olesen, J., Skinhoj, E., and Lassen, N. A.   Autoregulation of brain circulation in severe arterial hypertension. *Br. Med. J.* 1:507, 1973.
16. Sullivan, H. G., Miller, J. D., Griffith, R. L., III., and Becker, D. P.   CSF pressure gradients in response to epidural and ventricular volume loading. *Am. J. Physiol.* 234:R167, 1978.

2. Effect of Anesthesia on Cerebral Physiology and Metabolism

Judith Donegan

I. Inhalation anesthetics

A. Nitrous oxide

1. **Effect on cerebral blood flow and cerebral oxygen consumption.** The effect of nitrous oxide (N_2O) on cerebral blood flow (CBF) and metabolism is somewhat controversial (Smith, 1972). The variant results obtained probably reflect differences in species, methodology, and the effects of other drugs given concomitantly with N_2O.

   a. **Rat.** In the rat, 60% to 70% N_2O appears to have no effect on CBF and a minimally depressant effect on cerebral metabolic rate ($\sim$ 10%) (Carlsson, 1976).

   b. **Dog.** In dogs that were given high spinal anesthesia, protected from external stimuli, and paralyzed and artificially ventilated, inhalation of 70% N_2O and 30% O_2 produced an increase of 11% in the cerebral metabolic rate for oxygen ($CMRO_2$), as compared with 70% N_2 and 30% O_2 (Theye, 1968). The addition of the high spinal anesthesia, paralysis, and ventilation to the regimen was necessary, as N_2O is always administered at less than 1 MAC (minimal alveolar concentration). Therefore, the possibility existed that the effects of external stimuli and catecholamine release on CBF and $CMRO_2$ might have been misinterpreted as an N_2O effect unless these stimuli were blocked by other means. Other investigators found even larger increases in flow and metabolism when 60% N_2O was added to halothane and oxygen (Sakabe, 1978). Pretreatment with reserpine for two days before the experiment did not modify the responses, suggesting that the effect was not due to catecholamines. Prior administration of thiamylal attenuated the influence of N_2O both on flow and on metabolism.

   c. **Human beings.** The results of a study in humans in which 60% N_2O was added to 0.8% halothane showed that, during N_2O inhalation, the CBF equivalent ($CBF/CMRO_2$) increased by 67% (Sakabe, 1976). The authors theorized that decreases in $CMRO_2$ during N_2O should not be large enough to explain the findings completely. They felt the evidence was strongly suggestive of an increase in CBF resulting from N_2O. Other groups of investigators obtained no change in CBF and a 15% to 20% decrease in $CMRO_2$ with 70% N_2O (Smith, 1970; Wollman, 1965). Thus, it appears that the inhalation of 60% to 70% N_2O in humans is associated with at least a relative cerebral hyperemia.

2. **Effect on intracranial pressure.** Nitrous oxide raises intracranial pressure (ICP), the effect being most pronounced in patients who have intracranial disorders (Henriksen, 1973). The rise in pressure is thought to result from cerebral vasodilatation that leads to increases in CBF and cerebral blood volume (CBV). Increases may be attenuated or prevented by prior administration of thiopental or diazepam but, at least in one study, not by mild hyperventilation before introduction of N_2O (Pherman, 1977).

3. **Effect on autoregulation and carbon dioxide response.** Autoregulation is well-preserved during anesthesia with 70% N_2O in response to both hypotension and hypertension (Smith, 1970). In addition, the response of the cerebral vasculature to CO_2 is not altered by 70% N_2O (Wollman, 1965).

B. **Volatile anesthetics.** In general, the volatile anesthetics produce dose-dependent increases in CBF, thus increasing cerebral blood volume and ICP. Other dose-related effects of volatile anesthetics include a decrease in cerebral metabolic rate and abolition of autoregulation (Fig. 2-1).

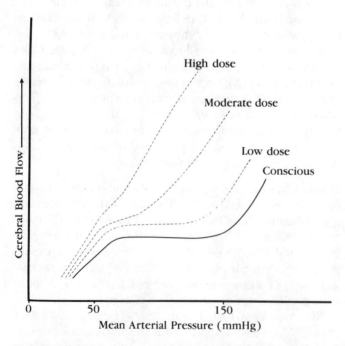

Fig. 2-1. Dose-dependent effect of the volatile anesthetics on cerebrovascular autoregulation.

1. Halothane

a. Effect on CBF and CMRO$_2$. Halothane in clinical doses increases CBF and decreases CMRO$_2$, thus uncoupling the normal relationship between metabolism and flow and increasing the CBF equivalent (Smith, 1972). The effect on CBF is a result of vasodilatation, presumably secondary to a direct effect of halothane on the cerebral vasculature. The decrease in cerebrovascular resistance is dose-dependent as halothane concentration is increased from 0.5% to 4.0% (McDowall, 1967). During inhalation of 1% halothane, the CBF is approximately 25% higher than in the awake state and CMRO$_2$ is decreased by about the same percentage. A study in goats examined the temporal relationship between the onset of anesthesia and the alterations in flow and metabolism (Albrecht, 1977). Two percent halothane produced an increase in CBF of 100%, and this increase occurred before there was a significant change in CMRO$_2$ or any evidence of anesthesia.

That CBF may actually be decreased by low inspired concentrations of halothane was demonstrated by a study done on monkeys (Morita, 1977). During the inhalation of 0.5% halothane, CBF decreased by 17% and CMRO$_2$ by 30%. In contrast, at 1% and 2% halothane, CBF increased by 26% and 97% respectively, although CMRO$_2$ continued to fall. The authors suggested that at low concentrations, the decrease in CBF might result from the marked reduction in CMRO$_2$, which the vasodilatory effect of halothane is unable to overcome. At higher concentrations, there is little further reduction in CMRO$_2$ (40% at 1% halothane, 50% at 2% halothane), and the direct dilator effects of halothane predominate. The cerebral metabolic rate for glucose (CMRgl) is decreased by halothane in proportion to the reduction in CMRO$_2$ (Shapiro, 1978). Regional differences in the reduction of glucose metabolism have been demonstrated; the greatest change occurs in the occipital lobes.

b. Effect on ICP. Because of its marked effect on CBF, halothane can produce profound increases in ICP. This increase can be devastating in a patient who has an intracranial disorder, particularly since, in addition to raising ICP, halothane often decreases mean arterial pressure (MAP). Thus, cerebral perfusion pressure (CPP) may be severely compromised (see Chap. 1, sec. **I.C.1**). The administration of thiopental or diazepam or hyperventilation before the introduction of halothane may prevent, or at least ameliorate, the increase.

c. **Effect on autoregulation and CO_2 response.** Impairment of autoregulation by halothane is dose-dependent. At 0.5%, it is partially intact, and at 1% to 2%, there is complete loss of autoregulation (Miletich, 1976; Morita, 1977). Carbon dioxide responsiveness is retained (Miletich, 1976).

2. **Enflurane (Ethrane)**

a. **Effect on CBF and $CMRO_2$.** Increases in CBF with enflurane are not quantitatively as great as increases with halothane. The maximum rise is approximately 12% to 20%. Enflurane is a potent depressor of $CMRO_2$ and CMRgl. At 1 MAC, cerebral metabolism is reduced by about 35%. In a canine study, this was found to be the maximal change (Michenfelder, 1974), but in a study in humans, metabolism was depressed 50% when 3% enflurane was inhaled (Wollman, 1969). In both studies, the appearance of a seizure pattern in the EEG, which may occur spontaneously during moderately deep levels of enflurane anesthesia, was associated with a reversal of the metabolic depression. A 48% increase in $CMRO_2$ was seen in the canine study when such an EEG pattern appeared.

b. **Effect on ICP.** Enflurane, like halothane, raises ICP, especially in patients who are at the limit of their compensatory ability. In addition, since hypocapnia increases the likelihood of seizure activity on the EEG during enflurane anesthesia, the use of hyperventilation in an attempt to attenuate the ICP response is not feasible.

c. **Effect on autoregulation and CO_2 response.** The autoregulatory response of the cerebral vasculature is at least partially effective at 0.5 MAC enflurane, whereas at 1 MAC it is abolished (Miletich, 1976). Responsiveness to CO_2 is maintained during enflurane anesthesia (Miletich, 1976).

3. **Isoflurane (Forane).** Isoflurane produces a significant increase in CBF (33% at 1 MAC) and a concomitant decrease in $CMRO_2$ (23% at 1 MAC) (Cucchiara, 1974). Isoflurane raises ICP but to a lesser extent than halothane and enflurane. Responsiveness to CO_2 is maintained.

II. Intravenous Anesthetics

A. Barbiturates

1. **Effect on CBF and $CMRO_2$.** Barbiturates, in doses large enough to produce unconsciousness, constrict cerebral vessels

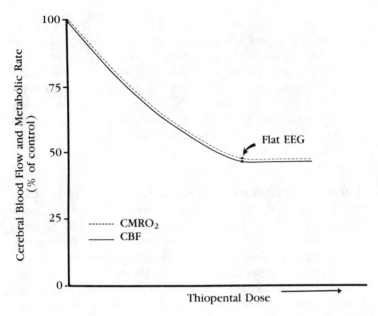

Fig. 2-2. Decrease in cerebral blood flow (CBF) and cerebral metabolic rate for oxygen (CMRO$_2$) produced by barbiturates. The change is dose-dependent until the EEG becomes isoelectric.

and increase cerebrovascular resistance, thereby decreasing CBF and CBV. The reduction in flow parallels a reduction in CMRO$_2$ and CMRgl, and the alteration in flow has been attributed entirely to metabolic changes (Michenfelder, 1974).The cerebral effects of barbiturates are dose-dependent; neither CBF nor metabolism is markedly altered by sedative doses. The onset of anesthesia with barbiturates, as defined by loss of response to pain in one study and by EEG changes in another, occurs when CBF and CMRO$_2$ have declined 25% to 30% (Albrecht, 1977; Stulken, 1977). With increasing doses of barbiturates, CBF and CMRO$_2$ are further decreased to the point at which the EEG becomes isoelectric. At this point, both flow and metabolism are approximately 50% of normal, and additional doses of drug have little effect on either (Fig. 2-2).

a. Analysis of tissue concentrations of phosphocreatine (PCr), ATP, and adenosine monophosphate during barbiturate anesthesia has demonstrated that the cerebral energy state is unchanged.

b. Acute tolerance to the anesthetic effects and the cerebral hemodynamic effects of barbiturates occurs. The plasma concentration of barbiturate at the time of awakening is dependent on the dose of the drug administered. The larger the dose, the higher the plasma concentration on awakening, suggesting that the CNS develops a resistance to the effects of the drug after a single administration. Acute tolerance to the reduction of CBF and $CMRO_2$ by thiopental has been demonstrated in dogs (Altenburg, 1969). In animals that received a single dose two hours before the start of an infusion of the drug, flow and metabolism did not decrease to the same extent as in animals that received only the infusion (17% vs. 40%).

2. **Effect on ICP.** Barbiturates, because they reduce CBF and CBV, can lower ICP significantly. This property has been used as a therapeutic measure in patients who have increased ICP secondary to head injury and encephalitis (Rockoff, 1979). Barbiturates may successfully lower pressure when other methods (e.g., hyperventilation, osmotic agents, or steroids) fail. The barbiturates are also valuable as induction agents in patients who have raised ICP who require anesthesia and surgery. The intravenous administration of barbiturates not only lowers ICP but may protect against the increases in ICP that often accompany laryngoscopy, intubation, suctioning, and head positioning.

3. **Effect on autoregulation, CO_2, and O_2 responses.** Barbiturates administered in sedative or anesthetic doses do not alter autoregulation or CO_2 responsiveness of the cerebral vasculature. The cerebrovascular response to hypoxia has not been studied in humans but has been demonstrated to remain intact in monkeys anesthetized with barbiturates.

B. **Narcotics.** Analgesic and premedicant doses of narcotics have little effect on either CBF or ICP unless arterial blood carbon dioxide tension ($PaCO_2$) increases secondary to respiratory depression.

1. **Morphine and meperidine (Demerol)**

   a. **Effect on CBF and $CMRO_2$.** In dogs, morphine was found to cause parallel, dose-related decreases both in $CMRO_2$ and in CBF (Takeshita, 1972). The maximum decrease occurred at 1.2 mg/kg which reduced $CMRO_2$ by 15% and CBF by 55%. In control dogs, CBF decreased 35% during the course of the experiment. Thus, the vasoconstrictor effect of morphine accounted for about 20% of the reduction in flow. The effect of meperidine on the $CMRO_2$ in dogs is similar to the effect of morphine (Messick, 1969). In contrast, CBF, $CMRO_2$, and CMRgl were essentially unchanged in human volunteers by the administration of a total of 3 mg/kg morphine combined with 70% N_2O and 30% O_2 (Jobes, 1977).

b. **Effect on ICP.** In normocapnic, normotensive individuals, morphine and meperidine in anesthetic doses do not affect ICP significantly. Since CO_2 responsiveness is maintained, an increase in $PaCO_2$ will be associated with a rise in ICP, whereas hyperventilation will decrease ICP.

c. **Effect on autoregulation and CO_2 response.** Under normocapnic conditions, autoregulation remains intact during anesthesia with morphine (2 mg/kg) and N_2O (Jobes, 1975). Cerebrovascular response to CO_2 is maintained with the narcotics.

2. **Fentanyl (Sublimaze)**

a. **Effect on CBF and $CMRO_2$.** Fentanyl, in a dose of 0.006 mg/kg, decreased CBF by 47% and $CMRO_2$ by 18% in dogs, both effects lasting approximately 30 minutes (Michenfelder, 1971). The reduction in CBF was primarily due to an increase in cerebrovascular resistance. Under normocapnic conditions in humans, however, fentanyl does not significantly influence CBF or $CMRO_2$ (Sari, 1972).

b. **Effect on ICP.** Fentanyl has little or no effect on ICP under conditions of normocapnia or hypocapnia (Artru, 1982; Misfeldt, 1976; Moss, 1978).

C. **Neuroleptics.** Neuroleptanesthesia is most commonly induced by combining fentanyl with droperidol (Inapsine). The two drugs may be given as a premixed combination (Innovar). The effects of fentanyl alone on cerebral hemodynamics and ICP have been described in section **B.2.** In this section the effects of droperidol alone and of the combination of the two drugs will be discussed.

1. **Effect on CBF and $CMRO_2$.** When administered to dogs in a dose of 0.3 mg/kg, droperidol decreased CBF approximately 40% without altering $CMRO_2$ significantly (Michenfelder, 1971). The reduction in CBF was due to cerebral vasoconstriction and a marked increase in cerebrovascular resistance. Innovar reduced CBF by 50% to 60% and $CMRO_2$ by 23%. Thirty minutes after injection, the effects on CBF and metabolism resembled the effects of droperidol alone. Thus, droperidol acted as a potent, long-lasting cerebral vasoconstrictor, and the effects of droperidol and fentanyl on CBF and $CMRO_2$ appeared to be additive in the first 30 minutes following injection but not thereafter. In a study performed on healthy patients, the administration of the combi-

nation drug (Innovar) was not associated with significant changes in either CBF or $CMRO_2$ (Sari, 1972). Similar results were obtained in humans in a study of regional hemispheric flow using droperidol and phenoperidine (Barker, 1968). Thus, while species differences exist, the neuroleptics appear to have little effect on CBF and metabolism in man.

2. **Effect on ICP.** The combination of droperidol, 5 mg, and fentanyl, 0.1 mg, has been shown to reduce ICP both in patients who have normal cerebrospinal fluid (CSF) pathways and in patients who have intracranial space-occupying lesions (Fitch, 1969). In a study in which droperidol was given in large doses (7.5 mg–12.5 mg), ICP was not reduced in normocapnic patients who had space-occupying lesions, but MAP was depressed and CPP was decreased significantly (Misfeldt, 1976). This blood pressure response is most likely related to the alpha-adrenergic blocking effect of droperidol. The addition of fentanyl, 0.2 mg to 0.3 mg, did not affect ICP but produced a further decrease in MAP and CPP. Hyperventilation reduced ICP, causing CPP to rise. Neuroleptanesthesia may be used safely in patients who have increased ICP, provided that hyperventilation is used concurrently and hypotension is avoided.

3. **Effect on autoregulation and CO_2 response.** The combination of droperidol and fentanyl produces marked cerebral vasoconstriction in dogs, and hypocapnia ($PaCO_2 = 20$ mmHg) has no further effect (Michenfelder, 1971). The vessels, however, respond to hypercapnia. Therefore, CO_2 responsiveness is not lost, but the vessels are maximally constricted by Innovar and unable to respond further when hypocapnia is induced. The cerebral autoregulatory response during Innovar anesthesia has not been examined.

D. Ketamine

1. **Effect on CBF and $CMRO_2$.** Ketamine is a potent dilator of the cerebral vasculature. Total increases in CBF of 60% with little change in $CMRO_2$ and CMRgl have been reported in humans (Takeshita, 1972). Marked regional differences in the increases in CBF have been found (Hougaard, 1974), leading some investigators to speculate that the change in CBF may be due to regional increases in metabolism that are not apparent when overall metabolism is measured. Ketamine may have direct vascular effects as well.

2. **Effect on ICP.** Ketamine produces a marked rise in ICP both in patients who have normal CSF pressures and in patients whose ICP is elevated (Gardner, 1972). This effect is presumably sec-

ondary to an increase in CBF and can be minimized, but not completely prevented, by concurrent hyperventilation (Sari, 1972). For this reason, it is best to avoid ketamine altogether in patients who have intracranial disorders.

3. **Effect on autoregulation and CO_2 response.** There is presumptive evidence to indicate that autoregulation remains intact during ketamine anesthesia. Cerebrovascular CO_2 responsiveness appears to be maintained, since hypocapnia lowers ICP during ketamine anesthesia, suggesting that it decreases CBF.

E. **Diazepam (Valium) and lorazepam.** Diazepam has been shown to decrease CBF and $CMRO_2$ to the same extent ($\sim 25\%$) in head-injured patients (Cotev, 1975). In normal dogs the reduction in CBF and metabolism was approximately 15% (Maekawa, 1974). Lorazepam, a benzodiazepine derivative resembling diazepam, produced a similar result in monkeys (Rockoff, 1980). CBF was reduced by 26%, $CMRO_2$ by 21% to 30%, and CMRgl by 42%. Presumably both of these drugs would lower ICP as a result of their effect on CBF.

References

1. Albrecht, R. F., Miletich, D. J., Rosenberg, R., and Zahed, B.   Cerebral blood flow and metabolic changes from induction to onset of anesthesia with halothane or pentobarbital. *Anesthesiology* 47:252, 1977.
2. Altenburg, B. M., Michenfelder, J. D., and Theye, R. A. Acute tolerance to thiopental in canine cerebral oxygen consumption studies. *Anesthesiology* 31:443, 1969.
3. Artru, A. A.   A comparison of the effects of isoflurane, enflurane, halothane, and fentanyl on cerebral blood volume and ICP. In *Society of Neurosurgical Anesthesia and Neurologic Supportive Care Proceedings*. Annual Meeting, Las Vegas, Nevada, Oct. 21, 1982. Pp. 98–101.
4. Barker, J., Harper, A. M., McDowall, D. G., et al.   Cerebral blood flow, cerebrospinal fluid pressure and e.e.g. activity during neuroleptanalgesia induced with dehydrobenzperidol and phenoperidine. *Br. J. Anaesth.* 40:143, 1968.
5. Carlsson, C., Hägerdal, M., and Siesjö, B. K.   The effect of nitrous oxide on oxygen consumption and blood flow in the cerebral cortex of the rat. *Acta Anaesthesiol. Scand.* 20:91, 1976.
6. Chapman, A. G., Nordström, C. H., and Siesjö, B. K.   Influence of phenobarbital anesthesia on carbohydrate and amino acid metabolism in rat brain. *Anesthesiology* 48:175, 1978.
7. Cotev, S., and Shalit, M. N.   Effects of diazepam on cerebral blood flow and oxygen uptake after head injury. *Anesthesiology* 43:117, 1975.
8. Cucchiara, R. F., Theye, R. A., and Michenfelder, J. D.   The effects of isoflurane on canine cerebral metabolism and blood flow. *Anesthesiology* 40:571, 1974.
9. Fink, B. R., and Haschke, R. H.   Anesthetic effects on cerebral metabolism. *Anesthesiology* 39:199, 1973.
10. Fitch, W., Barker, J., Jennett, W. B., and McDowall, D. G.   The influence of neuroleptanalgesic drugs on cerebrospinal fluid pressure. *Br. J. Anaesth.* 41:800, 1969.

11. Forster, A., Van Horn, K., Marshall, L. F., and Shapiro, H. M.   Anesthetic effects on blood-brain barrier function during acute arterial hypertension. *Anesthesiology* 49:26, 1978.
12. Gardner, A. E., Dannemiller, F. J., and Dean, D.   Intracranial cerebrospinal fluid pressure in man during ketamine anesthesia. *Anesth. Analg. (Cleve.)* 51:741, 1972.
13. Henriksen, H. T., and Jörgensen, P. B.   The effect of nitrous oxide on intracranial pressure in patients with intracranial disorders. *Br. J. Anaesth.* 45:486, 1973.
14. Hougaard, K., Hansen, A., and Brodersen, P.   The effect of ketamine on regional cerebral blood flow in man. *Anesthesiology* 41:562, 1974.
15. Jennett, W. B., Barker, J., Fitch, W., and McDowall, D. G.   Effect of anaesthesia on intracranial pressure in patients with space-occupying lesions. *Lancet* 1:61, 1969.
16. Jobes, D. R., Kennell, E. M., Bitner, R., et al.   Effects of morphine-nitrous oxide anesthesia on cerebral autoregulation. *Anesthesiology* 42:30, 1975.
17. Jobes, D. R., Kennell, E. M., Bush, G. L., et al.   Cerebral blood flow and metabolism during morphine-nitrous oxide anesthesia in man. *Anesthesiology* 47:16, 1977.
18. Maekawa, T., Sakabe, T., and Takeshita, H.   Diazepam blocks cerebral metabolic and circulatory responses to local anesthetic-induced seizures. *Anesthesiology* 41:389, 1974.
19. McDowall, D. G.   The effects of clinical concentrations of halothane on the blood flow and oxygen uptake of the cerebral cortex. *Br. J. Anaesth.* 39:186, 1967.
20. Messick, J. M., Jr., and Theye, R. A.   Effects of pentobarbital and meperidine on canine cerebral and total oxygen consumption rates. *Can. Anaesth. Soc. J.* 16:321, 1969.
21. Michenfelder, J. D.   The interdependency of cerebral functional and metabolic effects following massive doses of thiopental in the dog. *Anesthesiology* 41:231, 1974.
22. Michenfelder, J. D., and Cucchiara, R. F.   Canine cerebral oxygen consumption during enflurane anesthesia and its modification during induced seizures. *Anesthesiology* 40:575, 1974.
23. Michenfelder, J. D., and Theye, R. A.   Effects of fentanyl, droperidol and Innovar on canine cerebral metabolism and blood flow. *Br. J. Anaesth.* 43:630, 1971.
24. Miletich, D. J., Ivankovich, A. D., Albrecht, R. F., Reimann, C. R., et al.   Absence of autoregulation of cerebral blood flow during halothane and enflurane anesthesia. *Anesth. Analg. (Cleve.)* 55:100, 1976.
25. Miller, J. D.   Barbiturates and raised intracranial pressure. *Ann. Neurol.* 6:189, 1979.
26. Misfeldt, B. B., Jörgensen, P. B., Spotoft, H., and Ronde, F.   The effects of droperidol and fentanyl on intracranial pressure and cerebral perfusion pressure in neurosurgical patients. *Br. J. Anaesth.* 48:963, 1976.
27. Morita, H., Nemoto, E. M., Bleyaert, A. L., and Stezoski, S. W.   Brain blood flow autoregulation and metabolism during halothane anesthesia in monkeys. *Am. J. Physiol.* 233:H670, 1977.
28. Moss, E., Powell, D., Gibson, R. M., and McDowall, D. G.   Effects of fentanyl on intracranial pressure and cerebral perfusion pressure during hypocapnia. *Br. J. Anaesth.* 50:779, 1978.
29. Nilsson, L., and Siesjö, B. K.   Influence of anaesthetics on the balance between production and utilization of energy in the brain. *J. Neurochem.* 23:29, 1974.
30. Phirman, J. R., and Shapiro, H. M.   Modification of nitrous oxide-induced intracranial hypertension by prior induction of anesthesia. *Anesthesiology* 46:150, 1977.
31. Rockoff, M. A., Marshall, L. F., and Shapiro, H. M.   High dose barbiturate therapy in humans: A clinical review of 60 patients. *Ann. Neurol.* 6:194, 1979.

32. Rockoff, M. A., Naughton, K. V. H., Shapiro, H. M., et al.   Cerebral circulatory and metabolic responses to intravenously administered lorazepam. *Anesthesiology* 53:215, 1980.
33. Sakabe, T., Kuramoto, T., Kumagae, S., and Takeshita, H.   Cerebral responses to the addition of nitrous oxide to halothane in man. *Br. J. Anaesth.* 48:957, 1976.
34. Sakabe, T., Kuramoto, T., Inoue, S., and Takeshita, H.   Cerebral effects of nitrous oxide in the dog. *Anesthesiology* 48:195, 1978.
35. Sari, A., Okuda, Y., and Takeshita, H.   The effects of thalamonal on cerebral circulation and oxygen consumption in man. *Br. J. Anaesth.* 44:330, 1972.
36. Sari, A., Okuda, Y., and Takeshita, H.   The effect of ketamine on cerebrospinal fluid pressure. *Anesth. Analg. (Cleve.)* 51:560, 1972.
37. Shapiro, H. M.   Intracranial hypertension: Therapeutic and anesthetic considerations. *Anesthesiology* 43:445, 1975.
38. Shapiro, H. M., Greenberg, J. H., Reivich, M., et al.   Local cerebral glucose uptake in awake and halothane anesthetized primates. *Anesthesiology* 48:97, 1978.
39. Shapiro, H. M., Wyte, S. R., Harris, A. B., and Galindo, A.   Acute intraoperative intracranial hypertension in neurosurgical patients: Mechanical and pharmacologic factors. *Anesthesiology* 37:399, 1972.
40. Smith, A. L., and Marque, J. J.   Anesthetics and cerebral edema. *Anesthesiology* 45:64, 1976.
41. Smith, A. L., Neigh, J. L., Hoffman, J. C., and Wollman, H.   Effects of general anesthesia on autoregulation of cerebral blood flow in man. *J. Appl. Physiol.* 29:665, 1970.
42. Smith, A. L., and Wollman, H.   Cerebral blood flow and metabolism: Effects of anesthetic drugs and techniques. *Anesthesiology* 36:378, 1972.
43. Stulken, E. H., Jr., Milde, J. H., Michenfelder, J. D., and Tinker, J. H.   The nonlinear responses of cerebral metabolism to low concentrations of halothane, enflurane, isoflurane and thiopental. *Anesthesiology* 46:28, 1977.
44. Takeshita, H., Michenfelder, J. D., and Theye, R. A.   The effects of morphine and N-allylnormorphine on canine cerebral metabolism and circulation. *Anesthesiology* 37:605, 1972.
45. Takeshita, H., Okuda, Y., and Sari, A.   The effects of ketamine on cerebral circulation and metabolism in man. *Anesthesiology* 36:69, 1972.
46. Theye, R. A., and Michenfelder, J. D.   The effect of nitrous oxide on canine cerebral metabolism. *Anesthesiology* 29:1119, 1968.
47. Wollman, H., Alexander, S. C., Cohen, P. J., et al.   Cerebral circulation during general anesthesia and hyperventilation in man. *Anesthesiology* 26:329, 1965.
48. Wollman, H., Smith, A. L., and Hoffman, J. C.   Cerebral blood flow and oxygen consumption during electroencephalographic seizure patterns induced by anesthesia with Ethrane. *Fed. Proc.* 28:356, 1969.

3. Electrophysiologic Monitoring: Electroencephalography and Evoked Potentials

Betty L. Grundy

Electrophysiologic monitoring can help minimize neurologic damage during neurosurgical operations. When the function of neural elements at risk is measured intraoperatively, surgical manipulations can be altered or treatment can be instituted to reduce the chance of injury. In some cases, electrophysiologic mapping of functional or diseased areas may be critical. Because electroencephalographic (EEG) and evoked potential monitoring provides information otherwise obtainable only by clinical examination of awake patients, these methods may, in some cases, obviate the need to do major procedures under regional anesthesia or to waken patients intraoperatively for the assessment of neurologic function.

The past decade has seen important progress in automated aids to electrophysiologic monitoring of the nervous system, but many questions are still unanswered. Machines can only execute with literal faithfulness the instructions we give them, and our knowledge is still too limited for us to give perfect instructions. At present, EEG and evoked potential monitoring in clinical neuroanesthesia is limited less by hardware (the machines themselves) than by software (programming, or instructions for the machines); and less by software than by our clinical knowledge about what measurements are useful and what values are alarming.

I. **Applications in clinical neuroanesthesia.** Electrophysiologic monitoring of the nervous system is useful when some part of the nervous system amenable to monitoring is at risk or requires identification; when equipment and personnel are available to obtain technically satisfactory recordings and interpret them accurately; and when prompt responses to monitoring data with an appropriate treatment are possible.

Both the convexity of the cerebral cortex and specific sensory pathways can be monitored noninvasively using surface electrodes. EEG monitoring is useful when cerebral perfusion or oxygenation may be compromised, as during carotid endarterectomy or induced hypotension. Evoked potentials are useful when the surgical procedure might compromise a sensory pathway amenable to monitoring. For example, we monitor somatosensory evoked potentials during the resection of spinal cord lesions, brainstem auditory evoked potentials during operations in the posterior fossa, and visual evoked potentials during the resection of large pituitary tumors.

A. **Technical considerations.** Though Gibbs, Gibbs, and Lennox advocated EEG monitoring during surgery in 1937, and Dawson (1947) described sensory evoked potentials only ten years later, these methods are just now beginning to find clinical use in the op-

This work was supported in part by Grant Number GM 27942 from the National Institute of General Medical Sciences.

29

erating room. Barriers to effective application are rapidly giving way to advances both in technology and in the clinical neurosciences. Progress has been made in the following areas:

1. **Signal acquisition.** Meticulous recording technique may be somewhat more difficult to achieve in the operating room than in the laboratory, but it is no less essential. Currently available technology allows efficient and clinically useful recording of electrophysiologic signals during anesthesia and surgery.

   a. **Recording montage (electrode placement).** Measurements must be made where events of interest are occurring. Single-channel EEG displays reflect only global insults or drug effects, and have limitations even in these applications. Nevertheless, they can provide useful information during profound hypotension, cardiopulmonary bypass, or drug-induced coma. For single-channel EEG monitoring, biparietal or fronto-occipital electrode placements are popular. Other electrode positions may be indicated to avoid impinging on the surgical field.

   Use of two or four recording channels greatly increases the value of EEG monitoring. For example, electrical asymmetry is often the first indication of compromised cerebral function, and asymmetry can never be detected with single-channel recording. Sixteen or more channels unquestionably provide even more information than two or four channels, but both machines and personnel may be overloaded with data unless either a fully trained EEG technologist or an electroencephalographer is available to observe the record continuously.

   Electrodes should be placed according to the International Ten Twenty System. Scalp locations over particular cortical areas are estimated from measurements of head circumference, distance between the nasion and inion, and distance between the ears (Fig. 3-1). It is helpful to have an experienced EEG technologist measure the head and place the electrodes. Symmetrical placement is particularly important when signals are processed by computer. Signal amplitude varies with the distance between scalp electrodes; because voltage asymmetries are of diagnostic interest, unevenly spaced electrodes hinder accurate interpretation of signals and displays.

   For EEG monitoring during carotid endarterectomy, we use a full set of electrodes and a 16-channel strip-chart EEG monitored by an experienced EEG technologist. We also use four-channel power spectral analysis (F3–C3, C3–P3, F4–

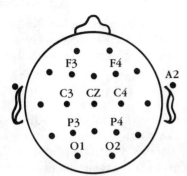

Fig. 3-1. Electrode positions designated by the International Ten Twenty System. The locations not labeled in this drawing also have standard letter and number designations. Note that all even numbers are to the right of the midline, all odd numbers to the left.

C4, C4–P4) and paired Cerebral Function Monitors (C3–P3, C4–P4). For single-channel EEG monitoring during hypotension or drug-induced coma, we suggest P3–P4, FpZ–OZ or reasonable *measured* approximations of these positions (see Fig. 3-1).

Montages for evoked potential monitoring vary according to sensory modality; they are discussed in section **III.**

b. **Application of electrodes.** We use 10-mm gold cup electrodes attached with collodion, filled with salt gel, and sealed with plastic tape. Silver–silver chloride or tin disk electrodes may also be used. The hair is parted but not cut. We tape electrode wires to the face to prevent strain on the electrodes, then twist the wires together at about two turns per inch and position them to avoid mechanical disturbance.

Electrodes can also be attached using conductive pastes. The application is simpler than with collodion, but electrodes are less secure and may be dislodged intraoperatively.

Sterile electrodes can be placed within the surgical field. We use platinum needle electrodes in subcutaneous tissue, ligament, or muscle. Wick electrodes, specially constructed metal electrodes, or electrode sets embedded in Silastic* sheets can be applied directly to the cerebral cortex or other neural structures.

Electrode impedances must be low and matched. Skin preparation with an abrasive gel minimizes the need for light skin abrasion with a blunt-tipped needle. Impedance should

*Dow Corning, Inc., Midland, Michigan

be measured at a frequency within the recording bandwidth, usually 20 or 30 Hz. We record electrode impedances before and after monitoring and at frequent intervals during the procedure, keeping them below 3000 ohm. With our method of electrode application, impedances remain stable for many hours.

The commercially available Electro-Cap* may facilitate electrode placement when electrodes can be placed anywhere on the head and only standard electrode placements are required. Tin disk electrodes in ceramic holders are mounted in stretchable nylon caps of various sizes. Application is quick and easy but positioning is less secure than with other methods, and movement of an electrode away from the prepared area of the scalp interrupts recording from that electrode.

c. **Electrical interference.** Electrical impulses generated by the nervous system are small. The usual calibration mark on a clinical EEG tracing is 50 μV, compared to the 1 mV standardization mark on an electrocardiogram. Some evoked potentials are less than 1 μV in amplitude. To see these small signals in an electrically hostile recording environment, such as the operating room or intensive care unit, special precautions are necessary.

(1) **Leakage currents from other electrical devices** attached to the patient present little difficulty if standard safety requirements for electrically sensitive patients are met: leakage current from each device to the patient should be less than 10 μamp; the electrical system should provide a common isolation grounding bus for all line-powered devices attached to a patient; and provision should be made for dissipating static electricity.

(2) **Ground-loop interference** picked up by cables between patient and machine can be minimized by initial signal amplification near the recording electrodes and eliminated by radiotelemetry or by fiberoptic transmission. Even without these special devices, adequate recording is usually possible if cables are electrically shielded and are kept away from other electrical cords and devices.

(3) **Interference from the electrosurgical machine** remains an unsolved problem. Recording must be inter-

*Electro-Cap, Dallas, Texas

rupted, either manually or automatically, during elec-
trocoagulation. Eventually, it may be possible to analyze
the activity produced by the electrosurgical machine and
subtract this activity from the total signal acquired, obviating the need to suspend monitoring.

2. **Signal processing and display.** Machines serve many functions in electrophysiologic monitoring of the nervous system.
Small electrical signals are filtered and amplified. Responses to
sensory stimulation are made apparent by summation, averaging, or other techniques. Data are compressed to make trends
stand out, or are stored for complex off-line analyses. Information of interest to the neuroanesthesiologist can be extracted
and displayed in a useful format, once the measurements required and the appropriate formats for presentation are developed. When quantitative measurements of interest and safe limits are defined, alarms can be generated.

Filter and amplifier settings vary according to the mode of
recording. Excessive filtering can provide beautiful but errone-
ous wave forms. Heavily filtered artifacts may resemble physiologic signals, but they bear no relationship to the neurophysiologic state of the patient. When electrophysiologic signals are
processed before display, the unprocessed wave form should be
monitored to insure adequate quality of the acquired data. Auto-
matic artifact rejection is helpful but can, like excessive filtering,
give misleading results.

II. Electroencephalogram

A. **Generators.** The EEG is generated by the pyramidal cells in the
granular layer of the cerebral cortex. These cells, with their long
dendritic trees oriented perpendicularly to the cortical surface, act
in concert to generate dipole fields measurable at the scalp. Voltage
fluctuations result not primarily from neuronal action potentials but
rather from graded summations of excitatory and inhibitory postsynaptic potentials. A single surface electrode detects the simultaneous electrical activity of many cells; signal strength falls as the
distance from the generator increases so that voltage is about $\frac{1}{20}$ of
its actual value at a distance of 2.5 cm.

B. **Traditional EEG recording.** The traditional EEG is a strip-chart
plot of voltage against time (Fig. 3-2). Sixteen channels are usually
recorded, but 8 or 32 channels may be used. Most often, 30 mm
horizontally on the strip chart represent 1 second and 7 mm verti-
cally represent 50 μV, but these parameters vary and must be de-

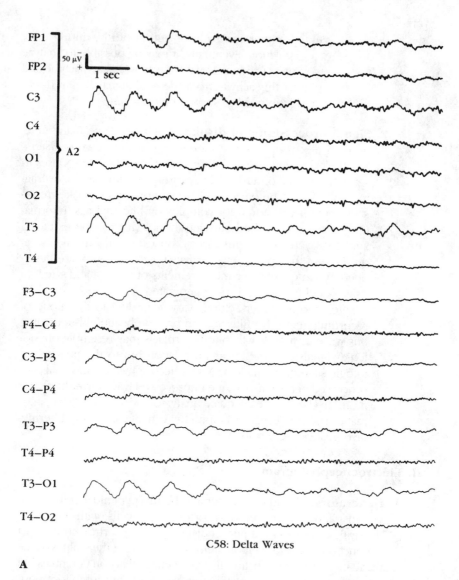

C58: Delta Waves

A

Fig. 3-2. Traditional strip-chart EEG recording, 16 channels, 10 seconds per page. *A.* Delta waves and loss of amplitude during test occlusion of the left carotid artery. Because of these EEG changes, a carotid artery shunt was inserted. *B.* Normal EEG after successful carotid endarterectomy. Note alpha spindles in occipital leads.

scribed. Records normally begin and end with calibration marks of known voltage (usually 50 μV) and "biocalibration," in which EEG activity from a single pair of electrodes is displayed on all channels simultaneously. Comments written on the strip chart by a well-trained technologist are an important part of the EEG record and are critical to subsequent interpretation.

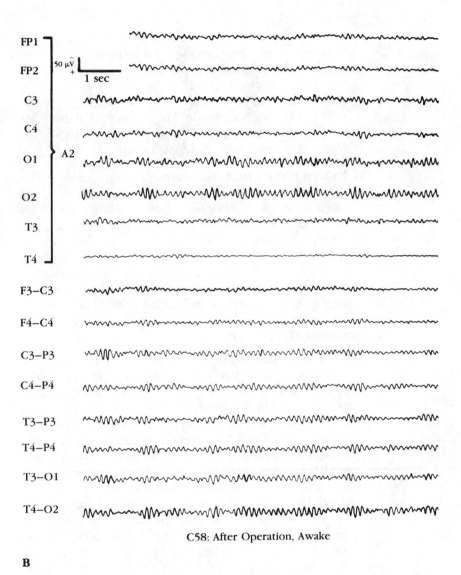

FP1

FP2 50 µV̄₊ ⌐ 1 sec

C3

C4

O1 A2

O2

T3

T4

F3–C3

F4–C4

C3–P3

C4–P4

T3–P3

T4–P4

T3–O1

T4–O2

C58: After Operation, Awake

B

1. Normal EEG patterns

a. Wave forms. Wave forms seen on traditional EEG records are described in terms of frequency, amplitude, distribution, regularity, and specific patterns. Delta waves (1–4 Hz) are normally seen in deep sleep (slow-wave sleep) or deep anesthesia; but during wakefulness or light anesthesia, delta waves suggest compromised neuronal function (Fig. 3-2A). Theta rhythms (4–8 Hz), normally seen during drowsiness, are common during general anesthesia. Alpha rhythm (8–13 Hz) is the characteristically dominant rhythm of the occipital

EEG during alert wakefulness with eyes closed (Fig. 3-2B). This rhythm may be seen over the entire scalp while the patient is under anesthesia. Frequencies in the beta range (13–30 Hz) are common in alert patients with eyes open and during light anesthesia. Beta activity is increased by barbiturates and benzodiazepines in doses given to ambulatory patients; characteristic patterns may persist as long as two weeks after withdrawal of chronic therapy.

b. **Pattern variations.** EEG patterns vary from person to person, with physiologic changes, and with anesthetic agents and other drugs. Effective EEG monitoring during anesthesia and surgery depends not only on recognition of specific EEG patterns, but also on detection of pattern changes during critical surgical or anesthetic manipulations. Anesthesia should be managed to provide a relatively constant electrophysiologic state so that acute EEG changes caused by surgical intervention or physiologic insult will be apparent.

2. **Abnormal EEG patterns**

a. **Cortical malfunction.** EEG signals can reflect impaired cortical function before irreversible tissue damage occurs. With sudden massive insult, such as cardiac arrest, the EEG becomes flat within seconds. Progressive ischemia produces slowing, then loss of amplitude. In 1145 cases of carotid endarterectomy with EEG monitoring, 321 patients had EEG changes when the carotid artery was clamped (Sundt, 1981). In 319 of these, the changes reverted to baseline with insertion of a shunt. All patients who had a regional cerebral blood flow (rCBF) of less than 10 ml/100 gm brain/min had rapid and severe EEG changes; flows of less than 15 ml/100 gm brain/min were usually associated with EEG alterations. Hypoxia, hypoglycemia, hypothermia, and extreme hypotension can also produce EEG slowing and loss of amplitude. These patterns are not specific to the type of injury, but indicate cortical malfunction from any of several causes.

b. **Anesthesia.** EEG patterns produced by different anesthetics are more specific; to some extent, they characterize particular drugs. Injury patterns, however, are recognizable during light general anesthesia with virtually all agents. With isoflurane, burst suppression occurs earlier than with most agents, and electrical silence is seen at approximately twice the minimum alveolar concentration (MAC) that produces immobility on skin incision in 50% of patients. In contrast, high voltage delta waves persist to four times MAC during halothane anesthesia. When EEG monitoring is required at deep levels of anesthesia, isoflurane should be avoided.

C. **Signal processing and display.** Traditional EEG interpretation depends on visual recognition of patterns in plots of voltage against time. This method is tedious and time-consuming. It is inherently limited by the sensitivity and precision of pattern recognition, and it depends on the personal experience, judgment, and attention level of the observer. The amount of data in a lengthy, multichannel EEG record can be overwhelming. Several attempts have been made to overcome these problems by using machines to process signals automatically and generate useful displays. We will confine this discussion to methods of EEG analysis and display performed by commercially available devices that have been used for monitoring neurosurgical patients in the operating room.

1. **Compressed spectral array.** Power spectral analysis converts EEG information from the time domain (strip-chart plot of voltage against time) to the frequency domain (plot of power against frequency for a given segment of EEG, usually 4–32 sec). Stockard and Bickford (1975) described the compressed spectral array (CSA), which is a display of serial power spectra plotted one above the other (with or without hidden-line suppression) to give a time-compressed "mountain and valley" representation of EEG patterns. The numerical data used to generate the CSA are available for further manipulation or for the generation of other displays. Digital computers using the Fast Fourier Transform (FFT) can plot power spectra and/or print digital values for several EEG channels on-line (Fig. 3-3). Although moment-to-moment changes in wave shape may be lost in the transform, there is little loss of data unless frequency components are averaged. The length of the EEG segment analyzed and the sampling rate of the analog-to-digital converter determine the frequency resolution possible.

   We find that the numerical values for power and predominant frequency in specific bandwidths of the EEG power spectrum are more valuable than the plotted CSA for monitoring in the operating room. Often, subtle changes become apparent in the CSA only after the lines representing power spectra for several epochs of EEG have been plotted; numerical values are more likely to show changes immediately.

   CSA programs have been developed for use on general purpose minicomputers. At least three monitoring units with fully developed software are commercially available.* We use the

*Nicolet Biomedical Instruments, Madison, Wisconsin; BIK Foundation, Inc., La Jolla, California; OTE Biomedica, Florence, Italy.

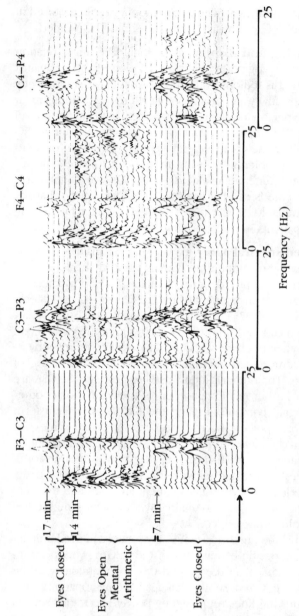

Fig. 3-3. Compressed spectral array (CSA), four channels. Activity in the alpha range, apparent when eyes are closed, diminishes markedly when subject opens eyes and does mental arithmetic.

Table 3-1. Compressed spectral array and evoked potential recording system: Hardware specifications

Nicolet MED-80 mainframe
12 K/20-bit memory
4 K/12-bit buffer memory
Dual display oscilloscopes (Tektronix, Inc., Beaverton, Oregon)
Data terminal (Silent 700, Texas Instruments, Inc., Houston, Texas)
High-speed paper-tape reader (Decitek, Westboro, Massachusetts)
Dual disk drives (8-sector discs, Diablo, Inc., Haywood, California)
Amplifiers and filters: 4 channels
Constant current stimulators
Click-noise stimulator
Visual stimulator (light-emitting diodes in opaque goggles)
X-Y plotter (Hewlett Packard, San Diego, California)
Isolation transformer

Note: This system was configured for the Division of Neuroanesthesia at University Health Center of Pittsburgh by Nicolet Biomedical, Madison, Wisconsin. All components are manufactured by Nicolet Biomedical, except as specified. Programs for CSA and evoked potential recording and analysis are supplied by Nicolet Biomedical.

Nicolet MED-80 (Table 3-1). Its "turn-key" (ready to use) software is particularly valuable. (Industrial sources now estimate the cost of developing computer software at 8 to 10 times the cost of hardware development.)

2. **Cerebral Function Monitor.** The Cerebral Function Monitor* is a single-channel device designed for trend recording of EEG amplitude and amplitude variability in the critical care unit or operating room. As it was originally designed, this unit heavily filtered the analog EEG to limit frequencies below 2 Hz and above 20 Hz, amplified higher frequencies more than lower ones to flatten the EEG spectrum, compressed amplitudes "semilogarithmically," rectified and smoothed the resulting signal, and traced it on a strip chart at either 6 or 30 cm/hr. The resulting records were easy to monitor, but they did not resemble the analog EEG and did not allow extraction of the unprocessed EEG signals for quality control purposes or for other analyses. A high, wide tracing indicated a relatively high EEG voltage with considerable variability in peak-to-peak amplitude; a low, narrow tracing reflected a low voltage with a relatively unchanging amplitude. A second channel on this device recorded electrode impedance, helping to identify segments of the

*Critikon, Inc., Tampa, Florida

record that should be disregarded because of heavy contamination with artifact.

In the operating room, the Cerebral Function Monitor has been used most commonly for patients requiring cardiopulmonary bypass or induced hypotension. Cucchiara (1979) used paired Cerebral Function Monitors during carotid endarterectomy. He found them useful for detecting decreased cerebral perfusion, but they were less useful than a traditional 16-channel EEG monitored by an experienced EEG technologist. Only a few anesthesiologists have attempted to monitor the depth of surgical anesthesia with the Cerebral Function Monitor, and its value for this purpose is doubtful. Quantitative representations of data can be obtained from this unit only by making tedious measurements manually or by using an optical scanner to measure the height and width of the tracing.

3. **CFM 870.** A new version of the Cerebral Function Monitor is now available—the CFM 870.* The CFM 870 is a simple, rugged piece of equipment, smaller than the original Cerebral Function Monitor, with quantitative output that is easy to interpret. For anesthesiologists without special training in electrophysiologic monitoring, it is probably the best alternative to traditional EEG monitoring when a traditional EEG unit and an experienced EEG technologist are not available. The quantitative representation of EEG power and frequency on the digital display are particularly useful. In providing convenience and ease of interpretation, however, these units sacrifice much information; and, because of the single-channel limitation, at least two units are required for monitoring during carotid endarterectomy.

This model differs from the original Cerebral Function Monitor in several respects although filtering, amplification, and much of the signal processing are similar. The CFM 870 provides a digital display of the average peak-to-peak microvoltage and average frequency. Its microprocessor samples the filtered EEG signal every 8 msec and calculates a running average of microvoltage. When the strip chart is set to run at 60 cm/hr, the digital display is refreshed every second, with backweighting over the preceding 14 seconds. When the strip chart runs at 30 cm/hr, the display is refreshed every 2 seconds and shows mean microvoltage for the previous 28 seconds. Each displayed value is plotted on the strip chart. In addition, minimum and maximum microvoltages are plotted at 1- or 2-second intervals with backweighting over 14 or 28 seconds. At the user's option, the

*Critikon, Inc., Tampa, Florida

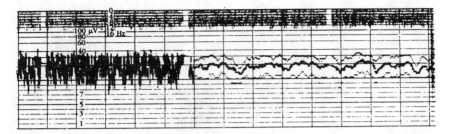

Fig. 3-4. Tracing from new Cerebral Function Monitor, CFM 870. Frequency histogram is at top of record; amplitude and amplitude variability are shown in each of the two available modes.

"actual real time CFM tracing" as seen on the original Cerebral Function Monitor, rather than the average, minimum, and maximum microvoltage, can be plotted (Fig. 3-4).

The CFM 870 determines EEG frequency by counting the positive zero crossings. The average frequency for each 2-second epoch is shown in 2-Hz increments on a strip-chart histogram that is updated every 2 seconds. The digital display shows the mean frequency for the last 14 seconds in 1-Hz increments, regardless of the strip-chart speed.

Like the original Cerebral Function Monitor, the CFM 870 has a separate "front-end" amplifier that is positioned near the patient's head. This unit is valuable in electrically noisy environments, such as the operating room, because artifacts picked up by the cable between patient and machine have less effect on the signal-to-noise ratio if the signal has been amplified before transmission.

Occasionally, when electrodes are near an open craniotomy and a salt bridge forms to the cerebral cortex, or when the scalp is sweaty, front-end amplifiers are overloaded, and the CFM 870 gives zero readings for both voltage and frequency despite normal cortical activity. This problem can usually be corrected by changing electrode montages, moving the "guard" electrode closer to the active electrodes, or choosing electrode sites farther away from the craniotomy site. Drying perspiration from the scalp around electrodes has been suggested, but this is usually effective only temporarily. A voltage divider could be added between electrodes and amplifier to solve the problem.

Because the CFM 870 has no impedance channel, a separate meter is necessary to check electrode impedances. The microprocessor will give an alarm if an electrode is pulled off or disconnected, however, and this condition is shown on the strip chart. Warning lights notify the anesthesiologist of system over-

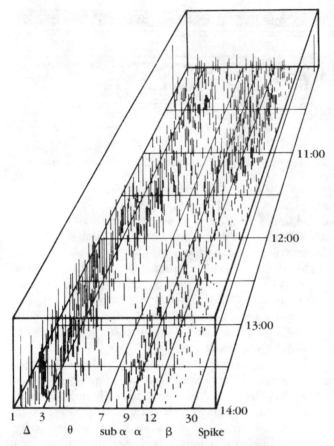

11:00

12:00

13:00

14:00

1   3   7 9 12   30

Δ   θ   sub α α   β   Spike

Fig. 3-5. EEG as displayed by Neurometrics Monitor by Diatek during enflurane anesthesia, light to deep.

load (often seen during use of the electrosurgical machine) or improper zero calibration. Both visual and audible alarms warn of microprocessor failure or EEG microvoltage below set limits.

4. **Neurometrics Monitor.** The Neurometrics Monitor* by Diatek is also a single-channel device for displaying processed EEG signals. Each wave in the analog EEG is recognized and plotted as a vertical line of height proportional to the wave's amplitude. Frequency is indicated by the position of this line on the horizontal axis of a three-dimensional display, and frequency bands are color-coded (Fig. 3-5). The display moves up a television screen with time, and 4 to 32 minutes of EEG pattern can be seen at once. The Neurometrics Monitor gives a potentially more complete representation of information in the analog EEG than

*Diatek, Inc., San Diego, California

does either the compressed spectral array or the Cerebral Function Monitor; but time compression is less than with the two other methods, and this limits the observation of trends.

Two special advantages of the Neurometrics Monitor, besides its relatively complete representation of EEG information, are (1) its preamplifier that can be positioned near the patient with a fiberoptic cable for transmitting signals to the processor, and (2) its electronic data storage capability. Fiberoptic transmission eliminates one of the common sources of artifact in the operating room: electrical noise picked up by the cable between patient and machine. Electronic data storage allows redisplay of EEG data after original recording. Text is entered by keyboard and displayed on a cathode-ray tube mounted beneath the television screen.

The Neurometrics Monitor has several disadvantages. No quantitative representation of data is accessible to the user, and no hard copy record of either EEG display or descriptive text is generated. (Hard copy records of designated data segments can be obtained by mailing the electronically stored EEG and text to the manufacturer.) As the method of wave form analysis and display has not been fully described in the literature, it cannot be conclusively evaluated. The recorded EEG can be redisplayed on the television screen, but there is no way of showing two different segments of analyzed EEG simultaneously for comparison. The single-channel limitation is a serious one; a dual channel machine is now being developed.

The Neurometrics Monitor may eventually prove useful for intraoperative monitoring. It has become available only recently, and its limitations are amenable to correction.

5. **Other methods of EEG analysis.** Several methods for processing EEG signals have been reported in the literature. The methods that allow automated pattern recognition and alarm generation appear very promising for use in the operating room, and it seems likely that several such devices will be marketed during the next few years. Inevitably, large, complex devices that require constant attention will become smaller, more rugged, and easier to use; and there will be less need to sacrifice information in facilitating display.

III. Evoked potentials

A. **General principles.** The neuroanesthesiologist who undertakes evoked potential monitoring in the operating room needs to understand not only the basic concepts of evoked potential monitoring but also the technical, pharmacologic, and physiologic factors that must be taken into account if monitoring is to be effective.

1. **The concept of evoked potential monitoring.** Sensory evoked potentials are the electrical responses of the nervous system to sensory stimulation. If a stimulus (e.g., a small electric pulse) is applied to one part of the nervous system (e.g., the posterior tibial nerve), and if the expected electrophysiologic response can be reproducibly recorded from another part of the nervous system (e.g., the corresponding somatosensory area of the cerebral cortex), then we can assume that the sensory pathways between the site of stimulation and the site of recording (e.g., posterior columns of the spinal cord) are functioning properly. When some part of the sensory pathway is at risk during a neurosurgical operation (e.g., resection of a spinal cord tumor), evoked potentials can be used to monitor neurologic function intraoperatively, guiding the surgeon in manipulation of neural structures (e.g., the spinal cord) and the anesthesiologist in management of physiologic parameters (e.g., arterial blood pressure).

2. **Signal processing.** Evoked potentials can sometimes be seen in traditional EEG recordings, but special techniques are required to make these responses reliably apparent. Although methods such as special filtering of single responses and non-linear analysis have been applied, most clinical evoked potential recording currently depends on summation or averaging of responses to repeated stimulation. Averaging increases the signal-to-noise ratio so that we can distinguish the signal (the evoked potential) from noise or, for potentials recorded from the scalp, from spontaneous EEG activity. Several devices for recording averaged evoked potentials are commercially available.

3. **Categorization of sensory evoked potentials.** The averaged sensory evoked potentials considered here can be categorized according to the distance separating electrodes from neural generators (near-field, far-field); according to poststimulus latency (short, intermediate, long); and according to sensory modality (auditory, visual, somatosensory).

   a. **Distance.** Near-field potentials recorded from the scalp originate primarily in the same pyramidal cells that generate spontaneous EEG signals. These cortical potentials have either intermediate or long latency. Their amplitudes at the scalp are greater than the amplitudes of far-field potentials (those arising at sites farther away from the recording electrode), so that fewer individual responses must be averaged to make them apparent.

   Electrophysiologic potentials generated at considerable distance from scalp electrodes can be recorded by averaging

Table 3-2. Applications of intraoperative evoked potential recording

Auditory evoked potentials
Resection of acoustic neurinoma
Posterior fossa procedures
Resection of temporoparietal lesions
Epilepsy surgery
Localization of specific auditory cortex
Somatosensory evoked potentials
Resection of peripheral nerve lesions
Resection of spinal cord lesions
Operative treatment of scoliosis or other spinal deformity
Posterior fossa procedures
Stereotactic thalamic procedures
Identification of rolandic fissure
Epilepsy surgery
Resection of parietal lesions
Visual evoked potentials
Hypophysectomy
Resection of retro-orbital lesions
Resection of suprasellar lesions
Procedures involving occipital cortex
Epilepsy surgery
Peripheral nerve potentials and evoked muscle potentials
Resection of acoustic neuroma or other posterior fossa lesions impinging on the facial nerve
Resection of lesions involving peripheral motor nerves
Resection of central lesions involving motor nerves

large numbers of individual responses. Potentials originating in the brainstem or in a peripheral nerve are transmitted to the scalp by volume conduction. These far-field potentials have shorter poststimulus latencies than do near-field potentials.

   b. Poststimulus latency. In general, short-latency potentials are less altered by drugs and reversible changes in physiologic state than are potentials of intermediate or long latency. Long-latency potentials change even with subanesthetic concentrations of anesthetic agents; they are of little use in the operating room. Short- and intermediate-latency potentials are useful for monitoring auditory, visual, and somatosensory function in neurosurgical patients.

   c. Sensory modality. For a discussion of sensory modalities, see sections **B, C,** and **D.**

  4. Applications in the operating room. Inviting applications of intraoperative evoked potential monitoring are summarized in Table 3-2. Of the applications now in clinical use, greatest experience has been gained with somatosensory evoked potential monitoring during surgical procedures on the spine and spinal cord. As experiments in animals and studies of human pathophysiology progressively clarify anatomic correlates of evoked potentials, the operating team can be increasingly confident that stable wave forms indicate intact neural function.

Technical difficulties, anesthetic agents, and physiologic changes can all interfere with evoked potential monitoring. If electrophysiologic measurements are to influence decision-making in the operating room, definitive answers are essential: Is the change produced by a loose electrode, by the anesthesiologist, or by the surgeon? Successful evoked potential monitoring requires meticulous recording technique, appropriate anesthetic management, and identification and constraint of variables other than surgical trespass on neural structures that might alter evoked potentials.

5. **Technical factors.** Each team must develop standard recording methods with built-in checks for quality control and must demonstrate reliability of evoked potential recording in the particular operating room environment in which monitoring is required. It is essential that standard electrode placement be based on measurement rather than estimation. Spontaneous EEG activity *must* be monitored continuously during averaging on either a strip chart or an oscilloscope. Artifact-reject options available on many machines are helpful; if the proportion of single responses rejected is excessive, however (e.g., greater than 25%), the averaged wave form is suspect. Baseline evoked potentials should be recorded in the operating room suite before anesthesia is induced to confirm adequate technical function of the recording system and to provide preanesthetic baseline records for comparison with wave forms recorded intraoperatively.

Several adequate systems for recording sensory evoked potentials are commercially available. We use a Nicolet MED 80 system specially configured for use in the operating room. (See Table 3-1 for hardware specifications.)

6. **Pharmacologic factors.** Rosner and Clark reviewed early descriptions of the effects of anesthesia on evoked potentials in 1973. The series reported since then have been small, and the evoked potential alterations produced by the combinations of drugs employed clinically have not been quantitatively evaluated. Virtually all anesthetics have some effect on evoked potentials, as do many drugs used as adjuncts to anesthesia. In general, short-latency potentials are more robust in the face of pharmacologic onslaughts than are later potentials.

The anesthesiologist should use drugs that only minimally modify the evoked potentials to be monitored. A relatively constant pharmacologic state must be maintained during the critical stages of the operative procedure so that changes in the wave form can be reliably attributed to surgical manipulation rather than to drug effects. New anesthetics and drugs that are not part of a group's established protocol should be avoided until their effects on evoked potentials have been defined.

Particular considerations apply to the following groups of drugs:

a. **Volatile anesthetics.** The volatile agents affect short-latency evoked potentials relatively little. Brainstem auditory evoked potentials, short-latency or "far-field" somatosensory evoked potentials, and evoked muscle potentials elicited by motor nerve stimulation can be reliably recorded during halothane or enflurane anesthesia. Sensory evoked potentials of intermediate latency can be recorded if very low concentrations of these agents are administered, but at MAC and higher concentrations, these potentials may be severely altered or abolished.

b. **Anesthetic gases.** Explosive agents are unacceptable; evoked potential monitoring equipment that is safe for use in the presence of flammable gases is not available. We therefore need consider only nitrous oxide (N_2O). This gas alters evoked potentials to a lesser extent than any agent in the anesthetic regimen. Clinically useful concentrations do affect long-latency evoked responses, but short- and intermediate-latency potentials can be recorded reliably.

N_2O can enlarge closed air spaces, diffusing into these spaces more rapidly than nitrogen can be removed. If the middle ear air space were to be enlarged, auditory evoked potentials might be delayed. The clinical importance of this problem is not clear, but any resulting latency changes should affect all peaks equally. Possible confusion could be avoided by measuring interpeak, as well as absolute, latencies.

c. **Intravenous anesthetics.** Short- and intermediate-latency potentials can be recorded after moderate doses of barbiturates, narcotics, or diazepam have been administered, but long-latency potentials are altered or abolished. Low doses of barbiturates and narcotics may enhance intermediate-latency somatosensory evoked potentials. Diazepam in low doses alters but does not abolish these responses. Droperidol is erratic in its effects and should be avoided when potentials of intermediate or long latency are to be recorded. The effects of other intravenous agents have yet to be established.

d. **Muscle relaxants.** Effects of neuromuscular blocking agents on sensory evoked potentials have not been fully examined, but they appear to be of little consequence. Although some observers have encountered difficulty in monitoring somatosensory evoked potentials during neuromuscular blockade, we have not found this to be a problem. That part of an evoked potential arising from the sensory impulses generated by motor activity would, of course, be lost during the period of neuromuscular blockade. Perhaps adequate direct stimulation of the sensory nerve was not achieved in those cases where muscle relaxants abolished the somatosensory evoked potential. Neuromuscular blockade must, of course, be allowed to dissipate when evoked muscle activity is to be monitored.

7. **Physiologic factors.** Variations in body temperature, arterial blood pressure, intracranial pressure (ICP), tissue perfusion, arterial tensions of oxygen and carbon dioxide, and body chemistry can alter evoked potentials. In general, potentials of longer latency (those further removed in time from stimulus) are more sensitive to such factors than are short-latency potentials, but all may be affected by physiologic changes commonly observed during anesthesia and surgery. For example, even short-latency potentials are delayed by modest hypothermia. Physiologic changes interact with drug effects to alter evoked potentials in complex ways that are not yet fully defined. The neuroanesthesiologist must monitor physiologic variables that can alter evoked potentials and keep them as constant as possible, particularly during critical phases of the surgical procedure.

B. Auditory evoked potentials

1. **Generators.** Generators of specific waves in the brainstem auditory evoked potential complex (Fig. 3-6) have been tentatively described on the basis of studies in animals and clinical-pathologic correlations in patients (Table 3-3). Although the identity of these generators has not been definitely established, the concepts are clinically useful. Clearly, each wave represents not isolated activity from a single source, but a composite of simultaneous activity at multiple sites. Both ascending volleys in axons and action potentials in brainstem nuclei are thought to contribute to the observed wave forms. The cortical components of intermediate- and long-latency auditory evoked potentials,

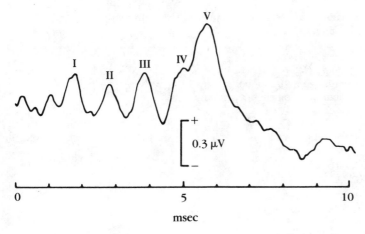

Fig. 3-6. Normal brainstem auditory evoked potential. Stimulation and recording parameters are shown in Table 3-4.

just as the spontaneous EEG recorded at the scalp, probably represent the graded summation of inhibitory and excitatory postsynaptic potentials in pyramidal cells.

2. **Methods.** The stimulation and recording parameters used for intraoperative monitoring of brainstem auditory evoked potentials at the University Health Center of Pittsburgh are shown in Table 3-4. For cortical auditory evoked potentials, we use the same stimulus and the same electrode montage; rates of stimulation and sampling, sweep times, and numbers of repetitions are set to record intermediate-latency evoked potentials (see Table 3-7).

The large shielded earphones used for auditory stimulation in the evoked potential laboratory are not appropriate for use during posterior fossa or temporoparietal craniotomy, because they

Table 3-3. Purported generators of brainstem auditory evoked potential waves

Wave	Purported generator
I	Extracranial auditory nerve
II	Intracranial auditory nerve and/or cochlear nucleus
III	Superior olive
IV	Lateral lemniscus
V	Inferior colliculus
VI	Thalamus
VII	Thalamocortical radiation

Table 3-4. Stimulation and recording parameters for brainstem auditory evoked potentials

---

Stimulation
    Ear insert transducer (Madsen Electronics, Inc., Buffalo, New York)
    Clicks: alternating rarefaction/condensation
    Volume: 60 decibels above patient's sensation level
    Duration: 100 μsec
    Rate: 11.2 Hz
    Masking contralateral ear: white noise, 35 decibels above average hearing level
Recording
    Channel 1: CZ–A1
    Channel 2: CZ–A2
    Ground: FpZ
    Filters: 30–3000 Hz
    Sensitivity: ±25 μV full scale
    Sweep time: 10.24 msec
    Sampling rate: 50,000 Hz
    Repetitions: 2000

---

would limit access to the surgical field. We use Madsen Electronics* speakers attached to ear inserts that fit into the external auditory canal like the earpieces of a stethoscope. With clicks of alternating polarity (rarefaction and condensation), stimulus artifact is minimal. Recording electrodes on the anterior surface of the earlobe are well away from the surgical field.

3. **Applications.** Auditory evoked potentials of both short and intermediate latency have been used to assess eighth nerve and brainstem function during neurosurgical operations in the posterior fossa. The patient who has an acoustic neuroma and intact function of the affected eighth nerve is a prime candidate for intraoperative monitoring. Auditory evoked potentials can also be used to monitor the effects of retractor pressure on the eighth nerve or brainstem, so that the appropriate adjustments can be made before irreversible damage occurs. Moreover, auditory evoked potential alterations may prove to be sensitive indicators of impending transtentorial brainstem herniation. Because they are less affected by anesthetic agents, brainstem auditory evoked potentials (see Fig. 3-6) are preferable to intermediate-latency potentials for intraoperative monitoring of eighth nerve and brainstem function. These short-latency potentials would not be useful for monitoring cortical function; however, potentials of intermediate latency may be helpful during

*Buffalo, New York

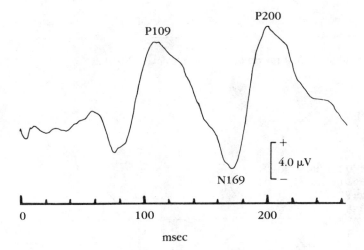

Fig. 3-7. Normal visual evoked potential. Stimulation and recording parameters are shown in Table 3-5. Peaks are labeled *P* for positive and *N* for negative, with numbers indicating poststimulus latency.

extracranial-intracranial bypass or resection of temporoparietal lesions when cortical function is at risk.

C. Visual evoked potentials

1. **Generators.** Intermediate-latency visual evoked potentials arise in the occipital poles of the cerebral cortex (Fig. 3-7). Whole-field stimulation of either eye normally produces potentials in both right and left occipital cortex. Satisfactory methods for hemifield stimulation during anesthesia and operation have not been developed. Far-field visual evoked potentials have received little attention.

2. **Methods.** Visual stimulation during anesthesia can be accomplished using light-emitting diodes embedded either in contact lenses or in opaque goggles for use over closed eyes. Only the latter are commercially available. Although pattern-reversal stimulation is usually preferable to flash stimulation in the diagnostic laboratory, in the operating room we are limited to flash stimulation; patterns would not be apparent through closed eyelids. We use the stimulation and recording parameters shown in Table 3-5.

3. **Applications.** Intraoperative monitoring of visual evoked potentials is most frequently used during operations on the pituitary gland, but monitoring can also be helpful during operations on retrobulbar lesions, lesions of the sphenoid wing, or

Table 3-5. Stimulation and recording parameters for visual evoked potentials

---

Stimulation
  Flash: light-emitting diode array on opaque goggles over closed eyelids
  Duration: 5 msec
  Rate: 1.9 Hz
Recording
  Channel 1: 01–A2
  Channel 2: 02–A1
  Ground: FpZ
  Filters: 1–1500 Hz
  Sensitivity: ±50 μV full scale
  Sweeptime: 262 msec
  Sampling rate: 3906 Hz
  Repetitions: 128

---

other lesions impinging on the optic nerves or tracts. In addition, visual evoked potentials may prove useful during operations on the occipital poles of the cerebral cortex or during neurovascular operations that might jeopardize the blood supply to this part of the brain. Ophthalmologists record electroretinograms (ERG) to evaluate retinal disorders, but we have not employed ERG monitoring in neurosurgical patients.

D. Somatosensory evoked potentials

1. Generators. Intermediate-latency somatosensory evoked potentials originate from pyramidal cells in the specific somatosensory areas of the postcentral gyrus (Fig. 3-8). Although genera-

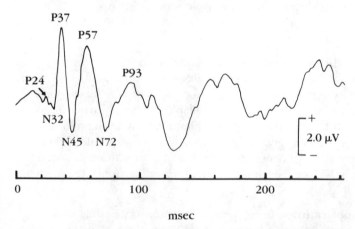

Fig. 3-8. Normal somatosensory cortical evoked potential. Stimulation (right posterior tibial nerve) and recording parameters are shown in Table 3-7. Peaks are labeled to show polarity and poststimulus latency.

Table 3-6. Purported generators of short-latency somatosensory evoked potentials to median nerve stimulation, recording CZ-knee

Wave	Purported generator
P9	Distal brachial plexus
P11	Entry to spinal cord
P13	Cervical cord
P14	Brainstem

tors of specific waves in short-latency somatosensory evoked potentials have not been conclusively identified, recent studies suggest the sources listed in Table 3-6.

2. Methods. We use subdermal platinum electrodes to stimulate peripheral nerves with brief electrical pulses. In our experience, surface electrodes give adequate stimulation only when pressure is applied, which seems undesirable during lengthy operations. Our stimulation and recording parameters for intermediate-latency somatosensory evoked potentials are shown in Table 3-7. Parameters suggested for recording short-latency somatosensory evoked potentials appear in Table 3-8.

Table 3-7. Stimulation and recording parameters for intermediate-latency somatosensory evoked potentials

Stimulation
 Posterior tibial nerve at ankle or median nerve at wrist
 Surface or subdermal electrodes
 Constant current square wave pulses slightly above motor threshold (usually 5–15 mamp)
 Duration: 250 μsec
 Rate: 0.9 Hz
Recording

	Channel 1	Channel 2	Ground
For right posterior tibial nerve	C1′–FZ	C1′–A2	right popliteal fossa
For left posterior tibial nerve	C2′–FZ	C2′–A2	left popliteal fossa
For right median nerve	C3′–FZ	C3′–A1	right antecubital fossa
For left median nerve	C4′–FZ	C4′–A2	left antecubital fossa

Filters: 1–1500 Hz
Sensitivity: ±50 μV full scale
Sweep time: 262 msec
Sampling rate: 3906 Hz
Repetitions: 128

Note: C1′ = 2 cm behind C1; C2′ = 2 cm behind C2; C3′ = 2 cm behind C3; C4′ = 2 cm behind C4.

Table 3-8. Stimulation and recording parameters for short-latency somatosensory evoked potentials (for right median nerve stimulation)

Stimulation
    Right median nerve at wrist
    Surface or subdermal electrodes
    Constant current square wave pulses slightly above motor threshold, usually
       5–15 mamp
    Duration: 250 μsec
    Rate: 5 Hz

Recording
    Channel 1: EPr–C3′
    Channel 2: FZ–C3′
    Channel 3: FZ–N2
    Channel 4: FZ–EPr
    Ground: right forearm

Back
    Filters: 30–3000 Hz
    Sensitivity: ±50 μV full scale
    Sweep time: 40 msec
    Repetitions: 1000

Note: EPr = Erb's point, right: C3′ = 2 cm behind C3: N2 = back of neck over second cervical vertebra

3. **Applications.** Because the somatosensory system has many available sites for stimulation and because this system traverses such a large proportion of the nervous system, somatosensory evoked potential monitoring finds many applications in neurosurgical patients. Spinal cord function has been monitored most frequently, but somatosensory function from peripheral nerve to cerebral cortex can be monitored equally well. If a sensory pathway is at risk during surgery, it can be monitored by stimulating distally and recording proximally. Most experience has been with intermediate-latency evoked potentials recorded from scalp electrodes (see Fig. 3-8); these potentials are altered if any part of the monitored pathway is compromised. Short-latency somatosensory evoked potentials are less affected by anesthetics, but more recording channels are required, and there is less cumulative intraoperative monitoring experience with short-latency somatosensory evoked potentials than with potentials of intermediate latency.

E. **Multimodality evoked potentials.** Present methods require that potentials produced by stimulation in each sensory modality be recorded separately, and the time needed to obtain full sets of multimodality evoked potential records is excessive for intraopera-

tive monitoring. Greenberg (1977) has described the use of multimodality evoked potentials in the critical care unit. These methods
may become valuable for monitoring in the operating room as
more rapid methods of signal analysis become available.

IV. **Corticography and stereotactic recording.** Corticography has
been important primarily for identifying epileptic foci that are to be
resected. Somatosensory evoked potentials recorded directly from the
cerebral cortex have been used for cortical mapping. Wick electrodes
or Silastic sheets with embedded electrodes are placed directly on the
exposed cortex, and the responses evoked by somatosensory stimulation are used to identify the sensorimotor strip for the surgeon.

Spontaneous EEG and evoked potential recordings are important for
identifying structures in the depths of the brain during stereotactic
operations when these operations are performed without the benefit of
intraoperative computerized tomography. Radiographic control of
stereotactic operations may largely replace control by EEG and
evoked potential recording, but advances in stereotactic neurosurgery
are likely to offer important new opportunities for electrophysiologic
monitoring.

V. **Guidelines for anesthetic care.** It is essential that surgeons, anesthesiologists, and neurophysiologists fully understand the requirements and constraints under which they mutually work. Reliably
functional protocols should be developed for electrophysiologic monitoring in specific situations, and necessary deviations from the protocol
should be communicated to team members immediately.

A. **Preoperative assessment.** The neuroanesthesiologist and neurosurgeon must jointly determine needs for intraoperative electrophysiologic recording.

1. Is EEG or evoked potential monitoring likely to provide information that can be acted on intraoperatively to improve the
outcome of anesthesia and surgery?

2. Which electrophysiologic measurements would be altered most
readily by the particular neurologic injury for which a patient
may be at risk?

3. What sites for stimulation and recording will be accessible during this procedure?

4. What physiologic manipulations might facilitate the surgical procedure, minimizing trauma to neural tissue, and how would
these physiologic manipulations affect the contemplated EEG or
evoked potential monitoring?

B. Pharmacologic management

1. **Monitoring requirements.** The anesthesiologist must select drugs that provide for the patient's safety and comfort, that maximally facilitate the operative procedure, and that minimally alter the EEG or the evoked potentials to be monitored. Once monitoring requirements are defined, the choice of anesthetic technique may be altered accordingly. For example, when intermediate-latency sensory evoked potentials are to be monitored, halogenated agents will not be used. If muscle activity evoked by motor nerve stimulation must be monitored, however, halogenated agents may be specifically chosen to ensure immobility of the patient in the absence of neuromuscular blockade. There are few situations in which individual patients require anesthetic regimens that interfere with intraoperative evoked potential monitoring.

   A relatively constant anesthetic state is needed to facilitate electrophysiologic monitoring, and patients should awaken rapidly at the conclusion of surgery to facilitate clinical neurologic assessment. Balanced anesthesia with nitrous oxide, thiopental, fentanyl, and muscle relaxants is usually suitable. Halothane or isoflurane can be added when neuromuscular blockade must be allowed to dissipate. These volatile agents do not interfere with monitoring of EEG or short-latency evoked potentials. Because early postoperative assessment is important in patients at risk for intraoperative neurologic injury, we avoid drugs with a long duration of action. Ketamine, scopolamine, and large doses of droperidol are particularly undesirable because of their prolonged and erratic effects on mental status in the postoperative period.

2. **Anesthetic regimen.** We premedicate patients with hydroxyzine and atropine, adding meperidine when patients are in pain or when additional sedation is indicated. Induction of anesthesia is with thiopental (2–7 mg/kg) in divided doses and N_2O (50%–70%) in oxygen. Pancuronium (0.1 mg/kg) provides muscle relaxation. Fentanyl (5 μg/kg) is given in divided doses before the skin incision. At the time of incision, thiopental (1 mg/kg) is given as a bolus and a constant infusion of thiopental is begun at 1 to 4 mg/kg/hr. Incremental doses of pancuronium and fentanyl are administered as necessary. The infusion of thiopental is terminated when wound closure begins or earlier if clinically indicated. Reversal of neuromuscular blockade and withdrawal of N_2O at the conclusion of the procedure produce prompt awakening of the patient.

C. **Physiologic management.** A primary goal of anesthetic care is maintenance of physiologic stability. However, specific physiologic manipulations are often used to facilitate neurosurgical operations or to minimize neurologic damage. The anesthesiologist can make evoked potential monitoring more effective by maintaining a relatively constant physiologic state during critical monitoring periods. With each change of state (e.g., hypothermia, hypotension, hemodilution), new "baseline" evoked potentials must be recorded for comparison with wave forms recorded during subsequent operative manipulation.

To induce hypotension we use nitroprusside or trimethaphan. Ephedrine and dopamine are drugs of choice to raise arterial blood pressure. Volume loading to minimize vasospasm is accomplished using albumin and a balanced salt solution. Packed red cells and whole blood are given to maintain an arterial hematocrit of 30% to 35%. Unintentional hypothermia is a common problem. To maintain normothermia, we use heated humidification of inspired gases, radiant and blanket heaters, and cotton webbing wraps for extremities. Elevation of room temperature is rarely necessary.

D. **Monitoring.** Arterial blood pressure, temperature, blood gas tensions, and hematocrit must be measured; changes in these parameters can alter evoked potentials. In addition, we routinely monitor the electrocardiogram, central venous pressure, urine output, inspired oxygen concentration, neuromuscular blockade, and serum electrolytes, albumin, and osmolality.

VI. **Perspective.** Intraoperative EEG and evoked potential monitoring are now practical, but some problems remain. Technical difficulties include cost, the lack of standardization in equipment and recording techniques, the need for a high level of operator training, the requirement for excessive operator-machine interaction, and the inability to record during use of the electrosurgical machine. We do not yet fully understand the anatomic correlates of evoked potential wave forms, and totally satisfactory methods of signal analysis have yet to be developed.

All of these problems are amenable to solution using currently available technology. Collaboration among neurophysiologists, clinicians, and manufacturers will facilitate standardization of equipment and recording methods. The levels of operator training and operator-machine interaction now required will be reduced by increasing automation. Anatomic correlates of evoked potential wave forms are being clarified in animal experiments and clinical studies. New developments in signal analysis and pattern recognition will facilitate EEG interpretation and characterization of evoked potential wave forms. Studies of the condition of patients after operative procedures are needed to define intraoperative EEG and evoked potential changes that are predictive of untoward neurologic sequelae.

The present state of EEG and evoked potential monitoring in the operating room resembles, in many respects, the state of electrocardiographic monitoring a generation ago. We know that loss of the signal is ominous, but quantitative description of. subtle wave form alterations that may have predictive value is lacking. Once technical problems and problems of interpretation are solved, EEG and evoked potential monitoring may, like electrocardiographic monitoring, enjoy widespread use. Cost-effective application of these new methods is now clearly within the realm of possibility. The anesthesiologist can facilitate intraoperative electrophysiologic monitoring by using those drugs that least alter EEG and evoked potentials, by giving careful attention to technical details, and by keeping the pharmacologic and physiologic state of the patient relatively constant during critical monitoring periods.

References

1. Clark, D. L., and Rosner, B. S. Neurophysiologic effects of general anesthetics: I. The electroencephalogram and sensory evoked responses in man. *Anesthesiology* 38:564, 1973.
2. Cooper, R., Osselton, J. W., and Shaw, J. C. *EEG Technology* (3rd ed.). London: Butterworths, 1980.
3. Cucchiara, R. F., Sharbrough, F. W., Messick, J. M., and Tinker, J. H. An electroencephalographic filter-processor as an indicator of cerebral ischemia during carotid endarterectomy. *Anesthesiology* 51:77, 1979.
4. Dawson, G. D. Cerebral responses to electrical stimulation of peripheral nerve in man. *J. Neurol. Neurosurg. Psychiatry* 10:137, 1947.
5. Demetrescu, M. The aperiodic character of the electroencephalogram (EEG): A new approach to data analysis and condensation. *Physiologist* 18:189, 1975.
6. Dolce, G., and Kunkel, H. (Eds.). *CEAN: Computerized EEG Analysis.* Stuttgart: Gustaf Fischer Verlag, 1975.
7. Gibbs, F. A., Gibbs, E. L., and Lennox, W. G. Effect on the electro-encephalogram of certain drugs which influence nervous activity. *Arch. Intern. Med.* 60:154, 1937.
8. Greenberg, R. P., Becker, D. P., Miller, J. D., and Mayer, D. J. Evaluation of brain function in severe human head trauma with multimodality evoked potentials. *J. Neurosurg.* 47:163, 1977.
9. Grundy, B. L. Monitoring of sensory evoked potentials during neurosurgical operations: Methods and applications. *Neurosurgery* 11:556, 1982.
10. Grundy, B. L. Intraoperative monitoring of sensory-evoked potentials. *Anesthesiology* 58:72, 1983.
11. Grundy, B. L., Brown, R. H., and Clifton, P. C. Effect of droperidol on somatosensory cortical evoked potentials (abs.). *Electroencephalogr. Clin. Neurophysiol.* 50:158P, 1980.

12. Grundy, B. L., Brown, R. H., and Greenberg, P. S.   Diazepam alters cortical evoked potentials (abs.). *Anesthesiology* 51:S38, 1979.
13. Grundy, B. L., Heros, R. C., Tung, A. S., and Doyle, E.   Intraoperative hypoxia detected by evoked potential monitoring. *Anesth. Analg.* (Cleve.), 60:437, 1981.
14. Grundy, B. L., Jannetta, P. J., Procopio, P. T., et al.   Intraoperative monitoring of brain-stem auditory evoked potentials. *J. Neurosurg.* 57:674, 1982.
15. Grundy, B. L., Lina, A., Procopio, P. T., and Jannetta, P. J.   Reversible evoked potential changes with retraction of the eighth cranial nerve. *Anesth. Analg.* (Cleve.) 60:835, 1981.
16. Grundy, B. L., Nash, C. L., and Brown, R. H.   Arterial pressure manipulation alters spinal cord function during correction of scoliosis. *Anesthesiology* 54:249, 1981.
17. Grundy, B. L., Nash, C. L., and Brown, R. H.   Deliberate hypotension for spinal fusion: Prospective randomized study with evoked potential monitoring. *Can. Anaesth. Soc. J.* 29:452, 1982.
17a. Grundy, B. L., Sanderson, A. C., Webster, M. W., et al.   Hemiparesis following carotid endarterectomy: Comparison of monitoring methods. *Anesthesiology* 55:462, 1981.
17b. Jasper, H. H.   The ten twenty electrode system of the International Federation. *Electroencephalogr. Clin. Neurophysiol.* 10:371, 1958.
18. Kooi, K. A., Tucker, R. P., and Marshall, R. E.   *Fundamentals of Electroencephalography* (2nd ed.). Hagerstown: Harper & Row, 1978.
19. Prior, P. F.   *Monitoring Cerebral Function: Long-term Recordings of Cerebral Electrical Activity.* Amsterdam: Elsevier, 1979.
20. Remond, A. (Ed.).   *EEG Informatics. A Didactic Review of Methods and Applications of EEG Data Processing.* Amsterdam: Elsevier, 1977.
21. Richey, E. T., and Namon, R.   *EEG Instrumentation and Technology.* Springfield, Ill.: Thomas, 1976.
22. Rosner, B. S., and Clark, D. L.   Neurophysiologic effects of general anesthetics: II. Sequential regional actions in the brain. *Anesthesiology* 39:59, 1973.
23. Stockard, J., and Bickford, R.   The Neurophysiology of Anaesthesia. In E. Gordon (Ed.), *A Basis and Practice of Neuroanaesthesia* (2nd ed.). Amsterdam: Excerpta Medica. 1981.
24. Sundt, T. M., Jr., Sharbrough, F. W., Piepgras, D. G., et al.   Correlation of cerebral blood flow and electroencephalographic changes during carotid endarterectomy: With results of surgery and hemodynamics of cerebral ischemia. *Mayo Clin. Proc.* 56:533, 1981.

4. Barbiturates for Intracranial Hypertension and Focal and Global Ischemia

Frederick G. Mihm

There are few areas of anesthesia or intensive care that are as controversial as barbiturate treatment of severe brain injuries. Differences of opinion exist because of limited useful information and because of different interpretations of the available data. Many clinicians caring for severely brain-damaged patients with poor prognoses are routinely using barbiturates, hoping that benefit will be gained in an otherwise hopeless situation. Meanwhile, researchers in the field, and those not directly involved with the care of severely brain-damaged patients, demand more solid experimental proof before endorsing the clinical use of barbiturates for brain protection. With these problems in mind, we will review the current state of barbiturate treatment for intracranial hypertension and focal and global ischemia, both from the researcher's perspective (potential beneficial and harmful effects, animals studies), and from the position of the clinician (current mortality, morbidity, and barbiturate experience in stroke, postcardiac arrest, head trauma, Reye's syndrome, and near-drowning).

I. **Potential beneficial effects.** Anesthetic barbiturates are unique in their ability to effect a significant decrease in cerebral metabolic requirement for oxygen ($CMRO_2$) and cerebral blood flow (CBF). Knowledge of these actions led to the barbiturates' initial use in animal models of cerebral ischemia. Barbiturates without anesthetic properties are unable to protect the brain, however (Steen, 1978). The potential beneficial effects of barbiturates, which may also result from other actions unrelated to changes in $CMRO_2$ and CBF, include the following: decreased free radical activity, decreased edema, beneficial anesthesia state, and anticonvulsant activity.

A. **$CMRO_2$.** Pierce (1962) documented in human beings that an anesthetic dose of thiopental will decrease the $CMRO_2$ by 52%. Since the brain has limited oxygen and energy reserves (with complete ischemia, oxygen and adenosine triphosphate [ATP] are exhausted in 10 sec and 5 min respectively), it is logical that an injured brain might benefit from a drug that reduces oxygen consumption. Michenfelder (1974) has shown in dogs that the flat EEG produced by administration of barbiturates provided a physiologic endpoint for maximal $CMRO_2$ depression. Additional barbiturates produced no further decrease in $CMRO_2$ (Michenfelder, 1974). This implies that barbiturates affect only the cells that are electrically active and not the severely ischemic cells that sacrifice electrical activity to preserve more vital cellular processes (e.g., sodium-potassium pump). Since other drugs that depress $CMRO_2$ do not protect the brain, other mechanisms of action have been sought to explain why barbiturates work.

B. **Increased cerebrovascular resistance (CVR).** Barbiturates are potent cerebral vasoconstrictors. Pierce (1962) has shown that anesthetic doses of thiopental will increase CVR and thereby decrease CBF by 48%. Barbiturates do not produce ischemia, however, because the decrease in $CMRO_2$ is always more profound than the decrease in blood flow. Cerebral vasoconstriction by barbiturates may produce two effects: a decrease in intracranial pressure (ICP) and a favorable redistribution of blood flow to more ischemic areas ("inverse steal").

1. **Decreased ICP.** The potent vasoconstriction induced by barbiturates will increase CVR, which decreases total cerebral blood volume (CBV), and thereby lowers ICP.

   Barbiturates $\rightarrow$ $\uparrow$ CVR $\rightarrow$ $\downarrow$ CBV $\rightarrow$ $\downarrow$ ICP

   Barbiturates have been effectively used to lower ICP in neurosurgical patients (Shapiro, 1973) and in patients who have head trauma (Collice 1976; Marshall, 1979), Reye's syndrome (Marshall, 1978), and near-drowning (Mickell, 1977). Many of these patients had failed to respond to routine therapy (hyperventilation, osmotic diuretics, and steroids).

   a. When barbiturates are used to treat increased ICP, care must be taken to **assure hemodynamic stability,** so that cerebral perfusion pressure (CPP) is not compromised. CPP is the difference between mean arterial pressure and intracranial pressure: CPP = MAP − ICP. Several studies show that CPP will increase while ICP decreases in most patients who are properly managed (Shapiro, 1973; 1974).

   b. The **response to thiopental** is rapid (1–10 min), but it is only of short duration (30–90 min) if administered by intermittent bolus (Collice, 1976). The dose of thiopental needed to maintain maximal cerebral vasoconstriction is not known, but suggested infusion rates range from 0.06 to 0.2 mg/kg/min. The exact infusion rate will be difficult to determine because of the nonlinear kinetics of this drug (see sec. **II.B.2**).

2. **"Inverse steal" or "Robin Hood phenomenon."** Another important effect of cerebral vasoconstriction is a beneficial redistribution of blood flow from normal (or near normal) areas of the brain to severely ischemic areas. This inverse steal or Robin Hood phenomenon can be easily understood by examining the effects of high and low $PaCO_2$ on a brain that has an area of focal ischemia (Fig. 4-1).

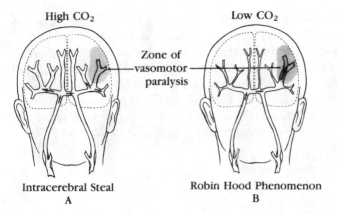

High CO$_2$ Low CO$_2$

Zone of
vasomotor
paralysis

Intracerebral Steal   Robin Hood Phenomenon
       A   B

Fig. 4-1. Effect of carbon dioxide (CO$_2$) on blood flow through ischemic brain. Ischemia causes a zone of vasomotor paralysis (shaded areas) in which the vessels are already maximally dilated. *A.* When the CO$_2$ is high, vessels in this ischemic area cannot dilate further and a condition of intracerebral steal results: blood is shunted *away* from the ischemic zone to areas of normal brain where vessels have dilated in response to the elevation in CO$_2$. *B.* Conversely, when the CO$_2$ is low, the Robin Hood phenomenon, or inverse steal, causes blood to go from areas of normally perfused brain where the vessels can constrict in response to a decrease in CO$_2$ to the zone of vasomotor paralysis in which the vessels do not respond to changes in CO$_2$.

    a. In the area of focal ischemia, the cerebral vessels are in a state of "vasomotor paralysis," where maximal vasodilation exists secondary to local tissue acidosis. Cerebral vessels in this area cannot respond further to vasodilators (e.g., high PaCO$_2$, halothane) and will not respond to vasoconstrictors (e.g., low PaCO$_2$, barbiturates). In a condition of high PaCO$_2$ (Fig. 4-1A), the normal areas of the brain will vasodilate, resulting in shunting of blood away from the ischemic area where the vessels were already maximally vasodilated ("intracerebral steal"). With a low PaCO$_2$ (Fig. 4-1B), which is analogous to barbiturate treatment, normal vessels vasoconstrict, shunting blood toward the ischemic area, which is unresponsive to other interventions (inverse steal).

    b. Barbiturates have been shown to cause an inverse steal in areas of focal ischemia and in areas of heterogeneous regional blood flow seen after global ischemia (Kofke, 1979). It is unclear what beneficial role cerebral vasoconstriction plays in some ischemic injuries, however, since hyperventilation after stroke in human beings has not been beneficial (Christensen, 1973).

C. Decreased free radical activity. Barbiturates can decrease free radical activity associated with ischemic brain injuries.

1. **Definition.** Free radicals are chemical forms containing an unpaired electron in their outer orbit. Whether or not they carry a charge, this unpaired electron makes the molecule highly reactive. Free radicals may represent a final common pathway of cell destruction. They are frequently intermediates of stable parent compounds, and they may be produced by a wide variety of agents or situations (Butterfield, 1978). The following are associated with free-radical activation:

   a. Adriamycin

   b. Bleomycin

   c. Daunorubicin

   d. Chloroform

   e. Halothane

   f. Paraquat

   g. Aging

   h. Granulocytes

   i. Hyperoxia

   j. Hypoxia

   k. Radiation

2. **Activators.** Radiation therapy (McCord, 1978) and chemotherapeutic agents (daunorubicin, bleomycin, Adriamycin) (Leibovitz, 1980) are known to damage tissue by forming free radicals. The liver toxicity produced by halogenated anesthetic drugs (chloroform, halothane) may be caused by reactive intermediate compounds (i.e., free radicals) (Brown, 1979). Granulocytes and macrophages phagocytize, "kill," and produce inflammation by release of the oxygen free radical, superoxide (Babior, 1973). The process of aging may actually be linked to a loss of control of free radical activity, which normally occurs in small amounts in aerobic cells (Leibovitz, 1980). Oxygen toxicity of the lung probably occurs secondary to superoxide formation, which is enhanced by the herbicide paraquat. Even ischemia with resultant hypoxia can produce oxygen free radicals that may ultimately destroy the cell (Fridovich, 1979; Flamm, 1978).

3. **Role of oxygen.** Oxygen has a key role in initiating free radical activity. Normally in the aerobic cell, most oxygen is consumed by a bivalent pathway in the respiratory chain (Fig. 4-2). This

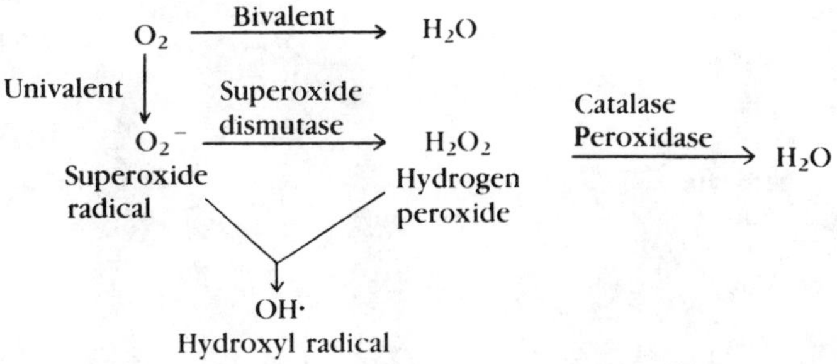

$$O_2 \xrightarrow{\text{Bivalent}} H_2O$$

Univalent |

$$O_2^- \xrightarrow[\text{dismutase}]{\text{Superoxide}} H_2O_2 \xrightarrow[\text{Peroxidase}]{\text{Catalase}} H_2O$$

Superoxide   Hydrogen
radical   peroxide

$$OH\cdot$$
Hydroxyl radical

Fig. 4-2. Oxygen free radicals. Oxygen picks up a bivalent charge and forms water (H_2O). When oxygen acquires a univalent charge, it is transformed into a superoxide radical that can be transformed by superoxide dismutase to hydrogen peroxide (H_2O_2) or can combine directly with H_2O_2 to form the hydroxyl radical ($OH\cdot$). Hydrogen peroxide is transformed to H_2O by the action of catalase and peroxidase.

means that two electrons are added simultaneously as water is formed. However, 5% is handled by a univalent pathway, where one electron is added at a time, creating the superoxide radical. All aerobic cells have the enzymes superoxide dismutase, catalase, and peroxidase, which convert superoxide first to hydrogen peroxide and then ultimately to water.

These enzyme systems are helped by various naturally occurring antioxidants, the so-called *free radical scavengers:* glutathione, alpha-tocopherol, ascorbic acid, and cholesterol. If the enzyme systems are overloaded (secondary to activators), superoxide and hydrogen peroxide will accumulate and combine to form the reactive hydroxyl radical. These free radicals destroy cells by attacking the lipid moieties within the cell wall. A chain reaction of lipid peroxidation (with production of lipid free radicals) will eventually disrupt the cell (Fridovich, 1979).

4. **Role of barbiturates.** Thiopental has been shown in vitro to decrease free radical lipid peroxidation induced by ultraviolet irradiation (Demopoulos, 1977). In a model of middle cerebral artery occlusion in cats, free radical activity was depressed by methohexital (Flamm, 1980). One of the few studies comparing different barbiturates demonstrated that thiopental was significantly more potent than phenobarbital and methohexital (Smith, 1980). The significance of barbiturate suppression of free radicals is unknown, although some authorities suggest that this suppression may be the main beneficial effect of these drugs.

D. **Decreased edema formation.** Barbiturates may affect edema formation after ischemic injuries. These brain injuries result in edema

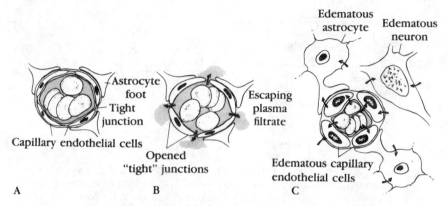

Fig. 4-3. Cerebral capillary endothelial cells. *A.* Endothelial cells of cerebral capillaries are joined by tight junctions. *B.* These tight junctions can open, permitting the escape of plasma filtrate into the surrounding brain parenchyma and causing vasogenic edema. *C.* In cytotoxic edema, the capillary endothelial cells, astrocytes, and neurons themselves become edematous from absorption of interstitial and intravascular fluid. (From R. A. Fishman. *N. Engl. J. Med.,* 293:708, 1975. Reprinted by permission.)

of two types: *vasogenic* edema, produced by infarction, and *cytotoxic* edema, produced by ischemia without infarction (Fishman, 1975; O'Brien, 1979).

1. **Vasogenic.** The normal anatomy of a cerebral capillary includes tight junctions between the endothelial cells that make up the blood-brain barrier (Fig. 4-3A). If an insult produces infarction, then these tight junctions fail, and *vasogenic* edema forms from leakage of protein-rich plasma into the interstitial spaces of the brain (Fig. 4-3B). This type of edema can increase total brain volume and frequently leads to increased ICP and further damage.

2. **Cytotoxic.** Ischemia, on the other hand, may not cause immediate cell death, but it may be so severe that the cellular energy stores (ATP) fall and the ATP-dependent sodium-potassium pump fails. In this situation, sodium (with water), which was maintained outside the cell, leaks intracellularly, causing the cellular swelling typical of *cytotoxic* edema (Fig. 4-3C). Note that the fluid shift with this kind of edema is primarily extracellular to intracellular, and, therefore, total brain volume may not increase. It is for this reason that vasogenic edema is associated with increased ICP and cytotoxic edema is not (Fishman, 1975).

Even though cytotoxic edema may not cause secondary brain damage by increasing ICP, it may be partly responsible for the "no-reflow" phenomenon. The no-reflow phenomenon refers to

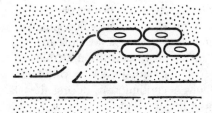

Fig. 4-4. No-reflow capillaries. Swelling of the cerebral capillary endothelial cells occurs after an ischemic insult, which prevents blood flow through that area once reperfusion has been established and exacerbates the initial injury. (From M. S. Christensen. *Acta Anaesthesiol. Scand.* [Suppl. 62]:8, 1976.)

regional nonperfusion of the brain in the postinsult period after systemic circulation has been reestablished. Other factors that may contribute to this phenomenon include viscosity changes, red cell and platelet aggregation, and potassium flux (Jamison, 1974; Nemoto, 1979; Wade, 1975). Capillary endothelial swelling from cytotoxic edema may "pinch" the capillary lumen in ischemic regions (Fig. 4-4). The increased resistance to flow caused by these capillary endothelial cells may occur while arterioles to the same region are maximally vasodilated (vasomotor paralysis).

In summary, ischemic injuries may result in two types of edema (Fig. 4-5). If necrosis occurs with the initial insult, vasogenic edema will form, with subsequent further injury from

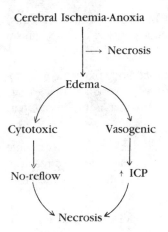

Fig. 4-5. Necrosis after cerebral ischemia or anoxia. The ischemic or anoxic insult causes necrosis both directly and indirectly through cytotoxic and vasogenic edema. Cytotoxic edema leads to necrosis because of the no-reflow phenomenon. Vasogenic edema causes necrosis by an increase in intracranial pressure (ICP).

increased ICP. In areas in which ischemia is not severe enough to cause infarction, cytotoxic edema and the no-reflow phenomenon may ensue, resulting in further, irreversible damage. Cerebral edema after ischemic injury peaks at 48 hours (O'Brien, 1974). It appears logical, then, that treatment (e.g., barbiturates) might be most effective if given continuously during the 48 hours after injury and not as a one-time administration.

3. **Barbiturates.** Barbiturates have been shown to decrease edema formation after cryogenic lesions (Smith, 1976; Clasen, 1976) and ischemic insults (middle cerebral artery occlusion in monkeys [Simeone, 1979] and carotid ligation in gerbils [Lawner, 1979]). Barbiturates also decrease potassium efflux from ischemic cells (Astrup, 1977), and this efflux may have a beneficial effect on cytotoxic edema. It is unclear if this effect of barbiturates has a separate mechanism or is simply a combined effect of decreased $CMRO_2$ (and thereby protection of ATP stores for the sodium-potassium pump) and the inverse steal (vasoconstriction of normal areas will increase regional perfusion pressure through "pinched" capillaries). Barbiturates may also decrease edema through an osmotic effect (Allman, 1980; Bandaranayake, 1978).

E. **Anesthesia.** The anesthetic state induced by high doses of barbiturates may be beneficial in several ways. Amnesia, immobilization, decreased total body oxygen consumption ($\dot{V}O_2$), and complete analgesia are part of this state. Nonanesthetic barbiturates have no cerebral protective effects (Michenfelder, 1978).

1. **Immobilization.** Immobilization by itself (muscle relaxants) has been shown to ameliorate ischemic injuries. The mechanism is not understood (Bleyaert, 1980).

2. **Decreased $\dot{V}O_2$.** The reduction of total body oxygen consumption may enhance oxygen delivery to more vital organs (e.g., brain, heart). This may be the reason that immobilization is effective.

3. **Analgesia.** High doses of barbiturates produce complete analgesia so that noxious stimuli, which can otherwise result in dangerous rises in ICP and catecholamines, are therefore avoided.

F. **Anticonvulsant.** Seizures are very expensive metabolic events. If seizures are controlled by barbiturates, then the oxygen supply to the brain will not be as severely taxed.

The potential beneficial effects of barbiturates remain controversial, particularly with regard to their effectiveness in protection from global ischemic injuries. Not all barbiturates share the same pharmacologic properties. Just as there are differences in the anticonvulsant activity of phenobarbital as compared to other commonly used barbiturates, there may be other important differences as well among these drugs and their potential beneficial effects.

II. **Potential harmful effects.** Barbiturates have no known direct tissue toxicity (Steen, 1979). In spite of this, the use of high doses of barbiturates is not necessarily a benign treatment. Hypotension, loss of the neurologic examination, pulmonary edema, allergic reactions, polyuria, and withdrawal symptoms may occur.

A. **Hypotension.** By far the most significant complication of the use of barbiturates results from inadequate management of the hemodynamic effects of these drugs. Hypotension may occur in any patient receiving barbiturates, and may be particularly harmful in head-injured patients because CPP may be compromised, even though ICP is reduced. Barbiturates act directly on the heart and on the arterial and venous circulations (Fig. 4-6).

1. **Systemic vascular resistance (SVR).** Traditionally, barbiturates were thought to constrict the arterial circulation, causing an increase in SVR (Etsten, 1955; 1960; Elder, 1955; Becker, 1978; Sonntag, 1975). However, in the high doses administered to critically ill patients, barbiturates may produce either no change or a decrease in SVR.

2. **Heart rate.** Chronotropic effects of barbiturates are variable. Heart rate can increase up to 15% to 30% in healthy persons, but may be variable or decrease in critically ill patients.

3. **Venous pooling, inotropic effects.** Regardless of their effect on systemic arterial tone and heart rate, hypotension may result after administration of barbiturates because of decreased inotropic effects and venous pooling of blood. Barbiturates cause dose-dependent depression of myocardial contractility as

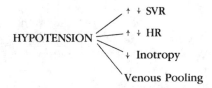

Fig. 4-6. Causes of hypotension after administration of barbiturates. These include an increase or decrease in systemic vascular resistance (SVR), an increase or decrease in heart rate (HR), a decrease in inotropy, and venous pooling.

measured by the changes in the first derivative of the left ventricular function curve (Sonntag, 1975; Siegel, 1964; Dwyer, 1969). Cardiac index may be decreased up to 15% to 25% by negative inotropic effects, but is equally influenced by venous pooling which can reduce right and left ventricular filling pressures.

4. **Assessment, treatment.** Both the venous pooling and negative inotropic effects of barbiturates can be reversed by the appropriate administration of fluids and positive inotropic agents (Siegel, 1964; Shubin, 1971). The rational management of hypotension caused by barbiturates depends on the measurement of intravascular filling pressures, cardiac output, and systemic vascular resistance with a thermodilution pulmonary artery catheter.

B. **Loss of neurologic examination.** Another effect of treatment with barbiturates is the loss of the neurologic examination because of drug-induced CNS depression. However, in most clinical circumstances where barbiturates have been used, the patient is *already* in a coma and the neurologic examination is either insensitive or already obviated by other routine therapy (e.g., muscle relaxants). In fact, for comatose patients who have increased ICP, an ICP monitor is a better indicator of the patient's course than the late neurologic findings associated with herniation of the brain.

1. **"Ultrashort" barbiturates.** The use of ultrashort-acting barbiturates should minimize the duration of drug-induced CNS depression. Unfortunately, the ultrashort barbiturates may be long-acting when given in large doses. For example, thiopental, like some other drugs metabolized by the liver, can be given in quantities sufficient to saturate the hepatic enzyme system. This saturation results in *zero-order* kinetics, which greatly increases the apparent half-life of the drug (Stanski, 1980).

2. **Nonlinear kinetics.** Thiopental in low doses behaves as a drug with *first-order* kinetics and has a half-life of about six hours. If we plot the log of the drug concentration ($\log C_p$) on the Y-axis, we find that drugs exhibiting first-order kinetics produce decreasing concentrations over time that fall along a straight line (Fig. 4-7). The slope of this line defines the rate of elimination (half-life) of the drug, and is constant at all concentrations of the drug. In high doses, however, the rate of decline of the concentration of thiopental is not linear, but falls very slowly over the range of zero-order kinetics. The apparent half-life of thiopental at these concentrations may be 50 to 60 hours. The rate of elimination progressively increases with time, however, and eventually returns to the first-order half-life of six hours (Stanski, 1980).

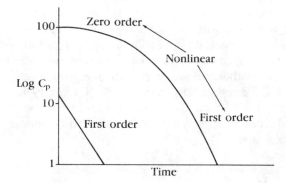

Fig. 4-7. Pharmacokinetics of drug metabolism. Most drugs follow first-order kinetics but the metabolism of large doses of barbiturates follows zero-order kinetics. (p = plasma concentration)

3. **Implications.** These findings have important implications for barbiturate therapy and the problem of obviating the neurologic examination. It may be possible to minimize the time for recovery from the effects of the drug as the pharmacokinetics of high doses of barbiturates are better understood and as we clarify the amount of drug needed for maximal benefit.

C. **Pulmonary edema.** In a preliminary report of a small controlled study, a noncardiogenic form of pulmonary edema (ARDS) was noted to occur in patients treated with barbiturates. This evidence is not conclusive, however, since appropriate fluid management was not documented. Pulmonary edema may occur in patients receiving barbiturates secondary to fluid overload, myocardial failure, allergic reactions (rare), or underlying disease states (e.g., head trauma, hypoxia, shock, myocardial infarction). Although giving some fluid may be appropriate in the treatment of drug-induced hypotension, fluid administration must be monitored closely to avoid fluid overload. Some patients will also require inotropic support. Only carefully controlled trials will reveal whether barbiturates, by themselves, can induce noncardiogenic pulmonary edema.

D. **Allergy.** Mild allergic reactions to barbiturates have occurred, but true anaphylaxis is a rare event. A few cases of thiopental anaphylaxis have been reported. It is treated by standard regimens (epinephrine, steroids, antihistamines) (Dolovich, 1980).

E. **Polyuria.** Purely anecdotal experience has led some investigators to associate polyuria with barbiturate treatment. Diabetes insipidus is a frequent secondary problem of neurosurgical patients, especially those who have head trauma, and is independent of barbiturate treatment.

F. Withdrawal syndrome. Barbiturate withdrawal syndrome may occur if a patient is treated with barbiturates for many days, although withdrawal symptoms associated with this type of barbiturate therapy have not been reported. In addition, there is evidence to suggest that neither withdrawal symptoms nor tolerance develops in patients treated for several days to two weeks (Carlon, 1978; Mihm, unpublished data). To avoid the possibility of seizures when discontinuing the barbiturates, another anticonvulsant drug (phenytoin) can be substituted.

III. Animal studies

A. Focal ischemia

1. **"Pro" studies.** Many experiments have demonstrated beneficial effects of barbiturates in focal ischemia. Barbiturate treatment before, or up to two hours after, middle cerebral artery (MCA) occlusion in monkeys (Michenfelder, 1975, 1976; Black, 1978; Hoff, 1975), dogs, cats, and baboons decreases neurologic morbidity as measured by neurologic function or infarction size (Smith, 1977; Hoff, 1978). Other studies of focal ischemia (middle cerebral and internal carotid artery occlusion in dogs [Smith, 1974; Hankinson, 1974], common carotid artery occlusion in gerbils [McGraw, 1977], embolization in monkeys [Moseley, 1975]) have produced similar results. An additional study suggests that delay of treatment for three or more hours after this type of injury reduces the effectiveness of barbiturates on neurologic injury (Corkill, 1976).

2. **"Con" studies.** There are few contradictory studies on focal ischemia, and most have significant methodologic errors. One such study showed increased mortality in treated animals (60% vs. 14%), but this may have been because of inadequately managed hypotension which offset the potential beneficial effect of barbiturates (Black, 1978).

B. Global ischemia.
Global ischemia is a difficult experimental model to create. The few studies carried out have generated much debate and conflicting opinion.

1. **"Pro" studies.** The first two studies reported impressive results. Wright (1964) found that intracarotid injection of pentobarbital or thiopental in cats significantly increased ischemic tolerance. Goldstein (1966) compared ischemic tolerance in dogs given local anesthesia (FiO_2 = .21 and 1.0), local anesthesia with 5% CO_2, morphine, or pentobarbital. Only animals anesthetized with pentobarbital tolerated global ischemia (aortic cross-clamp for 10 min) without severe morbidity or death. Recently,

thiopental given after global ischemia in monkeys was shown to ameliorate neurologic deficits over the seven-day period (Bleyaert, 1978). In a study of incomplete global ischemia and hypoxia (trimethaphan, 4% oxygen → flat EEG), methohexital treatment after the insult provided dramatic improvement as compared to control animals (Yatsu, 1972). In addition, there have been many global hypoxia (asphyxia) experiments that document the benefit of barbiturate pretreatment (Brann, 1970).

2. **"Con" studies.** Goldstein's ischemic model has recently been duplicated. Following the same protocol, pentobarbital did not have any beneficial effects (Steen, 1979). The explanation for the different results is not clear but certainly leaves the initial study in question. Since depression of $CMRO_2$ by barbiturates parallels decreased electrical activity (Michenfelder, 1974), it was postulated that barbiturates would not be beneficial in global injuries once electrical activity had ceased (Michenfelder, 1973; Nilsson, 1971). A study of global hypoxia (clamped endotracheal tube) attempted to prove this theory. Unfortunately, this protocol included inadequate management of the hemodynamic effects of barbiturates, which affected the results (Snyder, 1979). There is evidence, however, that, in spite of a flat EEG, barbiturates did appear to help (Yatsu, 1972), perhaps by another mechanism. The study by Bleyaert (1978) has been criticized for the ischemic model used and for the variable results reported. In this model, changing supportive care in the control group (immobilization and controlled ventilation) significantly decreased the group's neurologic deficit (Bleyaert, 1980). Finally, a recent animal model of cardiac arrest in cats showed no neurologic improvement with postarrest treatment with thiopental (Chadwick, 1980), although the treated group did survive longer, perhaps because of control of seizures (Todd, 1982).

C. **Problems in clinical application.** Animals studies of focal and global ischemia answer some questions, but leave many more unanswered. The clinical relevance of these studies deserves some discussion.

1. **General problems.** What animal models parallel a given clinical state? Some feel that data from focal ischemia models (e.g., MCA occlusions) can only be applied to humans who have clinical stroke, while global ischemia models relate only to human beings who have cardiac or respiratory arrest or near-drowning. However, it must be realized that MCA occlusion in a small animal produces a massive hemispheric infarction with increased ICP: the injury cannot be equated to the injury of a

patient who suffers a small ischemic injury in the internal capsule. It must also be remembered that human survivors of global
insults, such as cardiac arrest, commonly suffer focal neurologic
deficits (hemiparesis, cortical blindness, aphasia, etc.) while
many other areas of the brain function normally (Norris, 1971;
Caronna, 1978).

2. **Specific problems.** Additional problems in interpreting animal studies include the following:

   a. **Species.** Small animals have significant physiologic differences from large animals and human beings (P_{50} of hemoglobin, adaptation to hypoxia, etc.). They are also prone to
   unique diseases that may alter outcome (e.g., rodent respiratory disease) (Davis, 1979). In large animals, there are major
   anatomic differences in the blood supply to the brain that
   may influence results in nonprimate models (Michenfelder,
   1976).

   b. **Anesthesia.** Interactions of anesthetic drugs with drugs
   used as treatment must be evaluated and avoided when possible.

   c. **Neurologic examination.** Performing an adequate neurologic examination is difficult in animals. In rodents, even a
   hemiparesis is difficult to identify. In large animals including
   primates, higher cognitive function cannot be tested. In addition, the normal course of functional deficits may vary
   significantly from human injuries (Waltz, 1979).

   d. **Models.** Models of global cerebral ischemia vary (choke col-
   lar, ventricular fibrillation, aortic and vena caval occlusion)
   but all have problems of immediate survival. Many ischemia
   models require major surgical procedures that can add to
   morbidity and mortality. Less invasive models of ischemia
   need to be studied (Jackson, 1979).

   e. **Intensive care.** Inappropriate postinsult life support is a
   problem of many studies. Intensive care of a large animal is
   very demanding and requires significant expertise and man-
   power, particularly if the study period lasts for 3 to 7 days to
   allow appraisal of long-term neurologic outcome.

IV. **Human studies.** Although many questions remain, barbiturates are
being used to treat human brain injuries. The clinical experience with
barbiturates includes stroke, cardiac arrest, head trauma, Reye's syndrome, near-drowning, and various anesthetic situations.

A. Stroke

1. **General information.** Over 200,000 people suffer strokes every year in this country. **Stroke** is the general term for neurologic deficits in four major categories: thrombosis, embolism, intracerebral hemorrhage, and ruptured aneurysm. Over 80% of strokes are ischemic (thromboembolic) (Sahs, 1976).

2. **Current mortality and morbidity.** Treatment for a completed ischemic stroke is supportive, but short-term mortality is more than 40% (Shafer, 1973). Significant permanent neurologic deficits will occur in about 60% of the long-term survivors (Shafer, 1973). There is no specific therapy (including surgery) that will improve mortality or morbidity in patients who have completed strokes (Table 4-1) (Browne, 1969; Van Horn, 1973; Bauer, 1969).

3. **Barbiturate experience.** The use of barbiturates in stroke is limited. Since most stroke patients are conscious, barbiturate treatment not only results in loss of the neurologic examination, but also requires possibly unnecessary intubation and controlled ventilation. Many institutions use barbiturates for focal ischemia associated with neurosurgical procedures, particularly if there is an opportunity to treat patients before the insult. Three centers have published their limited experience in various stroke injuries.

   a. A randomized controlled study of 35 patients with thromboembolic stroke reported a 40% decrease in mortality in patients treated with thiopental, 10 gm (2 gm q8h for 5

Table 4-1. Outcome of stroke, cardiac arrest, head trauma, Reye's syndrome, near-drowning, and immersion accidents in 100 typical patients

	Thrombo-embolic stroke	Cardiac arrest (survivors in coma)*	Head trauma (Glasgow coma scale ≤ 8)	Reye's syndrome (stages IV and V)	Near-drowning (coma)	Immersion accidents (survivors of near-drowning)†
Normal	24	8	25		45	80
Permanent neurologic deficit	36	37	25		20	10
Death	40	55	50	60–100	35	10

*When 32 survivors in coma were treated with thiopental (30–50 mg/kg), the outcome was as follows: 15 (48%) normal; 1 (3%) permanent neurologic damage; 15 (48%) death.
†Out of 200 immersion accidents, 100 result in drowning, 100 in near-drowning.

doses). However, there were significant design problems with this study (control patients were treated with glycerol and dextran), and the control group had an unacceptably high mortality (80%) (Davis, 1979).

b. Seven patients undergoing cerebral aneurysm surgery requiring temporary or permanent occlusion of a major artery were treated with pentobarbital (15–20 mg/kg initially, then 15 mg/kg/day for 2 days). Although two patients died, four of the five survivors had no neurologic deficits, suggesting to the authors that these patients had benefited from barbiturate treatment (Hoff, 1977).

c. Four patients undergoing treatment of surgically inaccessible cerebral aneurysms were treated with pentobarbital after iatrogenic thrombosis occurred (stereotatic injection of a methyl methacrylate-iron mixture). All patients died with fatal ICP elevations after 5 days of barbiturate treatment (Rockoff, 1979).

B. Cardiac arrest

1. **General information.** With the expanded use of cardiopulmonary resuscitation (CPR) and advanced cardiac life support (ACLS), it is now possible to save 30% to 45% of the 350,000 people who will have a cardiac arrest each year (Myerburg, 1980). However, many "survivors" of cardiac arrest go on to die a cerebral death or survive with a significant neurologic deficit (Cobb, 1980).

2. **Current mortality/morbidity.** Approximately 30% of the survivors of cardiac arrests will die a cerebral death (i.e., they will never recover consciousness) (Snyder, 1977; Bell, 1974). The subgroup of patients who do not recover consciousness shortly after successful CPR have a particularly poor prognosis (see Table 4-1). Patients in a coma one hour after CPR have a high mortality (55%) and a very small chance (8%) of leaving the hospital with normal brain function (Snyder, 1977; Willoughby, 1974; Bates, 1977). At the present time, postcardiac arrest care is strictly supportive, maintaining cardiac and pulmonary function with a "watch and wait" attitude as far as the brain is concerned.

3. **Barbiturate experience.** Some authorities have expressed great enthusiasm for the treatment of survivors of cardiac arrest who remain in a coma after resuscitation. The results of animal studies suggest that this kind of brain insult should be treated

within 1 to 2 hours to achieve maximal benefit (Corkill, 1976; Bleyaert, 1978).

a. Other than several case reports, only one nonrandomized, noncontrolled study has been reported: a collection of 40 patients treated in four institutions (Breivick, 1978). Eight of these patients will be excluded from discussion because they did not have a clinical cardiac arrest and three of the eight were treated before their brain injury. In the remaining 32 patients who were in a coma after successful CPR, thiopental (30–50 mg/kg) was given as a single-dose treatment. The outcome of these patients was extraordinarily good (see Table 4-1) but must be interpreted with caution since some patients were treated immediately after cardiac arrest. If all cardiac arrest survivors are examined (not just those in coma one hour after CPR), long-term chances for normal brain recovery may be as good as in this series (30%–50%) (Snyder, 1977; Bell, 1974; Linko, 1967). This report is important because it demonstrated the feasibility of administering single, large-dose barbiturate treatment to patients after cardiac arrest.

b. A different feasibility trial was performed at Stanford in patients who had ischemic or traumatic brain injuries to evaluate a much more aggressive treatment regimen using thiopental as a 15-mg/kg loading dose and then as a continuous infusion for 2 to 3 days. The endpoints for dose and duration of treatment were specific. A continuous infusion of the drug was administered to keep the cortical EEG isoelectric (to achieve maximal $CMRO_2$ depression), since this represents the only known physiologic endpoint other than control of ICP. The duration of treatment of two to three days was chosen since this represents the time interval for accumulation of edema after ischemic and traumatic brain injuries (O'Brien, 1974; 1979).

Fourteen patients who had various brain injuries have been treated with total doses of thiopental ranging from 0.2 to 0.6 g/kg. Four of these patients were postcardiac arrest; two survived with complete neurologic recovery and two died (Rosenthal, 1978). Hemodynamic stability was maintained during the infusions by close monitoring and rational supportive care. There was no cardiac arrest or death during the drug infusion nor did the infusion have to be stopped because of intractable hypotension. This trial established the feasibility of continuous treatment of patients with large doses of barbiturates during the entire "postresuscitative disease" period (Negovskii, 1974).

c. No matter what dose of barbiturate is used, only controlled, randomized trials will answer the question of efficacy. The question now is, "*Should* we treat?", not, "Can we treat?"

C. Head trauma

1. General information

a. **Incidence.** An estimated 30,000 people die each year in the United States from head injuries (Miller, 1978). This number can be expected to increase with the growing popularity of motorcycles, mopeds, and bicycles.

b. **ICP.** Increased ICP, a frequent secondary event in the head-injured patient, may cause additional brain damage either by herniation with trauma to various parts of the brain (cingulate gyrus, temporal lobe, or cerebellar tonsils) or by decreasing CBF below the critical range necessary for neuronal viability. A progressive cycle of increasing cerebral compression may develop because of edema with resultant ischemia and necrosis. This secondary complication frequently leads to demise or severe disability. Although not always an accompaniment of severe head trauma (25% incidence of normal ICP) (Bruce, 1979), significant intracranial hypertension (> 30 mmHg) will almost double mortality (Langfitt, 1976). Increased ICP does not always correlate with detectable neurologic deterioration; however, most patients will suffer more brain damage when there is a significant rise in ICP (Collice, 1976). Therefore, controlling ICP has become the main goal in treating head-injured patients. Although the reason for using barbiturates is to decrease ICP, their other effects may also be important.

c. **Glasgow coma scale (GCS).** This scoring system (Jennett, 1975) has clarified the definition of severe head trauma as a score ≤ 8 (Table 4-2). Reasonable comparisons can be made among different series, since patient populations are comparable. The *Glasgow coma scale* is an attempt to standardize classification of outcome and will also help clarify the many unresolved issues in the management of head-injured patients (Langfitt, 1978).

2. Current mortality and morbidity.
The current mortality from severe craniocerebral trauma has been surprisingly constant at 50% (Jennett, 1977; Cooper, 1979). Approximately 25%

Table 4-2. Glasgow coma scale

Eye opening	
Spontaneous	4
To speech	3
To pain	2
None	1
Verbal response	
Oriented	5
Confused conversation	4
Incomprehensible words	3
Incomprehensible sounds	2
Nil	1
Best motor response	
Obeys	6
Localizes	5
Withdraws	4
Abnormal flexion	3
Extensor response	2
Nil	1

of severely brain-injured patients will fully recover to normal brain function (see Table 4-1).

a. A recent study reported a mortality of 32% (Becker, 1977). However, this study included a younger patient population and excluded patients with a coma score of 3. The morbidity in this study was also improved, suggesting that aggressive management had favorably affected the outcome.

b. Aggressive management is facilitated by monitoring ICP to direct therapeutic interventions. Treatment regimens for intracranial hypertension vary significantly among institutions, but all include some combination of the following modalities:

Controlled ventilation ($PO_2 > 80$ mmHg)
Blood pressure control
Hyperventilation ($PCO_2 = 25$–30 mmHg)
Steroids
Immobilization
Fluid restriction
Surgery (clot evacuation)
Osmotherapy
Diuretics
Normothermia/hypothermia
CSF drainage

Table 4-3. Outcome of three studies using barbiturates in head trauma

	n	Mortality (%)	Significant morbidity (%)	Good recovery (%)
Overgaard (1973)	139	40	30	30
Rockoff (1979)	45	36	20	44
Bruce (1979)	85	9	4	88

3. **Barbiturate experience.** Barbiturates received wide attention after they were shown to decrease ICP effectively in neurosurgical patients (Shapiro, 1973). Three studies have been published using barbiturates in head trauma (Table 4-3).

   a. Overgaard (1973) reported a series of 201 patients treated very unaggressively by today's standards (no steroids, intubation, osmotherapy, or ICP monitoring). All patients were treated with phenobarbital (150–400 mg/day). Since 62 patients were awake or able to obey commands (GCS > 8), only the results for the remaining 139 severely injured patients are listed in Table 4-3. It is interesting that the mortality and morbidity in this group of patients treated with barbiturates and without conventional therapy were as good or better than most conventional protocols.

   b. Rockoff (1979) reported on the use of pentobarbital in 45 of 172 patients who had ICP elevations of greater than 40 mmHg for 15 minutes. Aggressive conventional therapy (controlled hyperventilation, steroids, osmotherapy, paralysis) was also used. Pentobarbital was given over 3 to 10 days (3–5 mg/kg initially, then 100–200 mg q1h) and the resulting mortality (36%) in this group was excellent (Table 4-3). This group of patients had fewer mass lesions than those in other series, which might favor a better outcome; however, this does not entirely explain the good results (Marshall, 1979; Rockoff, 1979).

   c. Most impressive results in head trauma were reported by Bruce (1979) in 85 patients (aged 4 months to 18 years) who had severe brain injuries. Their complicated protocol included conventional therapy (ICP monitoring, hyperventilation, paralysis) for all patients and other additional therapy (steroids, mannitol, furosemide, hypothermia, pentobarbital, and thiopental) according to specific guidelines. The low mortality (9%) and morbidity (4%) are gratifying but may be due in part to the young population and the low incidence of mass lesions in this group (Table 4-3) (Langfitt, 1978).

D. Reye's syndrome

1. **General information.** Although Brian described a syndrome of encephalopathy and fatty liver in 1929, Reye and Johnson are credited with the description of a distinct clinical syndrome in 1963.

   More than 1000 cases from all over the world had been reported by 1976, but the true incidence is probably much higher than this number would indicate. A seasonal variation with peaks in January and June has been noted along with an association with certain viral infections (Safar, 1978). A significant outbreak of the disease occurred at the time of the influenza-B epidemic of 1973–1975 (one case of Reye's syndrome per 1700 cases of influenza B) (Hochberg, 1975; Bobo, 1975). Although the illness generally involves children aged 4 to 15 years, three adults have been reported to have the disease (Atkins, 1979).

   a. **Clinical course.** The clinical course begins with a mild antecedent illness (upper respiratory infection, gastroenteritis, varicella) followed within a week by persistent vomiting and a progressive encephalopathy. Over a period of hours to days, the encephalopathy can progress from combative behavior and hallucinations to decreased responsiveness, coma with abnormal posturing, and finally, loss of brainstem function and death (Nadler, 1974).

   b. **Diagnosis.** The diagnosis is made on the basis of a compatible clinical history and the following: hepatic injury evidenced by elevations of SGOT/SGPT to twice normal, negative toxicology screen, and normal CSF examination. Although they are not necessary for the diagnosis, prolonged prothrombin time, elevated blood ammonia, and hypoglycemia are also consistent with the diagnosis (Chin, 1974).

   c. **Clinical staging.** Two staging systems have been devised for Reye's syndrome (Lovejoy, 1974; Huttenlocher, 1972). The more elaborate classification of Lovejoy has been widely accepted and includes five stages with associated EEG findings (Table 4-4). Morbidity appears increased in patients who pass rapidly through stages I to III and who have high ammonia levels (> 200 $\mu g/ml$) and/or a metabolic acidosis.

2. **Current morbidity and mortality**

   a. Reye's syndrome frequently has an **unpredictable course,** making evaluation of various treatments confusing. In the first few years after its recognition, supportive therapy included administration of glucose, neomycin, and dexametha-

Table 4-4. Reye's syndrome staging

Stage	Symptoms
I	*Lethargy,* vomiting
II	*Disorientation,* combativeness, hyperventilation, hyperreflexia
III	*Coma,* decorticate rigidity, hyperventilation
IV	*Coma,* decerebrate rigidity, fixed pupils, brainstem signs
V	*Coma,* apnea, seizures, flaccidity

sone, resulting in an overall mortality of 60% to 100% (Bobo, 1975; Mickell, 1977; Samaha, 1974; Bradford, 1967).

b. **Aggressive therapy** developed along two lines: management of hepatic coma and treatment of cerebral edema. Soon a large list of specific treatment existed (Table 4-5). When the etiology of the encephalopathy was determined to be a direct insult to the brain and not an hepatic encephalopathy, treatment became focused on preventing an increase in ICP from the cerebral edema. None of the treatments has undergone controlled trials in Reye's syndrome. However, since the direct insult to the brain appears to be reversible, the effectiveness of aggressive therapy in reducing cerebral edema and ICP is currently believed responsible for the improved mortality and morbidity. Even with aggressive therapy, mortality for all patients varies from 0% to 82%, with a 3% to 15% incidence of neurologic morbidity (Nadler, 1974; Bobo, 1975; Lovejoy, 1974; Huttonlocker, 1972; Samaha, 1974; Shaywitz, 1977; Van Caille, 1977; DeVivo, 1975; Kindt, 1975; Boutnos, 1977; Lansky, 1977; Acki, 1973). In the subgroup of patients in stages IV and V coma, mortality is still high (see Table 4-1) (Van Caille, 1977; DeVivo, 1975; Lansky, 1977).

3. **Barbiturate experience**

a. The limited role of barbiturates in the treatment of Reye's syndrome dramatically changed when Marshall (1978) re-

Table 4-5. Aggressive therapy for Reye's syndrome

Hepatic coma	Cerebral edema
Citrulline	Intubation/hyperventilation
Arginine	Fluid restriction
L-Dopa	Osmotherapy
Exchange transfusion	Paralysis
Dialysis	CSF drainage
Total body washout	Hypothermia

ported seven patients with stages IV and V coma who were treated with pentobarbital after standard measures (hyperventilation, steroids, mannitol) had failed to control ICP. All seven patients had ICP $\geq$ 30 mmHg for at least 30 minutes before administration of barbiturates. Pentobarbital was given in a dose of 3 to 5 mg/kg initially, followed by 2 to 3.5 mg/kg every hour as long as the mean arterial pressure (MAP) was $\geq$ 60 mmHg and the pentobarbital blood level was < 25 μg/ml. Patients were treated for 5 to 13 days, and all made a complete recovery except one who had a neurologic deficit.

b. Currently, barbiturates have been given last place in the order of treatments for raised ICP in Reye's syndrome (Trauner, 1980).

E. Near-drowning

1. General information

a. Approximately 7000 to 9000 drowning-related deaths occur each year in the United States. Drowning is the second leading cause of death in young children. About 50% are under 16 years of age (Conn, 1978). By definition, near-drowning indicates at least temporary survival (24 hours) after asphyxia secondary to submersion in a fluid medium (Peterson, 1977).

b. Hypoxia occurs because of asphyxia, aspiration, and ischemia after cardiac arrest. Most persons aspirate, but the volume of water aspirated is generally small (< 20 ml/kg). Although there are differences between salt-water and fresh-water aspiration, the resultant hypoxemia and respiratory failure are clinically indistinguishable (Giammona, 1971). An important distinction can be made between warm- and cold-water drowning, however, since hypothermia associated with the latter offers some protection to the brain and may account for survival after prolonged submersion (Siebke, 1975).

2. Current morbidity and mortality

a. Serious immersion accidents (loss of consciousness in water) result in a mortality of 20% to 80% (Pearn, 1979). Mortality rates are highest in the adult population and in fresh-water immersions. About half of all immersion accidents are drownings (death within 24 hours). The other half are near-drownings in which the victims survive past the first day (see Table 4-1). Victims of near-drowning have a significantly lower morbidity and mortality, although the subgroup of patients who are comatose on arrival at the hospital has a poorer prognosis. Patients in deep coma who are areflexic and flaccid have a 70% mortality (Conn, 1980).

b. Current therapy for near-drowning victims reflects advances in cardiopulmonary resuscitation and brain-oriented intensive care. There is not much controversy about initial resuscitative efforts, subsequent controlled ventilation with positive end-expiratory pressure, and other general supportive measures. Patients who have significant brain dysfunction may be treated with steroids (not of value for the pulmonary lesion) and hyperventilation. Intracranial pressure monitoring has been recommended for severely affected patients, in combination with the use of osmotic agents, CSF drainage, and hypothermia to help prevent and control intracranial hypertension (Mickell, 1977; Conn, 1978; Hoff, 1979).

3. Barbiturate experience

a. Before the acceptance of the effectiveness of barbiturates for lowering ICP, their role in near-drowning was limited to treating seizures when they occurred (Giammona, 1971).

b. Conn (1980) recently reported a series of 96 children whose aggressive treatment after near-drowning was based on their neurologic function at the time of arrival at the hospital. Patients were categorized "A," awake; "B," blunted consciousness; and "C," coma. The treatment regimen for "C" patients included administration of barbiturates (phenobarbital) for four days, regardless of the ICP. The morbidity and mortality for this group were not better than for a smaller group reported by Modell (Hoff, 1979), in which no barbiturates were used. The groups in coma were not necessarily comparable, however, and only half of Conn's patients received barbiturates. Conn's study was prospective but not randomized or controlled.

c. The role of barbiturates in near-drowning is unclear, but many institutions use barbiturates in this clinical situation just as they do for head trauma and Reye's syndrome patients.

F. Anesthesia. Anesthesiologists may be involved in the care of patients who have a variety of brain injuries. They should be familiar with the special considerations for anesthetizing patients who have increased ICP and those who require cerebral protection.

1. ICP. Anesthesia for patients who have intracranial hypertension may involve the use of barbiturates. Because of its rapid action (within 60 sec), thiopental is most commonly used (Shapiro, 1973). The dose for maximal cerebral vasoconstriction is not known but measurement of ICP provides a valuable guide to therapeutic efficacy. Repeated doses may be necessary if increases in ICP persist or recur. There may be an advantage to continuous infusion of barbiturates to prevent elevations in ICP instead of treating increases after they occur, but this is not currently popular because of concern about hemodynamic instability and prolonged recovery from anesthesia.

2. Cerebral protection

  a. Patients frequently require anesthesia for a surgical procedure that may compromise oxygenation of the brain. Barbiturates are a reasonable choice of anesthetic, especially since this situation represents an opportunity to protect the brain before injury. Barring contraindications to its use, barbiturate anesthesia may be indicated in patients undergoing cerebral aneurysm clip-ligation, carotid endarterectomy, aortic arch repair, cardiopulmonary bypass (in patients who have cerebrovascular disease), mitral or aortic valve replacement (when there is increased risk for air embolism). Although the need to have an awake patient at the end of the operation will limit the amount of drug that can be given, this goal can be achieved in experienced hands (Hunter, 1972).

  b. In general, the anesthesiologist and the surgeon should agree beforehand that the potential benefits of barbiturate anesthesia will offset the anticipated need for invasive monitoring and postoperative ventilatory and circulatory support. The type of barbiturate, amount of drug, method of administration (single dose vs. continuous infusion), and duration of treatment (24–72 hr) are controversial. Many people use small single doses (e.g., thiopental 3–5 mg/kg) since this dose causes flattening of the EEG. No further reduction in $CMRO_2$ is achieved with the use of larger doses. The advantage of a small dose is the possible avoidance of hypotension, although this hemodynamic stability is not assured. Other clinicians recommend larger single doses (thiopental 30 mg/kg), but this ignores the fact that the period of postinsult injury may last from 24 to 72 hours. A more rational approach would be to adjust the dose to a physiologic endpoint (e.g., flat EEG) and to use a continuous infusion for 24 to 48 hours.

V. Treatment guidelines

A. Which barbiturate?

1. **Currently-used barbiturates.** Several drugs (thiopental, pentobarbital, phenobarbital, methohexital, thiamylal) have been used experimentally and clinically, but there are few comparative studies available. Therefore, the choice of drug must be based on the physical and pharmacologic properties of the individual drugs.

2. **Physical criteria and pharmacologic properties.** The passage of drugs across the blood-brain barrier requires low protein binding, low degree of ionization, and high lipid solubility. There are important differences among the pharmacologic properties of the three most commonly used barbiturates (phenobarbital, pentobarbital, thiopental; Table 4-6) (Sharpless, 1970; Scurr, 1974).

   a. **Phenobarbital.** Even though it has a low degree of protein binding, phenobarbital is highly ionized and has a comparatively low lipid solubility. Although it may not cross the blood-brain barrier as readily as pentobarbital and thiopental, phenobarbital has unique anticonvulsant properties, and this may be an important benefit to some patients.

   b. **Pentobarbital and thiopental.** Both pentobarbital and thiopental are significantly less ionized and more lipid soluble than phenobarbital. Thiopental has a more rapid onset of action than pentobarbital and although thiopental may not share the unique anticonvulsant actions of phenobarbital, its effectiveness in status epilepticus is well known (Brown, 1967).

   Thiopental is biotransformed to a pharmacologically active compound, pentobarbital (Fig. 4-8) (Mark, 1963). While thiopental's major metabolic pathway produces thiopental carboxylic acid, an inactive metabolite, significant (i.e., phar-

Table 4-6. Pharmacologic properties of the three most commonly used barbiturates

	Plasma protein binding (%)	pKa	% Nonionized (pH 7.4)	Partition coefficient (lipid/H_2O)
Phenobarbital	20	7.3	44	3
Pentobarbital	35	8.1	83	39
Thiopental	65	7.6	61	580

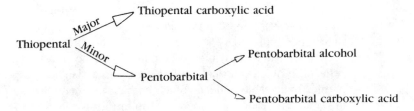

Fig. 4-8. Metabolism of thiopental along the major pathway to thiopental carboxylic acid and along the minor pathway to pentobarbital, which is then further metabolized to pentobarbital alcohol and pentobarbital carboxylic acid.

macologic) amounts of pentobarbital are produced when high doses of thiopental are used. Pentobarbital is metabolized exclusively to inactive compounds.

At the present time, thiopental appears to be the drug of choice because of its pharmacologic and physical properties. Pentobarbital is a reasonable alternative. Until we understand more about the mechanisms of their beneficial actions in specific brain injuries, the selection of a barbiturate will remain empiric.

B. Monitoring

  1. Blood levels. Blood levels of barbiturate should be measured every 6 to 8 hours during treatment. This is essential because of its nonlinear kinetics and the possibility of hepatic dysfunction in some persons. It should be clear that even with a constant rate of infusion, a steady-state condition cannot be achieved with a drug like thiopental. Therefore, serial blood levels provide essential feedback for proper adjustment of dose.

  2. ICP monitoring. ICP monitoring, a technique that offers a high degree of reliability and a low risk of infection, is essential in patients receiving barbiturates for control of increased ICP for the following three reasons:

  a. To detect neurologic deterioration when physical signs are obscured by barbiturates

  b. To guide therapeutic decisions

  c. To provide objective information (e.g., ICP, intracranial compliance) to support decisions about when to withdraw treatment

  3. Hemodynamic considerations

  a. Hemodynamic monitoring. Adequate hemodynamic monitoring of patients receiving high doses of barbiturates includes ECG, urinary catheter, and direct measurement of arterial pressure and central venous pressure (CVP). A thermodilution pulmonary artery catheter is indicated for any patient in whom CVP measurements would be unreliable reflections of left ventricular filling pressures and in hemodynamically unstable patients. Since barbiturates may directly affect all the major components of the cardiovascular system (heart rate, strength of contraction, preload, afterload), these parameters should be assessed individually to guide specific therapeutic interventions.

b. **Management of hypotension.** The management of hypotension is greatly facilitated by adequate monitoring (Shubin, 1971). It is not necessary to stop the barbiturate infusion.

   (1) The first step is to **restore intravascular volume.** This is particularly important in the patient who has been fluid-restricted.

   (2) If hypotension persists despite normovolemia, a **positive inotropic drug,** such as dopamine, can be used.

   (3) In rare instances, the addition of a **pure vasopressor,** such as phenylephrine, may be necessary.

   (4) As with any critically ill patient, the **adequacy of perfusion** should be assessed continually by physical examination, physiologic measurements (urine output, cardiac output), and biochemical tests (blood gases, pH, lactate).

C. **Drug administration**

1. **Dose versus efficacy.** The dosage of a drug can be determined when the pharmacology of the drug is understood and when there are clear endpoints indicating achievement of the desired therapeutic effect(s). With barbiturates, however, not only are the pharmacokinetics poorly understood, but the important therapeutic effects (except for the changes in $CMRO_2$ and ICP) are unknown or clinically unmeasurable.

   a. **Intracranial pressure** is easily measured, and, if reducing ICP is the only desired effect, then the dose can be adjusted according to response.

   b. Since the EEG becomes isoelectric when there is **maximal reduction of $CMRO_2$,** this monitor can be used to determine the dose needed for maximal metabolic depression.

   c. The dose to effect the **potential benefits of barbiturates** (free radical scavenging activity, improved perfusion) is unknown but may be equivalent to the large doses required to produce maximal depression of $CMRO_2$.

2. Dose regimens

a. Intraoperative control of ICP: thiopental, 1 to 3 mg/kg; may repeat every 20 to 30 minutes.

b. Prolonged control of ICP: pentobarbital.

(1) Loading dose: 3 to 5 mg/kg.

(2) Maintenance: 100 to 200 mg every 30 to 60 minutes or 2 mg/kg/hr as continuous infusion.

(3) Titrate to maximum blood level of 40 μg/ml.

(4) Stop treatment after 72 hours if ICP < 20 mmHg and compliance is normal.

c. "Maximal benefit" dose: thiopental.

(1) Loading dose: 15 mg/kg.

(2) Maintenance: 0.2 mg/kg/min as continuous infusion.

(3) Endpoints.

(a) Isoelectric EEG.

(b) Maximum blood level of 60 to 80 μg/ml.

(4) Stop treatment after 48 hours.

VI. Other drugs and techniques. The recent efforts to develop clinically useful techniques of cerebral protection (therapy before the ischemic episode) and amelioration (therapy after the episode) are based on experimental and anecdotal evidence that, under proper circumstances, the brain's tolerance to global and focal ischemia can be extended. Attempts to define these circumstances have been hampered, however, by the difficulty in applying animal data to the human situation and by the complexity, risk, and expense of certain of the therapeutic modalities. In addition to the barbiturates, a number of other drugs and procedures are currently under investigation.

A. Hypothermia. Hypothermia lowers the cerebral metabolic oxygen requirement by 7% to 13% for each degree centigrade that the temperature is reduced, thus enhancing the brain's ability to tolerate ischemia. Consequently, the brain can withstand complete ischemia for 4 minutes at 38°C, for 8 minutes at 30°C, for 16 minutes at 22°C, and for more than 30 minutes at 16°C. Few complications are associated with hypothermia of several hours' duration (as long as the temperature remains above 28°C to avoid arrhythmias), since brief periods of hypothermia do not entail significant metabolic alterations in the absence of shivering, poor tissue perfusion, or prolonged circulatory arrest. Liver, kidney, and endocrine function are decreased during hypothermia, but return to normal within 24 hours after rewarming. The action of narcotics and muscle relaxants is prolonged with cooling.

Shivering during cooling and rewarming increases oxygen consumption by 50% to 200%, and may be accompanied by anaerobic metabolism, progressive metabolic acidosis, and cardiac depression. Either thorazine (2.5 mg IV) or incremental doses of meperidine (10 mg IV) can be used to treat shivering in the postoperative period.

Rewarming after prolonged hypothermia for 1 to 3 days, however, has been accompanied by systemic acidosis, hemodynamic collapse, and death (Steen, 1979). Hypothermia to 29° for this period causes an increase in peripheral vascular resistance, areas of hypoperfusion of the skeletal muscle and cerebral cortex (Steen, 1980), and the accumulation of acid metabolites. The vascular beds that had closed down during hypothermia reopen with rewarming, introducing the previously sequestered acid metabolites to the systemic circulation and causing cardiovascular collapse. These events documented in animal models may represent the "rewarming shock" noted clinically after prolonged hypothermia (Fay, 1959).

Decreasing the body temperature also causes an increase in CO_2 solubility, pH, and CO_2-combining power, and a decrease in buffer capacity. The higher pH and lower temperature produce a leftward shift of the oxygen-hemoglobin dissociation curve. This greater affinity of oxygen for hemoglobin is partially counteracted by the increased solubility of oxygen at lower temperatures.

The desired temperature is attained by surface cooling. The blanket control is returned to the warm mode when the esophageal temperature falls to 33°C, because the temperature will drift downward another 2° to 3° to the desired level of 31°C. To achieve profound hypothermia, extracorporeal circulation is required.

The combination of barbiturates with a moderate degree of hypothermia (34° to 36°C) may be even more effective than either barbiturates or hypothermia alone, since a modest reduction in temperature has been shown in the hypoxic mouse model to retard depletion of adenosine triphosphate (ATP) and accumulation of lactic acid and to prolong survival time. The effects of barbiturates and hypothermia are additive in view of the fact that barbiturates affect cellular function as reflected by the EEG, while hypothermia preserves cellular integrity (protein synthesis, pump function).

B. Naloxone. Research continues to identify other drugs effective against focal ischemic insults. The neurologic deficit resulting from unilateral occlusion of the right common carotid artery in gerbils has been modified by the intraperitoneal or subcutaneous administration of the narcotic antagonist naloxone. Morphine given after ligation of the common carotid artery in gerbils that had not had a stroke was associated with development of a neurologic deficit that could be reversed by intraperitoneal injection of naloxone.

C. **Gamma-hydroxybutyrate, phenytoin.** Other drugs may exert a protective effect when given before or after a period of complete global ischemia. Gamma-hydroxybutyrate decreases the cerebral metabolic rate (Wolfson, 1977) and enhances hypoxic tolerance (in combination with glucagon), but it has been shown in dogs to reduce CBF to a greater extent than metabolic rate (Artru, 1980), limiting the degree of protection. In the hypoxic mouse model, phenytoin conferred protection that was greater than with gamma-hydroxybutyrate but less than with barbiturates. The mechanism of phenytoin's effect may be related to its limitation of potassium release from ischemic neurons due to membrane stabilization. This correlates with the postulated role released potassium plays in the irreversible neuronal damage that occurs during and after ischemia.

D. **Midazolam.** Midazolam depresses the cerebral metabolic rate in a dose-related fashion in dogs without a disproportionate reduction in CBF while maintaining hemodynamic stability. Brain biopsies taken after administration of midazolam revealed a normal cerebral energy state (phosphocreatine, ATP, ADP, and AMP) and normal glucose, lactate, and pyruvate concentrations. In the hypoxic mouse model ($FiO_2 = 0.05$), midazolam provided greater protection from hypoxia (2.8 times control survival time) than diazepam (1.6 times control survival time) but less than barbiturates (4.0 times control survival time).

Evidence that cerebral ischemic damage after stroke (Sundt, 1969) and cardiac arrest may be potentially reversible has spurred efforts to identify pharmacologic and mechanical means to avert infarction. While there has been progress, restraint is indicated in applying unsubstantiated and risk-laden modalities in the name of therapeutics.

References

1. Agnoli, A., Palesse, N., Ruggiersi, S., et al. Barbiturate Treatment of Acute Stroke. In M. Goldstein (Ed.), *Advances in Neurology*. New York: Raven, 1979. Pp. 269–274.
2. Alexander, S. C., Cohen, P. J., Wollman, H., et al. Cerebral carbohydrate metabolism during hypocarbia in man. *Anesthesiology* 26:625, 1965.

3. Allman, F. D., Talamo, J., and Rogers, M. C. Increased serum osmolality following pentobarbital anesthesia—A possible mechanism for lowering ICP. *Crit. Care Med.* 8:227, 1980.
4. Altura, B. T., and Altura, B. M. Barbiturates and aortic and venous smooth muscle function. *Anesthesiology* 43:432, 1975.
5. Ames, A., Wright, R. L., Kowada, M., et al. Cerebral ischemia: II. The no-reflow phenomenon. *Am. J. Pathol.* 52:455, 1968.
6. Aoki, Y., and Lembroso, C. T. Prognostic value of electroencephalography in Reyes Syndrome. *Neurology* 23:333, 1973.
6a. Artru, A. A., Steen, P. A., and Michenfelder, J. D. γ-Hydroxybutyrate: Cerebral metabolic, vascular, and protective effects. *J. Neurochem.* 35:1114–1119, 1980.
7. Astrup, J., Nordstorm, C. H., and Rehncrona, S. Rate of Rise in Extracellular Potassium in the Ischemic Rat Brain and the Effect of Preischemic Metabolic Rate. In O. H. Ingvar and N. Lassen (Eds.), *Cerebral Function, Metabolism and Circulation.* Copenhagen: Munksgaard, 1977. Pp. 376–377.
8. Atkins, J. N., and Haponik, E. F. Reyes syndrome in the adult patient. *Am. J. Med.* 67:672, 1979.
9. Babior, B. M., Kipnes, R., and Cornutte, J. Biologic defense mechanisms: The production by leukocytes of superoxide, a potential bactericidal agent. *J. Clin. Invest.* 52:741, 1973.
10. Bandaranayake, N. M., Nemoto, E. M., and Stezoski, S. W. Rat brain osmolality during barbiturate anesthesia and global brain ischemia. *Stroke* 9:249, 1978.
11. Bates, D., Caronna, J. J., Cartlidge, N. E. F., et al. A prospective study of nontraumatic coma: Methods and results in 310 patients. *Ann. Neurol.* 2:211, 1977.
12. Bauer, R. B., Meyer, J. S., Fields, W. S., et al. Joint study of extracranial arterial occlusion: Progress report of controlled study of long-term survival in patients with and without operation. *J.A.M.A.* 208:509, 1969.
13. Becker, D. P., Miller, J., Ward, J. D., et al. The outcome from severe head injury with early diagnosis and intensive management. *J. Neurosurg.* 47:491, 1977.
14. Becker, K. E., and Tonnesen, A. S. Cardiovascular effects of plasma levels of thiopental necessary for anesthesia. *Anesthesiology* 49:197, 1978.
15. Bell, J. A., and Hodgson, J. F. Coma after cardiac arrest. *Brain* 97:361, 1974.
16. Berman, W., Pizzi, F., Schut, L., et al. The effects of exchange transfusion on intracranial pressure in patient with Reyes syndrome. *J. Pediatr.* 87:887, 1975.
17. Black, K. L., Weidler, M. D., Jallad, N. S., et al. Delayed pentobarbital therapy of acute focal ischemia. *Stroke* 9:245, 1978.
18. Bleyaert, A. L., Nemoto, E. M., Safar, P., et al. Thiopental amelioration of brain damage after global ischemia in monkeys. *Anesthesiology* 49:390, 1978.
19. Bleyaert, A. L., Safar, P., Nemoto, E. M., et al. Effect of postcirculatory-arrest life support on neurological recovery in monkeys. *Crit. Care Med.* 8:153, 1980.
20. Bobo, R. C., Schubert, W. K., and Partin, J. C. Reyes syndrome: Treatment by exchange transfusion with special reference to the 1974 epidemic in Cincinnati, Ohio. *J. Pediatr.* 87:881, 1975.
21. Boutnos, A., Hoyt, T., Menezes, A., and Bell, W. Management of Reyes syndrome. A rational approach to a complex problem. *Crit. Care Med.* 5:234, 1977.
22. Bradford, W. D., and Latham, W. C. Acute encephalopathy and fatty hepatomegaly. *Am. J. Dis. Child.* 114:152, 1967.
23. Brann, A. W., and Montalvo, J. M. Barbiturates and asphyxia. *Pediatr. Clin. North Am.* 17:851, 1970.
24. Branston, N. M., Hope, T., and Symon, L. Barbiturates in focal ischemia of primate cortex: Effects on blood flow distribution, evoked potential and extracellular potassium. *Stroke* 10:647, 1979.
25. Breivik, H., Safar, P., Sands, P., et al. Clinical feasibility trials of barbiturate therapy after cardiac arrest. *Crit. Care Med.* 6:228, 1978.

26. Brian, W. R., Hunter, D., and Turnbull, H. M. Acute meningo-encephalitis of childhood. *Lancet* 1:221, 1929.
27. Brown, A. S., and Horton, J. M. Status epilepticus treated by intravenous infusions of thiopental sodium. *Br. Med. J.* 1:27, 1967.
28. Brown, B. R. Anesthetic Hepatic Toxicity: A Scientific Problem? *ASA Refresher Courses* number 106B, 1979.
29. Browne, T. R., and Roskanzer, D. C. Treatment of strokes. I and II. *N. Engl. J. Med.* 281:594 and 650, 1969.
30. Bruce, D. A., et al. Pathophysiology, treatment and outcome following severe head injury in children. *Childs Brain* 5:174, 1979.
31. Butterfield, J. D., and McGraw, C. P. Free radical pathology. *Stroke* 9:443, 1978.
32. Carlon, G. C., Kahn, R. C., Goldiner, P. L., et al. Long-term infusion of sodium pentothal: Hemodynamic and respiratory effects. *Crit. Care Med.* 6:311, 1978.
33. Caronna, J. J., and Finkelstein, S. Neurological syndromes after cardiac arrest. *Stroke* 9:517, 1978.
34. Chadwick, H. S., Todd, M. M., Shapiro, H. M., et al. Neurologic outcome following cardiac arrest in thiopental treated cats. *Anesthesiology* (Suppl.) 53:156, 1980.
35. Chin, J. Influenza surveillance: Reye's Syndrome and viral infections—United States. *Morbid. Mortal.* 23:58, 1974.
36. Christensen, M. S. Prolonged artificial hyperventilation in cerebral apoplexy. *Acta Anaesthesiol. Scand.* (Suppl. 62):8, 1976.
37. Christensen, M. S., Paulson, O. B., Olesen, J., et al. Cerebral apoplexy (stroke) treated with or without prolonged artificial hyperventilation: Cerebral circulation, clinical course, and cause of death. *Stroke* 4:568, 1973.
38. Clasen, R. A., Pandolfii, S., and Casey, D. Furosemide and pentobarbital in cryogenic cerebral injury and edema. *Neurology* 24:642, 1974.
39. Cobb, L. A., Warner, J. A., and Trobaugh, G. B. Sudden cardiac death: Outcome of resuscitation, management, and future directions. *Mod. Concepts Cardiovasc. Dis.* 69:37, 1980.
40. Collice, M., et al. Management of head injury by means of ventricular fluid pressure monitoring. In J. W. F. Beks, D. A. Bosch, and M. Breck (Eds.), *Intracranial Pressure III.* New York: Springer, 1976. Pp. 101–109.
41. Conn, A. W., Edmonds, J. F., and Barker, G. A. Near-drowning in cold freshwater: Current treatment regimens. *Can. Anaesth. Soc. J.* 25:259, 1978.
42. Conn, A. W., Montes, J. E., Barker, G. A., and Edmonds, J. F. Cerebral salvage in near-drowning following neurological classification by triage. *Can. Anaesth. Soc. J.* 27:201, 1980.
43. Cooper, P. R., Moody, S., Clark, K., et al. Dexamethasone and severe head injury: A prospective double-blind study. *J. Neurosurg.* 51:307, 1979.
44. Corkill, G., Chikovani, O. K., McLeish, I., et al. Timing of pentobarbital administration for brain protection in experimental stroke. *Surg. Neurol.* 5:147, 1976.
45. Coté, J., Simard, D., and Rouillard, M. Repercussion sur le debit sanguin cerebral d'une perfusion de thiopental. *Can. Anaesth. Soc. J.* 26:269, 1979.
46. Davis, J. N. The use of small animals to study the effects of hypoxia. *Adv. Neurol.* 26:167, 1979.
47. Demopoulos, H. B., Flamm, E. S., Seligman, M. L., et al. Antioxidant effects of barbiturates in model membranes undergoing free radical damage. *Acta Neurol. Scand.* 56 (Suppl. 64):7, 1977.
48. DeVivo, D. C., Keating, J. P., and Haymond, M. W. Reye's syndrome: Results of intensive supportive care. *J. Pediatr.* 87:875, 1975.
49. Dolovich, J., Evans, S., Rosenbloom, D., et al. Anaphylaxis due to thiopental sodium anaesthesia. *Can. Med. Assoc. J.* 123:292, 1980.
50. Dwyer, E. M., and Wiener, L. Left ventricular function in man following thiopental. *Anes. Analg.* 48:499, 1969.

51. Eckstein, J. W., Hamilton, W. K., and McCammond, J. M.   The effect of thiopental on peripheral venous tone. *Anesthesiology* 22:525, 1961.
52. Elder, J. D., Nagono, S. M., Eastwood, D. W., and Harnagel, D.   Circulatory changes associated with thiopental anesthesia in man. *Anesthesiology* 16:394, 1955.
53. Etsten, B., and Li, T. H.   Hemodynamic changes during thiopental anesthesia in humans: Cardiac output, stroke volume, total peripheral resistance, and intrathoracic blood volume. *J. Clin. Invest.* 34:500, 1955.
54. Etsten, B., and Li, T. H.   Effects of anesthesia upon the heart. *Am. J. Cardiol.* 6:706, 1960.
54a. Fay, T. Early experiences with local and generalized refrigeration of the human brain. *J. Neurosurg.* 16:239, 1959.
55. Fishman, R. A.   Brain edema. *N. Engl. J. Med.* 293:706, 1975.
56. Flamm, E. S., Demopoulos, H. B., Seligman, M. L., et al.   Free radicals in cerebral ischemia. *Stroke* 9:445, 1978.
57. Flamm, E. S., Seligman, M. L., and Demopoulos, H. B.   Barbiturate Protection of the Ischemic Brain. In J. E. Cottrell and H. Turndorf (Eds.), *Anesthesia and Neurosurgery*. St. Louis: Mosby, 1980. Pp. 248–266.
58. Frank, L., and Massaro, D.   The lung and oxygen toxicity. *Arch. Intern. Med.* 139:347, 1979.
59. Fridovich, I.   Hypoxia and Oxygen Toxicity. In S. Fahn (Ed.), *Advances in Neurology*. New York: Raven Press, 26:255, 1979.
60. Giammona, S. T.   Drowning pathophysiology and management. *Curr. Probl. Pediatr.* 1:1, 1971.
61. Goldstein, A., Wells, B. A., and Keats, A. S.   Increased tolerance to cerebral anoxia by pentobarbital. *Arch. Int. Pharmacodyn. Ther.* 161:138, 1966.
62. Hankinson, H., Smith, A. L., Nielsen, S. L., et al.   Effect of thiopental on focal ischemia in dogs. *Surg. Forum* 25:445, 1974.
63. Hochberg, F. H., Nelson, K., and Janzen, W.   Influenza type B related encephalopathy: The outbreak of Reyes syndrome in Chicago. *J.A.M.A.* 231:817, 1975.
64. Hoff, B. H.   Multisystem failure: A review with special reference to drowning. *Crit. Care Med.* 7:310, 1979.
65. Hoff, J. T.   Resuscitation in focal brain ischemia. *Crit. Care Med.* 6:245, 1978.
66. Hoff, J. T., Pitts, L. H., Spetzler, R., et al.   Barbiturates for protection from cerebral ischemia in aneurysm surgery. In D. H. Ingvar and N. Lassen (Eds.), Cerebral Function, Metabolism and Circulation. *Acta Neurol. Scand.* 56 (Suppl. 64) 56:158, 1977.
67. Hoff, J. T., Smith, A. L., Hankinson, H. L.   Barbiturate protection from cerebral infarction in primates. *Stroke* 6:28, 1975.
68. Hunter, A. R.   Thiopentone supplemented anaesthesia for neurosurgery. *Br. J. Anaesth.* 44:506, 1972.
69. Huttenlocher, P. R.   Reyes syndrome: Relation of outcome to therapy. *J. Pediatr.* 80:845, 1972.
70. Jackson, D. L., and Dole, W. P.   Total cerebral ischemia: A new model system for the study of post cardiac arrest brain damage. *Stroke* 10:38, 1979.
71. Jamison, R. L.   The role of cellular swelling in the pathogenesis of organ ischemia. *West. J. Med.* 120:205, 1974.
72. Jennett, B., and Bond, M.   Assessment of outcome after severe brain damage: A practical scale. *Lancet* 1:480, 1975.
73. Jennett, G., Teasdale, S., Galbraith, J., et al.   Severe head injuries in three countries. *J. Neurol. Neurosurg. Psychiatry* 40:291, 1977.
74. Johnson, G. M., Scurletis, T. D., and Carroll, N. B.   A study of sixteen fatal cases of encephalitis-like disease in North Carolina children. *N. C. Med. J.* 24:464, 1963.

75. Keenan.   Personal communication.
76. Kennealy, J. A., McLennan, J. E., Loudon, R. G., and McLaurin, R. L.   Hyperventilation-induced cerebral hypoxia. *Am. Rev. Respir. Dis.* 122:407, 1980.
77. Kindt, G. W., Waldman, J., Kohl, S., et al.   Intracranial pressure in Reye's syndrome: Monitoring and control. *J.A.M.A.* 231:822, 1975.
78. Kofke, W. A., Nemoto, E. M., Hossman, K. A., et al.   Brain blood flow and metabolism after global ischemia and post-insult thiopental therapy in monkeys. *Stroke* 10:554, 1979.
79. Langfitt, T. W.   The Incidence and Importance of Intracranial Hypertension in Head-Injured Patients. In J. W. F. Beks, D. A. Bosch, and M. Breck (Eds.), *Intracranial Pressure III*. New York: Springer, 1976. Pp. 67–72.
80. Langfitt, T. W.   Measuring the outcome from head injuries. *J. Neurosurg.* 48:673, 1978.
81. Lansky, L. L., Kalavsky, S. M., Brackett, C. E., et al.   Hypothermic total body washout and intracranial pressure monitoring in stage IV Reye's syndrome. *J. Pediatr.* 90:634, 1977.
82. Lawner, P., Lourent, J., Simeone, F., et al.   Attenuation of ischemic brain edema by pentobarbital after carotid ligation in the gerbil. *Stroke* 10:644, 1979.
83. Leibovitz, B. E., and Siegel, B. V.   Aspects of free radical reactions in biological systems—Aging. *J. Gerontol.* 35:45, 1980.
84. Linko, E., Koskinen, P. J., Sitonen, L., and Ruosteenoja, R.   Resuscitation in cardiac arrest: An analysis of 100 consecutive medical cases. *Acta Med. Scand.* 182:611, 1967.
85. Lovejoy, F. H., Bresnan, M. J., Lombroso, C. T., and Smith, A. L.   Anticerebral edema therapy in Reye's syndrome. *Arch. Dis. Child.* 50:933, 1975.
86. Lovejoy, F. H., Smith, A. L., Bresnan, M. J., et al.   Clinical staging in Reye's syndrome. *Am. J. Dis. Child.* 128:36, 1974.
87. Mark, L. C.   Metabolism of barbiturates in man. *Clin. Pharmacol. Ther.* 4:504, 1963.
88. Marshall, L. F., Shapiro, H. M., Ranscher, A., and Kaufman, N. M.   Pentobarbital therapy for intracranial hypertension in metabolic coma: Reye's syndrome. *Crit. Care Med.* 6:1, 1978.
89. Marshall, L. F., Smith, R. W., and Shapiro, H. M.   The outcome with aggressive treatment in severe head injuries: Part II. Acute and chronic barbiturate administration in the management of head injury. *J. Neurosurg.* 50:26, 1979.
90. McCord, J. M., and Fridovich, I.   The biology and pathology of oxygen radicals. *Ann. Intern. Med.* 89:122, 1978.
91. McGraw, C. P.   Experimental cerebral infarction effects of pentobarbital in Mongolian gerbils. *Arch. Neurol.* 34:334, 1977.
92. Michenfelder, J. D.   The interdependency of cerebral functional and metabolic effects following massive doses of thiopental in the dog. *Anesthesiology* 41:231, 1974.
93. Michenfelder, J. D.   Cerebral protection with barbiturates: Relation to anesthetic effect. *Stroke* 9:140, 1978.
94. Michenfelder, J. D., and Milde, J. H.   Influence of anesthetics on metabolic functional and pathological response to regional cerebral ischemia. *Stroke* 6:405, 1975.
95. Michenfelder, J. D., Milde, J. H., and Sundt, T. M.   Cerebral protection by barbiturate anesthesia. *Arch. Neurol.* 33:345, 1976.
96. Michenfelder, J. D., and Theye, R. A.   Cerebral protection by thiopental during hypoxia. *Anesthesiology* 39:510, 1973.
97. Mickell, J. J., Reigel, D. H., Cook, D. R., et al.   Intracranial pressure: Monitoring and normalization therapy in children. *Pediatrics* 59:606, 1977.

98. Mihm, F.   Unpublished data.
99. Miller, J. D., Sweet, R. C., Narayan, R., and Becker, D. P.   Early insults to the injured brain. *J.A.M.A.* 240:439, 1978.
100. Modell, J. H., Graves, S. A., and Kuck, E. J.   Near-drowning: Correlation of level of consciousness and survival. *Can. Anaesth. Soc. J.* 27:211, 1980.
101. Moseley, J. I., Laurent, J. P., and Molinari, G. F.   Barbiturate attenuation of the clinical course and pathologic lesions in a primate stroke model. *Neurology* 25:870, 1975.
102. Myerburg, R. J., Conde, C. A., Sung, R. J., et al.   Clinical, electrophysiologic, and hemodynamic profile of patients resuscitated from prehospital cardiac arrest. *Am. J. Med.* 68:568, 1980.
103. Nadler, H.   Therapeutic delirium in Reye's syndrome. *Pediatrics* 54:265, 1974.
104. Negovskii, V. A.   Introduction: Reanimatology—The Science of Resuscitation. In H. E. Stephenso (Ed.), *Cardiac Arrest and Resuscitation.* St. Louis: Mosby, 1974. Chap. 1.
105. Nemoto, E. M., Erdman, W., Strong, E., Rao, G. R., et al.   Regional brain PO_2 after global ischemia in monkeys: Evidence for regional differences in critical perfusion pressures. *Stroke* 10:44, 1979.
106. Nilsson, L.   The influence of barbiturate anesthesia upon the energy state and upon acid-base parameters of the brain in arterial hypotension and in asphyxia. *Acta Neurol. Scand.* 47:233, 1971.
107. Norris, J. R., and Chandrasekar, S.   Anoxic brain damage after cardiac resuscitation. *J. Chronic. Dis.* 24:585, 1971.
108. O'Brien, M. D.   Ischemic cerebral edema—A review. *Stroke* 10:623, 1979.
109. O'Brien, M. D., Waltz, A. G., and Jordan, M. M.   Ischemic cerebral edema: Distribution of water in brains of cats after occlusion of the middle cerebral artery. *Arch. Neurol.* 30:456, 1974.
110. Overgaard, J., et al.   Prognosis after head injury based on early clinical exam. *Lancet* 2:631, 1973.
111. Pearn, J.   Survival rates after serious immersion accidents in childhood. *Resuscitation* 6:271, 1979.
112. Peterson, B.   Morbidity of childhood near-drowning. *Pediatrics* 59:364, 1977.
113. Pierce, E. C., et al.   Cerebral circulation and metabolism during thiopental anesthesia and hypoventilation in man. *J. Clin. Invest.* 41:1664, 1962.
114. Reye, R. D. K., Morgan, G., and Baral, J.   Encephalopathy and fatty degeneration of the viscera: A disease entity in childhood. *Lancet* 2:749, 1963.
115. Rockoff, M. A., Marshall, L. F., and Shapiro, H. M.   High-dose barbiturate therapy in humans: A clinical review of 60 patients. *Ann. Neurol.* 6:194, 1979.
116. Rosenthal, M. H., and Larson, C. P.   Protection of the brain from progressive ischemia. *West. J. Med.* 128:145, 1978.
117. Safar, P.   Brain resuscitation in metabolic-toxic infectious encephalopathy. *Crit. Care Med.* 6:68, 1978.
118. Sahs, A. L. (Ed.).   Stroke Unit: Patient Evaluation, Treatment, and Followup. In *Fundamentals of Stroke Care.* U.S. Government Printing Office, 1976. Pp. 330–339.
119. Samaha, F. J., Balu, E., and Berardinelli, J. L.   Reye's syndrome: Clinical diagnosis and treatment with peritoneal dialysis. *Pediatrics* 53:336, 1974.
120. Scurr, C., and Feldman, S. (Eds.).   *Scientific Foundations of Anesthesia.* Chicago: Year Book, 1974. P. 410.
121. Shafer, S. Q., Bruun, B., and Richter, R. W.   The outcome of stroke at hospital discharge in New York City blacks. *Stroke* 4:782, 1973.
122. Shapiro, H. M., Galindo, A., Wyte, S. R., and Harris, A. B.   Rapid intraoperative

reduction of intracranial pressure with thiopentone. *Br. J. Anaesth.* 45:1057, 1973.

123. Shapiro, H. M., Wyte, S. R., and Loeser, J.   Barbiturate augmented hypothermia for reduction of persistent intracranial hypertension. *J. Neurosurg.* 40:90, 1974.

124. Sharpless, S. K.   Hypnotics and Sedatives—The Barbiturates. In L. S. Goodman and A. Gilman (Eds.), *The Pharmacological Basis of Therapeutics* (4th Ed.). New York: Macmillan, 1970. Pp. 98–120.

125. Shaywitz, B. A., Leventhal, J. M., Kramer, M. S., and Venes, J. L.   Prolonged continuous monitoring of intracranial pressure in severe Reye's Syndrome. *Pediatrics* 54:595, 1977.

126. Shubin, H., and Weil, M. H.   Shock associated with barbiturate intoxication. *Crit. Care Med.* 215:263, 1971.

127. Siebke, H., Rod, T., Breivik, H., and Lind, B.   Survival after 40 minutes submersion without cerebral sequelae. *Lancet* 1:1275, 1975.

128. Siegel, J. H., and Sonneblick, E. H.   Quantification and prediction of myocardial failure. *Arch. Surg.* 89:1026, 1964.

129. Simeone, F. A., Frazer, G., and Lawner, P.   Ischemic brain edema: Comparative effects of barbiturates and hypothermia. *Stroke* 10:8, 1979.

130. Smith, A.   Barbiturate protection in cerebral hypoxia. *Anesthesiology* 47:285, 1977.

131. Smith, A. L., Hoff, J. T., Nielsen, S. L., and Larson, C. P.   Barbiturate protection in acute focal cerebral ischemia. *Stroke* 5:1, 1974.

132. Smith, A. L., and Margue, J. J.   Anesthetics and cerebral edema. *Anesthesiology* 45:64, 1976.

133. Smith, D. S., Rehncrona, S., and Siesjo, B. K.   Inhibitory effects of different barbiturates on lipid peroxidation in brain tissue in vitro: Comparison with the effects of promethazine and chloropromazine. *Anesthesiology* 53:186, 1980.

134. Snyder, B. D., Ramirez-Lassepas, M., and Lippert, D. M.   Neurologic status and prognosis after cardiopulmonary arrest: A retrospective study. *Neurology* 27:807, 1977.

135. Snyder, B. D., Ramirez-Lassepas, M., Sukhaum, P., et al.   Failure of thiopental to modify global anoxic injury. *Stroke* 10:135, 1979.

136. Sonntag, H., Hellerberg, K., Schesk, H. D., et al.   Effects of thiopental (trapanal) on coronary blood flow and myocardial metabolism in man. *Acta Anaesthesiol. Scand.* 19:69, 1975.

137. Stanski, D. R., Mihm, F. G., Rosenthal, M. H., and Kalman, S. M.   Pharmacokinetics of high dose thiopental used in cerebral resuscitation. *Anesthesiology* 53:169, 1980.

138. Steen, P. A., and Michenfelder, J. D.   Cerebral protection with barbiturates: Relation to anesthetic effect. *Stroke* 9:140, 1978.

139. Steen, P. A., and Michenfelder, J. D.   Neurotoxicity of anesthetics. *Anesthesiology* 50:437, 1979.

140. Steen, P. A., Milde, J. H., and Michenfelder, J. D.   No barbiturate protection in a dog model of complete cerebral ischemia. *Ann. Neurol.* 5:343, 1979.

140a. Steen, P. A., Milde, J. H., and Michenfelder, J. D.   The detrimental effects of prolonged hypothermia and rewarming in the dog. *Anesthesiology* 52:224, 1980.

140b. Steen, P. A., Soule, E. H., and Michenfelder, J. D.   Detrimental effects of prolonged hypothermia in cats and monkeys with and without regional cerebral ischemia. *Stroke* 10:522, 1979.

140c. Sundt, T. M., Jr., Grant, W. C., and Garcia, J. H.   Restoration of middle cerebral artery flow in experimental infarction. *J. Neurosurg.* 31:311, 1969.

140d. Todd, M. M., Chadwick, H. S., Shapiro, H. M., et al.   The neurological effect of thiopental therapy following experimental cardiac arrest in cats. *Anesthesiology* 57:76, 1982.

141. Toman, J. E. P.   Drugs Effective in Convulsive Disorders. In L. W. Goodman and A. Gilman (Eds.), *The Pharmacological Basis of Therapeutics* (4th Ed.). New York: Macmillan, 1970. P. 209.

142. Trauner, D. A.   Treatment of Reye's Syndrome. *Ann. Neurol.* 7:2, 1980.

143. Van Caille, M., Morin, C. L., Roy, C. C.,   Reye's Syndrome: Relapses and neurological sequelae. *Pediatrics* 59:244, 1977.

144. Van Horn, G.   Cerebrovascular Disease. In *Disease-A-Month*. Chicago: Year Book, 1973. Pp. 1–35.

145. Venes, J. L., Shaywitz, B. A., and Spencer, D. D.   Management of severe cerebral edema in the metabolic encephalopathy of Reye-Johnson syndrome. *J. Neurosurg.* 48:903, 1978.

146. Wade, J. G., Amtorp, O., and Sorensen, S. C.   No-flow state following cerebral ischemia: Role of increase in potassium concentration in brain interstitial fluid. *Arch. Neurol.* 32:381, 1975.

147. Waltz, A. G.   Clinical relevance of models of cerebral ischemia. *Stroke* 10:211, 1979.

148. Willoughby, J. O., and Leach, B. G.   Relation of neurological findings after cardiac arrest to outcome. *Br. Med. J.* 3:437, 1974.

148a. Wolfson, L. T., Sakurado, O., and Sokoloff, L.   Effects of γ-butyrolactone on local cerebral glucose utilization in the rat. *J. Neurochem.* 29:777, 1977.

149. Wright, R. L., and Ames, A.   Measurement of maximal permissible cerebral ischemia and a study of its pharmacologic prolongation. *J. Neurosurg.* 21:567, 1964.

150. Yatsu, F. M., Diamond, I., Graziano, C., and Lindquist, P.   Experimental brain ischemia: Protection from irreversible damage with a rapid-acting barbiturate (methohexital). *Stroke* 3:726, 1972.

II. Intensive Care

5. Respiratory Care of the Neurosurgical Patient

Robert L. Iverson, Jr.
Neal H. Cohen
Elizabeth A. M. Frost

The hospital course of patients who have neurosurgical disorders is adversely affected by pulmonary complications. If untreated, these secondary complications can contribute significantly to morbidity and mortality. Intensive respiratory care to reverse the abnormalities of gas exchange will improve survival.

I. Clinical physiology

A. Oxygen transport and consumption

1. **Oxygen delivery.** The presence of adequate ventilation and oxygenation, as indicated by an acceptable arterial oxygen tension (PaO_2) and carbon dioxide tension ($PaCO_2$), does not guarantee sufficient oxygen transport and delivery at the cellular level. Oxygen loading into and release from the hemoglobin molecule depend on the configuration of the oxyhemoglobin dissociation curve (Fig. 5-1). Shifting the oxyhemoglobin dissociation curve to the right increases the P_{50} (PaO_2 at which hemoglobin is half-saturated with oxygen) and decreases hemoglobin's affinity for oxygen. There is thus greater cellular unloading of oxygen. A shift of the curve to the left has the opposite effect, and peripheral delivery of oxygen is decreased.

   a. **Factors that shift the curve to the right** include

      (1) Hyperthermia

      (2) Hypercapnia

      (3) Acidosis

      (4) Increased red cell 2,3-diphosphoglyceric acid (2,3-DPG) concentration

   b. **A leftward shift** is associated with

      (1) Hypothermia

      (2) Hypocapnia

      (3) Hypophosphatemia

      (4) Alkalosis

      (5) Reduction in red cell 2,3-DPG concentration (as from administration of old blood)

      (6) Anemia

2. **Oxygen consumption.** The normal rate of oxygen consumption at basal metabolic rate (BMR) for the average 70-kg adult is

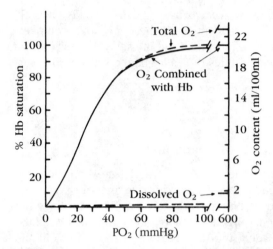

Fig. 5-1. Oxyhemoglobin dissociation curve. The oxyhemoglobin curve in graphic form describes the affinity of hemoglobin for oxygen. It depicts the percent of hemoglobin that exists as HbO_2 at various levels of O_2 tension. For example, when PO_2 is 50 mmHg, Hb is 85% saturated with O_2. (This standard curve is applicable when pH is 7.4, PCO_2 40 mmHg, temperature 37°C.) Oxygen content is also shown. This assumes the hemoglobin level is 15 gm/100 ml, and that each gram of hemoglobin when fully saturated combines with 1.34 ml O_2. The dotted line represents O_2 content (HbO_2 plus dissolved O_2). Note that dissolved O_2 contributes little to O_2 content at ordinary levels of PaO_2. (From H. A. Braun, F. W. Cheney, Jr., and C. P. Loehnen, *Introduction to Respiratory Physiology* (2nd ed.). Boston: Little, Brown, 1980.)

250 ml O_2/min (150 ml O_2/min/m^2). Oxygen consumption is increased by fever, tissue trauma, and sepsis.

Arterial oxygen saturation must be greater than 80% to provide adequate oxygen content. Any decrease in cardiac output, hemoglobin, or oxygen saturation will decrease oxygen delivery unless compensatory mechanisms occur. In the presence of either anemia or hypoxia, cardiac output will increase to maintain oxygen delivery at a constant level. If either the heart is failing or cardiac output is reduced by shock, this compensation cannot occur. As cardiac output decreases and circulation time slows, the oxygen extraction by the tissues increases, resulting in an increased arterial-venous (A-V) oxygen difference. When all compensatory mechanisms fail, anaerobic metabolism at the cellular level causes lactic acidosis.

B. Interpretation of arterial blood gases. A clear understanding of the significance of arterial blood gas values is essential. Assessment of respiratory and acid-base status may be made by application of a few basic concepts. Data from arterial blood gas measurement should always be interpreted in the light of the patient's age, past medical history, and current clinical condition.

1. Normal arterial blood gas values

PaO_2	80–100 mmHg
$PaCO_2$	37–43 mmHg
pH	7.37–7.43
HCO_3^-	23–28 mEq/L

2. Definition and rules

a. The patient is acidemic if the pH is less than 7.37.

b. The patient is alkalemic if the pH is greater than 7.43.

c. The patient has respiratory acidosis if the $PaCO_2$ is greater than 43 mmHg.

d. The patient has respiratory alkalosis if the $PaCO_2$ is less than 37 mmHg.

e. The patient has metabolic acidosis if the bicarbonate (HCO_3^-) is less than 23 mEq/L.

f. The patient has metabolic alkalosis if the HCO_3^- is greater than 28 mEq/L.

3. Primary vs. compensatory acid-base imbalance. A primary acid-base disturbance moves the pH *away* from normal and is the consequence of an underlying disease process. The compensatory response of the body is to move the pH back *toward* normal (Table 5-1). A *mixed* acid-base imbalance occurs when more than one *primary* acid-base imbalance coexist. For example, a mixed imbalance exists in the patient who has acute respiratory acidosis owing to hypoventilation and CO_2 retention and a coexisting metabolic acidosis, such as lactic acidosis, from hemorrhagic shock. A situation in which the primary pathologic processes would move the pH in opposite directions and tend to normalize the pH occurs in the patient in respiratory failure from pulmonary edema (respiratory acidosis) who is treated by prolonged nasogastric suction (metabolic alkalosis).

a. Primary respiratory acidosis

(1) Causes. Primary respiratory acidosis occurs during hypoventilation with CO_2 retention. Retention of CO_2 increases the concentration of carbonic acid (H_2CO_3) and

Table 5-1. Compensatory responses to primary acid-base imbalances

Imbalance	Compensatory response
Primary respiratory acidosis (acute)	HCO_3^- rises 3–4 mEq/L to 32 mEq/L
Primary respiratory acidosis (chronic)	HCO_3^- rises 0.4 mEq/L for each 1 mmHg increase in $PaCO_2$
Primary respiratory alkalosis (acute)	HCO_3^- decreases 0.2 mEq/L for each 1 mmHg decrease in $PaCO_2$
Primary respiratory alkalosis (chronic)	HCO_3^- decreases 0.5 mEq/L for each 1 mmHg decrease in the PCO_2 to 15 mEq/L
Primary metabolic acidosis	PCO_2 decreases 1–1.3 mmHg for each 1 mEq/L decrease in HCO_3^-
Primary metabolic alkalosis	$PaCO_2$ increases 0.5–1.0 mmHg for each 1 mEq/L increase in HCO_3^-

causes acidemia. Hypoventilation can be caused by the following:

(a) Central nervous system (CNS) depression from drugs or lesions affecting the respiratory center

(b) Neuromuscular disorders

(c) Acute or chronic parenchymal lung disease

(d) Airway obstruction

(e) Thoracic cage disorders

(f) Cardiorespiratory arrest

(g) Abnormal lung motion caused by pleural effusion or pneumothorax

(h) Ventilator malfunction

(2) **Compensation.** Secondary compensation for primary respiratory acidosis does occur. Acutely, acidosis causes

an increase in HCO_3^- of only 3 to 4 mEq/L. No significant renal compensation occurs initially. In the chronic phase, however, the kidney compensates after 6 to 12 hours, and renal retention of HCO_3^- occurs. There will be an increase of 0.4 mEq/L in the serum HCO_3^- for each 1.0 mmHg rise in the $PaCO_2$. Hypochloremia is also associated with renal compensation since, during HCO_3^- retention, chloride is excreted by the tubule to preserve electroneutrality.

b. Primary respiratory alkalosis

(1) **Causes.** Primary respiratory alkalosis occurs during hyperventilation because of increased CO_2 excretion by the lungs. Hyperventilation can be caused by the following:

(a) Hypoxia

(b) CNS injury

(c) Fever

(d) Sepsis

(e) Inappropriate mechanical ventilation

(f) Parenchymal lung disease

(g) Drugs

(h) Hepatic insufficiency

(i) Hyperthyroidism

(2) **Compensation.** Hypocapnia results in an alkalosis, which titrates tissue buffers and causes an immediate decrease in the serum HCO_3^- of 0.2 mEq/L for each 1 mmHg fall in the $PaCO_2$. Renal compensation, sufficient to restore the pH to normal, is marked by acid retention; excretion of HCO_3^- occurs after 7 to 9 days. Chronic respiratory alkalosis is the *only* primary acid-base disturbance in which the secondary compensatory reactions will return the pH to normal.

c. Primary metabolic acidosis

(1) **Causes.** Metabolic acidosis occurs when a strong acid is externally or endogenously added to the body or when alkali (HCO_3^-) is lost from body fluids by way of the kidney or gastrointestinal tract.

(2) Compensation. Acidemia is immediately buffered, causing a decrease in the serum HCO_3^-. Respiratory compensation occurs rapidly through hyperventilation and a decrease in $PaCO_2$. Carbonic acid (H_2CO_3) concentration is reduced and returns the pH toward normal. The respiratory compensation does not reach a steady state until 12 to 24 hours after the onset of metabolic acidosis, and pH is never restored to the previous normal level.

d. Primary metabolic alkalosis

(1) Causes. Metabolic alkalosis occurs when there is an increase in the serum HCO_3^- owing to the following:

(a) Endogenous or exogenous addition of alkali

(b) Loss of acid

(c) Increased excretion of chloride that exceeds the loss of HCO_3^-

(2) Compensation. The respiratory compensation for alkalemia is hypoventilation and retention of CO_2, which increases the concentration of H_2CO_3 and moves the pH toward normal. The degree of hypoventilation is limited by the development of hypoxia, such that the upper limit of CO_2 retention usually will not exceed 55 mmHg, making compensation incomplete.

e. Mixed acid-base disturbances.
Mixed acid-base disturbances occur when two or more primary disorders exist simultaneously, each eliciting its own compensatory response. Metabolic alkalosis and metabolic acidosis may occur together, just as respiratory acidosis or alkalosis may coexist with metabolic acidosis or alkalosis. A *triple* mixed disorder may occur when one primary respiratory disorder is superimposed on a coexisting metabolic acidosis and alkalosis (e.g., a patient on continuous gastric suction who has chronic obstructive lung disease and develops central hyperventilation and hemorrhagic shock after head injury and multiple trauma). This situation emphasizes the importance of analyzing the blood gas values in the setting of the patient's past and present medical condition.

II. Respiratory disorders

A. Blunt chest trauma

1. Pulmonary contusion. Pulmonary contusion caused by blunt chest trauma is frequently associated with head injuries, especially after automobile accidents. The high mortality (up to 50%) from pulmonary contusion reported several years ago in a large series of patients was due primarily to the unrecognized onset of respiratory failure, which usually occurs within six hours after injury and often progresses to the adult respiratory distress syndrome (ARDS) (Kirsh, 1977). Contusion may also result from blast injury or any other nonpenetrating chest trauma and is associated with rib fractures, pneumothorax, myocardial contusion, and aortic laceration. Pulmonary contusion may also occur alone without obvious external evidence of chest trauma.

Characteristics of pulmonary contusion include alveolar capillary damage with intra-alveolar and interstitial hemorrhage and edema; this is followed by a parenchymal inflammatory response. Radiographically, there are ill-defined infiltrates in the area of trauma to the chest wall. The patient is dyspneic, complains of chest wall pain, and may have hemoptysis. Arterial blood gases indicate hypoxia and a widened alveolar-arterial oxygen gradient. Initial hypocapnia is a common feature. As the work of breathing increases, the patient may develop hypercapnia.

Therapy includes supplemental oxygen, analgesics, and close monitoring of respiratory function. Any deterioration warrants early endotracheal intubation. Administration of steroids is of doubtful value. Isolated pulmonary contusion commonly begins to improve radiographically in 48 to 72 hours, but two to three weeks may be required for complete resolution.

2. **Rib fractures and flail chest.** Rib fractures, common after blunt chest trauma, often go undiagnosed on chest x-ray films. Meticulous physical examination of the chest wall is required in each patient who has sustained blunt chest trauma. Complications of nondisplaced rib fractures include pneumothorax, laceration of intercostal arteries, and flail chest (usually in the lateral part of the chest).

Flail chest of the anterior type occurs when the ribs become separated at their costochondral junction, with or without an associated fracture of the sternum. The characteristic paradoxical chest movement may not be seen in this area because of tissue edema or hematoma formation. Mechanical ventilation with intermittent mandatory ventilation (IMV) for 7 to 10 days with the addition of positive end-expiratory pressure (PEEP) as necessary is effective therapy.

3. **Pneumothorax.** Pneumothorax is most often caused by laceration of the lung by a fractured rib. It can also result from the disruption of alveoli when the limits of intra-alveolar pressure are exceeded during chest wall impact or from rupture of the

esophagus or tracheobronchial tree. In simple pneumothorax, the initial air leak will seal and be self-limiting. If the defect is too large and cannot seal spontaneously, tension pneumothorax, which is a life-threatening situation, will develop. Chest tube insertion and underwater drainage are required immediately.

If the pneumothorax is caused by a *penetrating* chest injury that has caused a large open wound (sucking chest wound), the defect should be covered immediately to seal the air leak. A chest tube is inserted in an area removed from the chest wall defect. After hemodynamic stabilization and adequate oxygenation have been assured, surgical exploration and revision of the chest wound can be performed.

4. **Hemothorax.** Hemothorax can occur with any form of blunt chest trauma. Respiratory embarrassment may result from the accumulation of sufficient blood to impair lung inflation. Immediate placement of a chest tube in a dependent position should provide adequate drainage, but persistent or massive hemorrhage requires prompt surgical exploration. Coagulation studies should be performed to rule out a hemostatic defect. To avoid laceration of intercostal arteries, any involuntary movements, such as seizures, must be prevented in neurosurgical patients who have rib fractures.

5. **Ruptured tracheobronchial tree.** Tears within the tracheobronchial tree cause pneumothorax and are usually promptly fatal. Placement of a chest tube with suction will not correct the situation because of the continuing air leak. Massive mediastinal and subcutaneous emphysema, dyspnea, cyanosis, and hemoptysis develop.

Auscultation of the anterior chest reveals a mediastinal crunching sound synchronous with cardiac rhythm (Hamman's sign). In rare instances, there may be no communication with the pleura and no pneumothorax. The lesion usually heals within one to three weeks, but granulation tissue may obstruct the airway and cause atelectasis. This is a difficult lesion to correct surgically. Fiberoptic bronchoscopy should be performed whenever disruption of the tracheobronchial tree is suspected.

6. **Diaphragmatic rupture.** Automobile accidents are responsible for more than 80% of traumatic diaphragmatic ruptures. The left diaphragm is involved in 95% of cases. Rupture is secondary to the abrupt elevation of intra-abdominal pressure at the time of impact, which causes herniation of stomach, bowel, spleen, or omentum into the chest. Associated rupture of an intestinal vis-

cus is not uncommon. A clinical picture of respiratory distress and shock develops. On chest x-ray film, the normal stomach gas bubble is seen above the diaphragm. Strangulation of the herniated abdominal contents may occur if the rupture is overlooked. Management of the airway is critical in these patients since regurgitation and aspiration from the fluid-filled stomach may occur during induction of anesthesia. Therefore, either precautions against aspiration (rapid intravenous induction) or intubation of the trachea in the awake state is recommended.

B. **Adult respiratory distress syndrome.** ARDS (noncardiac pulmonary edema) frequently occurs after severe chest trauma or shock. It may be difficult to distinguish this syndrome from neurogenic pulmonary edema associated with head injury.

1. **Pathophysiology.** The syndrome of ARDS is characterized by increased capillary permeability, pulmonary edema, and a low or normal pulmonary capillary wedge (PCW) pressure. Unlike acute cardiogenic pulmonary edema, the colloid osmotic pressure of the edema fluid is at least 60% of the plasma colloid osmotic pressure. Chest x-ray study reveals patchy or confluent pulmonary infiltrates throughout the lung fields. The arterial blood gases indicate significant hypoxia with an extremely wide alveolar-arterial gradient. Hypercapnia is seldom present (in contrast to cardiogenic pulmonary edema) unless there is associated hypoventilation from flail chest, head injury, hemopneumothorax, or high cervical spinal cord injury.

2. **Treatment.** The clinical evidence of ARDS is not always present immediately after injury but can develop within 12 to 24 hours. Endotracheal intubation and ventilatory support with continuous positive airway pressure (CPAP) or PEEP at high inspired oxygen concentration (FIO_2) and a large tidal volume are usually essential. Although evidence for the efficacy of steroids is conflicting, methylprednisolone, 30 mg/kg, may be given intravenously as soon as possible and continued every four hours for 48 hours. Pulmonary artery (PA) catheterization provides invaluable information regarding appropriate fluid therapy. Ideally, the pulmonary capillary wedge (PCW) pressure should be maintained at 5 to 8 mmHg. Vasoactive drugs may be needed. Their use must be carefully monitored, however, since they increase myocardial oxygen demand and may aggravate intrapulmonary shunting.

C. **Chronic obstructive lung disease.** Chronic obstructive lung disease presents greatly increased risks to the neurosurgical patient. Pulmonary function testing is impossible before emergency surgery and frequently only vague accounts of smoking, emphysema, or bronchitis are obtained. Physical findings, chest x-ray films, electrocardiogram, and arterial blood gases must be carefully reviewed. An elevated total CO_2 may suggest underlying lung disease with CO_2 retention.

When they can be obtained, pulmonary mechanics can be helpful in assessing underlying respiratory reserve. For example, a forced expiratory volume at one second (FEV_1) of less than 500 ml before an elective procedure usually represents insufficient pulmonary reserve to sustain life without mechanical ventilation.

Postoperatively, patients who have chronic lung disease require supplemental oxygen and careful observation. The importance of control of oxygen therapy for these patients should be recognized in the recovery room since excessive oxygen concentration may remove the stimulus for spontaneous ventilation and cause respiratory arrest. Patients who are known to depend on the "hypoxic drive" for breathing may not tolerate an FiO_2 of greater than 24% to 28% unless mechanical ventilation is used.

D. Other pulmonary problems

1. **Central neurogenic hyperventilation.** Patients who have head injuries occasionally demonstrate sustained deep and rapid breathing. The lesion within the CNS associated with these abnormal ventilatory patterns is usually bilateral and involves the brainstem. Prognosis is poor. Problems arising from central neurogenic hyperventilation include (a) a pH greater than 7.60, which predisposes the patient to malignant ventricular arrhythmias and cerebral lactic acidosis; (b) increased ICP; (c) increased metabolic rate, oxygen consumption, and hypoxia in patients who are already in an extremely hypermetabolic state; and (d) inability to produce positive nitrogen balance.

   Management of the patient who has central neurogenic hyperventilation includes endotracheal intubation for airway protection and pulmonary toilet. Careful monitoring of respiratory function for signs of fatigue and hypercapnia is essential. Addition of dead space is contraindicated because it merely increases the work of breathing. If either the metabolic demands become too great or the pH becomes too alkalotic, then paralysis, sedation, and maintenance of $PaCO_2$ between 25 and 30 mmHg by controlled ventilation are indicated to reduce the metabolic rate and the alkalosis. Muscle relaxation, controlled ventilation, and sedation may also help treat intracranial hypertension.

2. **Neurogenic pulmonary edema.** Acute pulmonary edema may develop in association with anterior hypothalamic compres-

sion, intraventricular hemorrhage, rupture of an anterior communicating artery aneurysm, or intracranial lesions remote from the hypothalamus. Intracranial hypertension may or may not be present. A possible mechanism involves catecholamine release caused by cerebral hypoxia, which increases peripheral vascular resistance and shifts blood to the relatively low-pressure pulmonary vascular system. This shift causes an increase in left atrial and pulmonary venous pressures with disruption of pulmonary capillary endothelial integrity and efflux of protein-rich fluid into the alveoli. Therapy of neurogenic pulmonary edema includes fluid restriction, diuretic administration, mechanical ventilation (usually with additional PEEP), and control of intracranial hypertension.

3. **Cardiogenic pulmonary edema.** Congestive heart failure occasionally develops in either elderly or very young patients or after high cervical spinal cord injury during over-zealous fluid resuscitation or mannitol administration.

   Management of cardiogenic pulmonary edema includes inotropic support (dopamine, dobutamine, digoxin), diuretics (furosemide), and vasodilators (sodium nitroprusside, nitroglycerin, hydralazine). In addition, hypokalemia, acid-base imbalance, and hypoxia should be corrected.

4. **Aspiration pneumonitis.** Acute ingestion of alcohol and gastric distention often accompany head injury. Aspiration may occur immediately after the injury or during transfer or endotracheal intubation. Aspiration pneumonitis is defined as chemical pneumonitis resulting from aspiration of fluid gastric contents with a pH of 1.2 to 2.5.

   The clinical picture of hypoxia, tachycardia, cyanosis, and expiratory rhonchi and wheezing develops within six hours. Radiographic evidence of either an infiltrate or atelectasis may or may not be present. Serial measurement of arterial blood gases provides a more reliable indicator of the extent and progression of the disease process.

   Initial treatment should include prevention of further aspiration by protection of the airway by endotracheal intubation. Appropriate mechanical ventilation and oxygen supplementation are also necessary. Prophylactic antibiotics have not been shown to decrease mortality or prevent secondary infection and may increase the risk of development of a nosocomial pneumonia from resistant organisms. Bacterial pneumonia does not usually develop. The use of steroids remains controversial since they probably do not alter the clinical course unless given within the first few minutes after aspiration. If obstructive pulmonary atelectasis develops, fiberoptic bronchoscopy must be performed to clear the obstruction.

5. **Respiratory failure in high cervical cord injuries.** Successful resuscitation at the scene of the accident has increased the number of survivors after high cervical cord injuries. The prognosis is poor for long-term survival and rehabilitation of patients who have cord injuries at the level of C-6 or higher. Initial aggressive supportive care must be provided, however, since resolution of spinal cord edema and return of ventilatory function may occur in a small percentage of patients.

Adequate nutrition through either nasogastric feedings or total parenteral nutrition must be provided to maintain positive nitrogen balance. Supportive efforts are directed to the early removal of mechanical ventilation. Quantitative ventilatory assessment is performed periodically to detect evidence of progressive return of voluntary ventilatory effort. Once such function is evident, the use of IMV or intermittent periods of spontaneous ventilation with the T-piece apparatus may assist in the weaning process. Alternate phrenic nerve stimulation techniques have been used successfully on several occasions.

Autonomic instability, manifested by hypotension, bradycardia, and hypothermia, occurs during the first two weeks after injury. Care must be taken to prevent pulmonary edema when giving intravenous fluids to treat hypotension, since fluctuation in sympathetic tone may cause wide variations in vascular resistance and cardiac filling pressures.

6. **Pulmonary embolism.** Pulmonary emboli usually originate from venous thrombosis in the lower extremities and complicate the course in 20% of multiple trauma victims. Less commonly, emboli arise from the pelvic or prostatic venous plexus or the right ventricle. The pathophysiology of pulmonary embolism includes obstruction of pulmonary blood flow, acute pulmonary hypertension and right ventricular failure, reduction of cardiac output, and hypoxia. Hemorrhagic necrosis and infarction of lung tissue may also occur.

Massive pulmonary embolism causes immediate acute respiratory failure, shock, cyanosis, tachycardia, extreme anxiety, and occasionally, anterior chest pain. On physical examination, there is jugular venous distention with hepatojugular reflux, wheezing, a right ventricular S_3 gallop, and an accentuated P_2 sound. The electrocardiogram is nonspecifically abnormal in 85% of cases and occasionally will show changes of left or right bundle branch block or suggest acute cor pulmonale. Sinus or ventricular rhythm disturbances are common. Positive radioactive isotope ventilation and perfusion lung scans are confirmatory. If the results of the lung scan are equivocal, then the patient should undergo pulmonary angiography.

The diagnosis of smaller pulmonary emboli is more difficult but should be suspected in any critically ill patient who has unexplained hypoxia, tachypnea, chest pain, or new electrocardiographic changes. Arterial blood gas measurement, isotopic lung scans, and pulmonary arteriograms usually confirm the diagnosis.

Treatment requires maintenance of adequate oxygenation. Anticoagulation is relatively contraindicated after intracranial or spinal cord operation or injury.

7. **Fat embolism.** Fat embolism syndrome, characterized by hypoxia, respiratory distress, neurologic changes, and coagulation abnormalities, occurs in victims of multiple trauma who have long bone fractures. Pathologically, small vessels, particularly in the lungs and the brain, are occluded by lipid particles and fibrin clots. The respiratory abnormality is indistinguishable from ARDS and can occur as late as 48 to 72 hours after the initial trauma.

Neurologic signs include confusion, delirium, or frank coma, focal or global deficit, or seizures. Petechiae occur in approximately 90% of cases. Lipid deposits may be seen in the retinal vessels. Disseminated intravascular coagulation (DIC), manifested by thrombocytopenia, elevated fibrin degradation products, and prolongation of prothrombin, partial thromboplastin, and thrombin times, is a further complication. Treatment is supportive and depends mainly on correction of hypoxia and establishment of cardiovascular stability. The syndrome usually resolves in 4 to 5 days.

III. Respiratory care

A. **Administration of oxygen.** All head-injured victims are hypoxic until proven otherwise. Although a PaO_2 of 60 mmHg may be adequate in healthy persons, laboratory evidence has confirmed a clinical impression that higher levels are essential to maintain adequate cerebral oxygenation in brain-injured patients.

Thus, although the danger of pulmonary oxygen toxicity from administration of high inspired oxygen concentrations exists, supplemental oxygen should be given to all neurosurgical patients. Several delivery devices are available.

1. **Nasal prongs.** Nasal prongs can deliver inspired oxygen concentrations of 24% to 44%. They are comfortable, inexpensive,

and need not be removed during eating. A low-flow system is maintained, but accurate continuous concentrations of oxygen cannot be guaranteed since the FIO_2 changes significantly with fluctuations of the patient's ventilatory pattern. Patients who have rapid inspiratory flow rates receive a lower FIO_2 than patients who have slow inspiratory flow rates.

When using nasal prongs, the oxygen flow rate should not exceed 6 L/min, since no increase in FIO_2 occurs at higher flows.

2. **Venturi mask.** The Venturi mask, a high-flow system, provides an accurate and constant concentration of oxygen delivery (F_DO_2) of 24% to 40% but is less comfortable and more expensive than nasal prongs. The exact F_DO_2 can be specified when ordering the use of a Venturi mask. It is the preferred means of oxygen administration in patients who have chronic obstructive lung disease until it has been determined that either nasal prongs or some other low-flow device can be safely tolerated.

Because of the narrow-bore tubing used with these devices, humidification of inspired gas is inadequate for prolonged use.

3. **High oxygen concentrations.** Other masks are available for patients who require a high FIO_2 without endotracheal intubation. Face tents and mist masks with or without oxygen reservoirs can be used to provide humidified oxygen concentrations of 60% to 95%. The amount of oxygen delivered varies with the patient's respiratory pattern. Therefore, elective intubation is often required when a high FIO_2 must be maintained.

4. **Endotracheal intubation**

   a. **Indications.** Indications for endotracheal intubation in the neurosurgical patient include the following:

      (1) Inability to clear secretions or protect the airway

      (2) PaO_2 less than 60 mmHg in spite of supplemental oxygen

      (3) $PaCO_2$ greater than 45 mmHg

      (4) pH less than 7.2

      (5) Respiratory rate greater than 40/min or less than 10/min

      (6) Tidal volume less than 3.5 ml/kg

      (7) Ratio of dead space to tidal volume (V_D/V_T) greater than 0.5

      (8) Vital capacity less than 10 to 15 ml/kg

b. **Nasotracheal intubation.** Intubation may be accomplished by either the nasal or oral route. Advantages of nasotracheal intubation include improved tolerance and better stabilization. Disadvantages are (1) pressure necrosis of the external nares; (2) obstruction of sinus drainage; (3) difficulty in suctioning owing to small tube diameter and position; and (4) otitis. An absolute contraindication to nasotracheal intubation is either facial fracture or fracture of the base of the skull with possible disruption of the cribriform plate.

c. **Orotracheal intubation.** In the emergency situation, orotracheal intubation is preferable and can be accomplished with minimal trauma by experienced personnel. In the hemodynamically stable patient, sodium thiopental, 3 to 5 mg/kg, and a short-acting muscle relaxant such as succinylcholine, 1.5 mg/kg (after pretreatment with a nondepolarizing muscle relaxant), prevent coughing and intracranial hypertension. Suction equipment and precautions to avoid aspiration are mandatory.

5. **Tracheotomy**

   a. **Indications.** Endotracheal intubation is well tolerated for prolonged periods of time. There are, however, indications for tracheotomy:

      (1) High spinal cord injury (C3–4)

      (2) Multiple facial fractures

      (3) Persistent vegetative state

      (4) Patient comfort during prolonged ventilatory failure

   b. **Advantages.** Advantages of tracheotomy include

      (1) Efficient suctioning

      (2) Reduction of dead space

      (3) Relative convenience in awake patients

   c. **Complications.** Complications involve

      (1) Damage to tracheal mucosa and subsequent infection

      (2) Ulceration

      (3) Hemorrhage

      (4) Granuloma formulation

      (5) Stenosis

B. Mechanical ventilation. Unless intubation is performed solely for tracheal suctioning or airway protection, some form of mechanical ventilation is indicated to improve gas exchange.

Ventilator parameters to be defined include (1) respiratory rate; (2) FiO_2; (3) mode (controlled, assisted, assist-control, or intermittent mandatory ventilation); (4) tidal volume; (5) peak flow; (6) inspiratory pressure limit; and (7) PEEP.

Vital signs should be carefully monitored and arterial blood gases should be measured within 30 minutes of either establishment of, or change in, ventilatory pattern to assure optimal oxygenation and acid-base balance.

1. **Controlled ventilation.** Patients who require controlled ventilation include those who have

   a. High spinal cord injury

   b. Drug overdose

   c. Absent ventilatory drive

   d. Neurologic death and are awaiting organ transplantation

2. **Intermittent mandatory ventilation.** Intermittent mandatory ventilation (IMV) is appropriate for patients who may have some spontaneous ventilatory activity. With IMV, the patient receives a preset number of breaths at a preset tidal volume, but is allowed to breathe spontaneously between mandatory breaths at a rate and tidal volume that are voluntarily generated.

   Although IMV was originally introduced as a method of weaning patients from the ventilator, it has become a widely accepted mode of primary ventilatory support and may have advantages over assisted or controlled modes. The advantages of IMV may be (a) fewer hemodynamic complications; (b) maintenance of spontaneous respiratory activity; and (c) better patient acceptance.

C. Positive airway pressure. Use of either PEEP with controlled ventilation or continuous positive airway pressure (CPAP) with spontaneous ventilation increases functional residual capacity, improves the ventilation-perfusion ratio, and may reverse hypoxia in patients who have abnormal intrapulmonary shunting. Application of PEEP may decrease the need to give high, potentially toxic concentrations of oxygen.

Expiratory pressure should be added in increments of 3 to 5 cmH_2O, while the hemodynamic response, ICP, and neurologic status are monitored carefully. The aim is to achieve a PaO_2 of close to 100 mmHg without exacerbation of neurologic dysfunction. During application of either PEEP or CPAP, patients should be nursed in a 30-degree head-up position. If ICP increases with PEEP, methods to improve intracranial compliance should be instituted, including cerebrospinal fluid (CSF) drainage through an intraventricular catheter and administration of mannitol, steroids, or barbiturates.

Owing to overexpansion of the lungs, use of high levels of PEEP (greater than 10 cm H_2O) can cause discrepancies from the central venous pressure (CVP) and PCWP levels observed before the addition of expiratory pressure. Overexpansion causes alveolar distention and compression of the alveolar capillaries, which increases alveolar capillary hydrostatic pressure and leads to an artifactual rise in PCWP. "Super" PEEP (greater than 25 cm H_2O) also allows transmission of positive pressure through the lung parenchyma to the intrapleural space. As the intrathoracic pressure increases, the intrathoracic vessels and cardiac chambers are externally compressed, resulting in elevation of PA and PCWP without necessarily reducing cardiac output.

D. **Weaning.** Before attempted weaning from mechanical ventilation, the patient should be (1) in normal acid-base balance; (2) hemodynamically stable; (3) well oxygenated; (4) free of major lung disease; (5) aseptic; and (6) in normal metabolic balance. A vital capacity of greater than 15 ml/kg allows adequate gas exchange and ventilatory reserve, permits coughing, and prevents atelectasis. An FiO_2 of 0.4 should be well tolerated. Resting minute ventilation must not exceed 10 L/min.

The alert patient should be able, on command, to produce a maximal minute ventilation of at least twice the resting minute ventilation and a maximal inspiratory force of at least -20 to -30 cm H_2O. The average tidal volume should be at least 5 ml/kg, and the spontaneous respiratory rate should not be greater than 30 breaths/min. The alveolar-arterial oxygen tension gradient must be less than 300 to 350 mmHg on 100% oxygen, and the V_D/V_T should be less than 0.5.

The patient's dependence on the ventilator can be reduced by use of the IMV mode when the patient is stable. Progressive reductions of the IMV rate are made as rapidly as tolerated until the patient no longer requires mechanical support. CPAP may be continued, as dictated by the adequacy of oxygenation, once the patient is breathing spontaneously.

E. **Monitoring.** Monitoring of the patient who has respiratory failure should include continuous electrocardiogram, direct arterial blood pressure, respiratory rate, temperature, heart rate, and fluid balance. Use of an apnea monitor is valuable in the spontaneously

Table 5-2. Glasgow coma scale

Best verbal response	
None	1
Incomprehensible sound	2
Inappropriate words	3
Confused	4
Oriented	5
Eyes open	
None	1
To pain	2
To speech	3
Spontaneously	4
Best motor response	
None	1
Abnormal extensor	2
Abnormal flexion	3
Withdraws	4
Localizes	5
Obeys	6

breathing patient. Hypotensive patients require CVP monitoring. If there is coexisting cardiopulmonary disease, PA catheterization is highly desirable.

Assessment of neurologic status should be ongoing. ICP may be measured through a cannula in the lateral ventricle or by a subdural catheter or bolt. Hourly recording of the Glasgow coma scale score affords a sequential indication of neurologic improvement or deterioration (Table 5-2).

The critically ill neurosurgical patient is at particular risk. Not only does he have severe intracerebral pathology, but surgical intervention may cause additional trauma. Many of the drugs and maneuvers employed also compromise intracranial dynamics, as does multisystem failure. Treatment is directed at correction of these conditions while providing for neurologic recovery.

References

1. Bryan-Brown, C. W.   Oxygen transport and the oxyhemoglobin dissociation curve. In J. L. Berk and J. E. Sampliner (Eds.), *Handbook of Critical Care* (2nd ed.). Boston: Little, Brown, 1982. Pp. 557–578.
2. Corman, L. C., and Bolt, R. J. (Eds.).   Medical evaluation of the preoperative patient. *Med. Clin. North Am.* 63:1979.
3. Frost, E.   The physiopathology of respiration in neurosurgical patients. *J. Neurosurg.* 50:699, 1979.
4. Hedley-Whyte, J., Burgess, G. E., III, Feeley, T. W., and Miller, M. G.   *Applied Physiology of Respiratory Care.* Boston: Little, Brown, 1976.

5. Kaehny, W. D.   Pathogenesis and Managment of Respiratory and Mixed Acid-Base Disorders. In R. W. Schrier (Ed.), *Renal and Electrolyte Disorders* (2nd ed.). Boston: Little, Brown, 1982. Pp. 159–181.
6. Kaehny, W. D., and Gabow, P. A.   Pathogenesis and Management of Metabolic Acidosis and Alkalosis. In R. W. Schrier (Ed.), *Renal and Electrolyte Disorders* (2nd ed.). Boston: Little, Brown, 1982. Pp. 115–157.
7. Kirsh, M. M., and Sloan, H.   *Blunt Chest Trauma.* Boston: Little, Brown, 1977.
8. Narins, R., and Emmet, M.   Simple and mixed acid-base disorders: A practical approach. *Medicine* 59:161, 1980.
9. Parfitt, A. M., and Kleerekoper, M.   Clinical Disorders of Calcium, Phosphorus, and Magnesium Metabolism. In M. H. Maxwell and C. R. Kleeman (Eds.), *Clinical Disorders of Fluid and Electrolyte Metabolism.* New York: McGraw-Hill, 1980.
10. Proceedings of the Conference on the Scientific Basis of In-Hospital Respiratory Therapy, Part 2. *Am. Rev. Respir. Dis.* 122:1980.
11. Richards, J. R., and Kinney, J. M. (Eds.).   *Nutritional Aspects of Care in the Critically Ill.* Edinburgh: Churchill Livingstone, 1977.
12. Rose, J., Valtonen, S., and Jennett, B.   Avoidable factors contributing to death after head injury. *Br. Med. J.* 2:615, 1977.
13. Shibel, E. M., and Moser, K. M. (Eds.).   *Respiratory Emergencies.* St. Louis: Mosby, 1977.
14. Shinozuka, T., and Nemoto, E. M.   Dynamics of cerebrovascular responses to oxygen. *Anesthesiology* 55:235, 1981.
15. Thompson, R. A., and Green, J. R.   *Critical Care of Neurologic and Neurosurgical Emergencies.* New York: Raven, 1980.
16. Weil, M. H., and Henning, R. J.   *The Handbook of Critical Care Medicine.* New York: EM Books, 1979.

6. Cardiovascular Therapy

J. G. Reves
Robert D. McKay

I. **Basic considerations.** Tissues of the central nervous system (CNS), like tissues of other organ systems, depend on an adequate supply of oxygen to meet their metabolic requirements. The cardiovascular system (CVS) supplies the CNS with oxygen and other substrates for metabolism. Preservation of cardiovascular function is essential for normal CNS function. Some fundamental considerations regarding the relationship of the CVS and CNS influence the ability of vasoactive drugs to affect the cerebral circulation.

   A. **Autoregulation.** Normal cerebral blood flow (CBF) in conscious adults is approximately 45 to 50 ml/100 gm brain tissue/min. CBF is maintained at this level over a wide range of cerebral perfusion pressures by autoregulation (Fig. 6-1). The cerebral perfusion pressure (CPP), mean arterial pressure (MAP) minus intracranial pressure (ICP), may be reduced without decreasing CBF until a perfusion pressure of 50 mmHg is reached. At this point, the cerebral vasculature can no longer compensate by dilatation, and further reductions in CPP lead to decreases in CBF with the potential for ischemia. Increases in CPP beyond the upper limit of 150 mmHg lead to increases in CBF with the possibility of edema formation. The entire autoregulation curve is shifted to the right with chronic hypertension. As a result of this shift, the brain is better protected at high CPP but is made more vulnerable to ischemia at low CPP. Autoregulation may become impaired in a variety of intracranial disorders. In the absence of autoregulation, CBF varies linearly with CPP: the higher the CPP, the higher the CBF. The importance of distinguishing between CPP and MAP will be even more apparent when conditions that increase the ICP are encountered.

   B. **Interrelationships among central nervous system fluid compartments.** There are three fluid compartments in the CNS: brain tissue water, cerebrospinal fluid (CSF), and cerebral blood volume (CBV). These three compartments are contained within the semiclosed, rigid confines of the skull. The Munro-Kellie doctrine describes the relationship between these three compartments: a volume increase in one of the intracranial fluid compartments must be matched by a volume decrease in one or both of the other compartments or ICP will increase. This doctrine is graphically shown in Figure 6-2. Of the three fluid compartments, CBV is most likely to be altered by vasoactive drugs.

   C. **The blood-brain barrier.** A barrier exists between the blood and the CNS. The blood-brain barrier is a continuous layer of endothelial cells lining the vascular lumen. These cells are connected by tight junctions, which restrict the intercellular passage of water-soluble drugs, proteins, and ions from blood to brain. The phys-

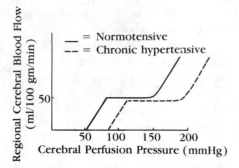

Fig. 6-1. Cerebral autoregulation in both normotensive and chronic hypertensive patients whose actual limits of CPP depend on the degree of hypertension. Autoregulation occurs normally from a cerebral perfusion pressure of about 50 to 150 mmHg and keeps cerebral blood flow relatively constant at about 50 ml/100 gm/min over this range.

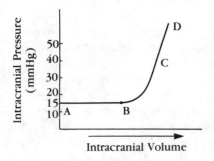

Fig. 6-2. The relationship between changes in intracranial volume and intracranial pressure. The line between A and B on the curve shows that the increase in volume of one of the three intracranial compartments (blood, brain, cerebrospinal fluid) was compensated successfully by a decrease in volume of one or both of the other two compartments. The line between B and C is the knee of the curve; intracranial compliance is decreased. Between C and D, a relatively small increase in intracranial volume leads to a large increase in intracranial pressure. The slope of the curve from B to C is also influenced by the rate at which the intracranial volume is increased.

iochemical properties that govern the ability of a given drug to cross the blood-brain barrier include lipid solubility, ionization, molecular size, and degree of protein binding.

Although alpha-adrenergic, beta-adrenergic, and dopaminergic receptors can be demonstrated in the cerebral circulation, vasoconstricting drugs and inotropic agents seem to have less effect on cerebral vasculature than on other vascular beds. Vasodilators, however, can have a profound effect on the cerebral vasculature. Presumably, the blood-brain barrier is more effective at restricting passage of the vasoconstricting drugs and inotropic agents than it is for the vasodilators. The following is a list of some of the conditions that can lead to a disruption in the blood-brain barrier, a development that may alter the usual responses of the cerebral circulation to vasoactive agents.

1. Increased blood pressure

2. Lead encephalopathy

3. Trauma

4. Stroke

5. Large increase in CO_2

6. Radiation

7. Angiography

8. Tumor

9. Infection

10. Convulsions

D. **Cardiac output and the central nervous system**

1. **Determinants of cardiac output.** Cardiac output is the product of heart rate and stroke volume (CO = HR × SV), but the determinants of cardiac output are a complex interrelation of the positive and negative influences of preload, afterload, heart rate, contractility, and synergy of myocardial contraction (Fig. 6-3). Blood pressure is the product of cardiac output and systemic vascular resistance (BP = CO × SVR).

2. **Cardiac failure**

a. **Cardiovascular causes** of pump failure are multifold (e.g., hypovolemia, tachyarrhythmia, decreased contractility, increased afterload), but most often a progressive cycle occurs that involves the major determinants of cardiac function and

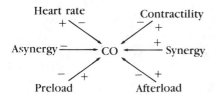

Fig. 6-3. Determinants of myocardial performance affect the cardiac output both positively and negatively. CO = cardiac output.

leads to heart failure (e.g., with ischemic heart disease, my-ocardial ischemia develops → decreased contractility → asynergy of contraction → increased preload → compensatory tachycardia → increased afterload → decreased cardiac output, worsened ischemia, forming a vicious circle).

Reduced preload (hypovolemia) is a common cause of reduced cardiac output in the neurologic intensive care unit (ICU). Hypotension (and presumably decreased cardiac output) in association with head injury almost always results from some other injury, rarely from the head injury per se. Common sites of injury associated with systemic hypotension include intra-abdominal hemorrhage, hemothorax, retroperitoneal hematoma, and hematoma forming from pelvic or femoral fractures. Blood loss from scalp and facial lacerations may be substantial enough to cause hypovolemia and reduced cardiac output. In a child, bleeding into a subgaleal or intracranial hematoma may be of sufficient magnitude to cause low cardiac output on a hypovolemic basis. To assess the patient's intravascular volume, cardiac filling pressure should be measured. With normal heart function, measuring the right atrial pressure is adequate. If there is left ventricular disease and dysfunction, the filling pressure should be assessed with a pulmonary artery catheter to measure the pulmonary artery diastolic or pulmonary artery occluded pressure.

b. **CNS causes** of reduced cardiac output include paralysis of the vasomotor center and subsequent hypotension from cerebral trauma. This hypotension is usually accompanied by bradycardia, agonal, gasping respirations, and death. Cardiac dysrhythmias may result from head injury, subarachnoid hemorrhage, or cerebrovascular insufficiency with potential alteration of cardiac output. Spinal cord injury, on the other hand, often causes neurogenic hypotension by sympathetic blockade and predominance of the parasympathetic autonomic system. However, spinal cord injury, like head injury, may be associated with other causes of hypotension (such as hypovolemia) and these causes must be ruled out. (Of assistance in the differential diagnosis is the usual association of neurogenic hypotension with bradycardia, whereas hypovolemic hypotension is usually accompanied by tachycardia.) In cases in which the cardiac output is depressed by both neurogenic and hypovolemic mechanisms, accurate assessment of preload is mandatory.

3. **Effect of low CO on the CNS.** The effect of reduced cardiac output on the CNS is apparently not pronounced until CPP falls

below the autoregulatory threshold value of approximately 50
mmHg. CBF is better preserved during pharmacologically induced hypotension than with decreased cardiac output from
hemorrhage. Data from anesthetized patients undergoing
carotid endarterectomy with continuous EEG monitoring and
periodic measurements of CBF show that a regional CBF (rCBF)
of less than 18 ml/100 gm/min is almost invariably accompanied
by EEG changes of ischemia. The EEG becomes isoelectric at
rCBF of 15 ml/100 gm/min, and cell death occurs when rCBF is
less than 10 ml/100 gm/min (Shapiro, 1981). Data from unanesthetized monkeys suggest that when CBF is less than 12 ml/100
gm/min for two hours or longer, infarction results (Morawetz,
1978).

II. **Pharmacologic intervention for cardiovascular dysfunction.**
Pharmacologic intervention is necessary to augment cardiovascular
function when it is suboptimal in the neurologic ICU patient. Vasoactive drugs may be broadly classified *by use* into four groups: vasoconstrictors, vasodilators, positively inotropic drugs, and negatively inotropic and/or chronotropic drugs. Commonly encountered cardiovascular
complications requiring therapy with these drugs are presented in
section **III.**

A. **Vasoconstrictors**

1. **Mode of action.** Generally speaking, the most commonly used
   vasoconstrictors are phenylephrine and methoxamine, which
   cause vasoconstriction by their primary alpha-adrenergic agonist
   action (Table 6-1). Both are sympathomimetic amines (so named
   because they mimic the action of norepinephrine and epinephrine) whose spectrum of activity is shown in Figure 6-4. The
   other sympathomimetic amines that have significant alpha-
   adrenergic actions are norepinephrine, metaraminol, ephedrine, mephentermine, and, in higher dosages, epinephrine and
   dopamine. The relative degree of alpha and beta effects of most
   sympathomimetic amines depends on the dosage: small doses
   have less alpha-adrenergic agonism than large dosages. An-
   giotensin (not readily available in the United States) is a potent
   nonadrenergic vasoconstrictor. It acts directly on vascular
   smooth muscle, even in the face of alpha-adrenergic blockade. A
   comparison of the pharmacologic characteristics of the commonly used vasoconstrictors is shown in Table 6-2.

2. **Hemodynamic effect.** The hemodynamic effects of vasoconstrictors depend on two factors: the specific drug chosen (relative degree of alpha and beta agonism) and the clinical setting
   (vascular resistance, cardiac function, and integrity of barorecep-

Table 6-1. Receptor stimulation by catecholamines

Adrenergic receptor	Site	Action
Alpha*	Smooth muscle arterioles (systemic and pulmonary circulation)	Vasoconstriction (increased impedance)
	Iris	Dilatation
	Myometrium	Contraction
Beta-1	Myocardium	Increased atrial and ventricular contraction
	Sinoatrial node	Increased heart rate
	Atrioventricular conduction	Increased conduction velocity or rate of conduction
	Kidney	Renin release
Beta-2	Smooth muscle arterioles (systemic and pulmonary circulation)	Vasodilatation (decreased impedance)
	Bronchi	Bronchodilatation
	Myometrium	Relaxation

* Alpha-adrenergic receptors may be further divided into two groups: alpha-2 "presynaptic" receptors blocked by phentolamine and phenoxybenzamine, and alpha-1 "postsynaptic" receptors blocked by prazosin. Stimulation of alpha-2 receptors results in a decrease of neuronal release of the neurotransmitter norepinephrine. Thus, an alpha-2 agonist such as clonidine causes a decrease in blood pressure by decreasing the neuronal release of norepinephrine. The alpha-1 receptors are adrenoceptors that are the "classic" alpha receptors that, when stimulated, cause the effects listed following alpha, as seen with phenylephrine.

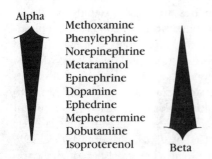

Alpha

Methoxamine
Phenylephrine
Norepinephrine
Metaraminol
Epinephrine
Dopamine
Ephedrine
Mephentermine
Dobutamine
Isoproterenol

Beta

Fig. 6-4. The spectrum of adrenergic activity of sympathomimetic amines. Drugs toward the top of the list possess more alpha-adrenergic agonist properties and those toward the bottom exert beta-adrenergic agonist effects. The proportion of alpha and beta activity changes according to dose: some drugs exhibit more alpha-adrenergic activity than beta-adrenergic activity as dose increases.

Table 6-2. Comparison of pharmacologic characteristics of commonly used vasoconstrictors

| Generic name | Trade name | Receptor Activity | | | Onset | Duration | Adult dose (IV) |
| | | Vascular | | Cardiac | | | |
		Alpha	Beta-2	Beta-1			
Methoxamine	Vasoxyl	++++	0	0	++	+++	0.2–0.5 mg bolus
Phenylephrine	Neo-Synephrine	++++	0	+	++	++	0.1–0.5 µg/kg/min infusion
Norepinephrine	Levophed	++++	0	++	++++	+	0.05–0.15 µg/kg/min infusion
Ephedrine	Ephedrine	+++	+	++	++	++++	2.5–5 mg bolus

The number of + denotes increasing activity or time; 0 = no activity.

tor reflexes). All vasoconstrictors increase vascular resistance, which usually results in an increase in systemic and pulmonary artery pressures, particularly when systemic vascular resistance is low. Depending on the original myocardial ventricular function and the amount of beta-1 agonism of the drug, cardiac output may decrease, increase, or remain unchanged. A pure alpha-adrenergic agonist (e.g., phenylephrine) may reduce cardiac output owing to increased resistance, whereas drugs with mixed alpha and beta-1 activity (e.g., ephedrine) increase systemic resistance as well as cardiac output. The response of the heart rate is also variable; it is more likely to decrease if a pure alpha drug is given because of reflex slowing from baroreceptor responses to increased systemic blood pressure, but may increase if the particular drug has significant beta-1 activity.

3. **Cerebral effect.** There is in vitro evidence that cerebral arteries possess alpha-adrenergic receptors. However, clinical doses of alpha-agonist drugs cause little or no cerebrovasoconstriction nor a decrease in CBF, perhaps because of their failure to cross the blood-brain barrier. If autoregulation is lost, or if these drugs are given in sufficient doses to raise the mean arterial blood pressure beyond the upper limits of autoregulation, CBF may increase significantly. This increase may be associated with a breakdown in the blood-brain barrier, which enhances vasogenic edema formation.

4. **Indications**

   a. The primary indication for the use of a vasoconstrictor is *decreased* **vascular resistance.** This is often an iatrogenic problem caused by the administration of either anesthetics , or other drugs with vasodilatory properties.

   b. Alpha drugs are often given to increase blood pressure and therefore correct **low CPP** during and after carotid endarterectomy when BP falls.

   c. Occasionally vasoconstrictors are essential in the treatment of **hypovolemia** (e.g., uncontrolled hemorrhage) to support blood pressure while volume deficits are being corrected with intravenous fluid therapy.

   d. Rarely, **anaphylactic** and other drug or blood **reactions** necessitate the use of vasoconstrictors to restore systemic resistance and perfusion pressure.

   e. Vasoconstrictors with both alpha and beta-1 agonism are used to **improve cardiac output** and resistance when both are diminished.

5. **Contraindications**

   a. The primary contraindication to the use of pure alpha-adrenergic drugs is the combination of **elevated vascular resistance** and **myocardial left ventricular failure.** Although the blood pressure may transiently improve in this setting, the increased work of the heart (oxygen consumption) and decreased cardiac output (oxygen supply) will inevitably result in deterioration of cardiac function.

   b. Vasoconstrictors, although effective, are relatively contraindicated in the presence of slight to **moderate hypovolemia** because the degree of actual hypovolemia is masked by the elevated arterial and venous pressure.

   c. With the exception of dopamine, the alpha-adrenergic stimulation by vasoconstrictors causes renal arterial constriction and reduced renal perfusion; therefore, **impaired renal function** is another contraindication.

B. **Vasodilators**

   1. **Mode of action.** There are three primary modes of action of vasodilators: direct smooth muscle relaxation (e.g., the calcium channel–blocking drugs verapamil and nifedipine), interruption of peripheral alpha-adrenergic stimulation (including ganglionic blockade, catecholamine depletion, prevention of catecholamine release, and competitive blockade), and conversion of CNS neurotransmitters (e.g., alpha-methyldopa conversion to alpha-methylnorepinephrine, which causes decreased peripheral nerve firing).

      The predominant site of vasodilator action (arterial vs. venous) is of paramount importance. Although this is not completely established for all drugs in human beings, and overlap exists among the drugs, generally the alpha-adrenergic blocking drugs are mixed arterial and venous dilators, the nitrates are venous dilators, and the other direct-acting drugs are arteriolar dilators. A comparison of the pharmacologic characteristics of commonly used vasodilators is shown in Table 6-3.

   2. **Hemodynamic effect.** The hemodynamic effects of vasodilators depend on the site of action of the drug and the status of the circulation. The drugs that cause arteriolar dilatation (e.g., diazoxide and hydralazine) decrease systemic resistance with little change in cardiac preload. Cardiac output will remain unchanged or increase (if a decrease had occurred because of increased systemic resistance), and heart rate will remain constant or increase (reflexly if the blood pressure drops significantly and the baroreceptors are functional). Drugs that

Table 6-3. Comparison of pharmacologic characteristics of commonly used vasodilators

Generic name	Trade name	Mode of action	Prominent vasodilatation	CBF	Onset (min)	Duration	Adult dosage (IV)
Sodium nitroprusside	Nipride	Direct	Arteriovenous	↑	0.5	2–4 min	0.2–1.0 μg/kg/min infusion
Nitroglycerin	Nitrostat	Direct	Venous	↑	1–2	10 min	0.4–0.8 mg sublingual or 0.5–5 μg/kg/min infusion
Diazoxide	Hyperstat	Direct	Arterial	↑	1–2	4–12 hr	3–5 mg/kg bolus
Trimethaphan	Arfonad	Ganglionic blockade	Arteriovenous	NC	1–2	4–8 min	10–50 μg/kg/min infusion
Hydralazine	Apresoline	Direct	Arterial	↑	10–20	3–4 hr	5.0–7.5 mg bolus
Phentolamine	Regitine	Alpha-1 and alpha-2 adrenergic blockade	Arteriovenous	?	1–2	20 min	0.5–? μg/kg/min infusion
Prazosin	Minipress	Alpha-1 adrenergic blockade	Arteriovenous	?	Not available in a parenteral formulation		
Droperidol	Inapsine	Alpha-adrenergic blockade	Arteriovenous	→	1–2	5–30 min	1.25–2.5 mg bolus
Chlorpromazine	Thorazine	Alpha-adrenergic blockade	Arteriovenous	→	1–2	5–30 min	2.5–5 mg bolus

NC = no change.

cause venous dilatation (e.g., nitroglycerin) decrease left ventricular filling pressure, as manifested by reduced pulmonary artery occluded (PAO) pressure. There can be concomitant decreases in cardiac output unless optimal filling pressures are maintained. Drugs that have mixed arterial and venous dilatation (e.g., nitroprusside and phentolamine) decrease systemic vascular resistance and blood pressure, and often cause a reflex tachycardia. Cardiac output may or may not decrease depending on whether the filling pressure is maintained. Reflex tachycardia is less of a problem with nitroglycerin (because of venous dilatation), trimethaphan (because of ganglionic blockade), and prazosin (because of maintenance of negative feedback presynaptically).

3. **Cerebral effect.** The direct-acting vasodilators, sodium nitroprusside, nitroglycerin, diazoxide, aminophylline, hydralazine, and papaverine, all produce cerebral vasodilatation. In the absence of hypotension, CBF will increase (Table 6-4). Intracerebral steal may be induced and autoregulation may be impaired with these drugs. Cerebral blood volume may increase and elevate ICP, altering the patient's neurologic status (see Fig. 6-2). However, the increase in ICP observed with sodium nitroprusside, and possibly other cerebral vasodilators, may be attenuated by a technique of slow administration under hypocapnic and hyperoxic conditions. Trimethaphan and alpha-blocking agents do not demonstrate this cerebrovasodilating property to the same extent.

4. **Indications**

   a. Treatment of **hypertension** that occurs during or after surgery.

   b. Treatment of **cerebral arterial spasm.**

   c. Reduction of the usual increase in systemic vascular resistance associated with **low cardiac output** and heart failure. Frequently vasodilators are combined with positively inotro-

Table 6-4. Effects of vasodilators on cerebral blood flow

Increase	Decrease or no change
Sodium nitroprusside	Droperidol
Nitroglycerin	Chlorpromazine
Diazoxide	Trimethaphan
Hydralazine	

pic drugs to treat heart failure, but vasodilators can work alone in some cases.

d. Vasodilators, specifically nitroglycerin, are indicated for treatment of **myocardial ischemia** associated with an imbalance in oxygen supply and demand, particularly when the filling pressure is elevated. The calcium channel–blocking drugs (verapamil and nifedipine) are effective coronary artery vasodilators useful in preventing coronary artery spasm.

e. Vasodilators improve forward flow or enhance forward cardiac output in cases of **aortic** and **mitral valvular insufficiency.** In these instances, vasodilator therapy increases cardiac output by lowering the afterload (decreasing impedance). As with administration of all vasodilators, care must be taken to preserve coronary artery perfusion pressure (diastolic blood pressure) to prevent myocardial ischemia, and to maintain ventricular filling pressure to preserve cardiac output.

5. Contraindications

a. The greatest contraindication to vasodilators is the presence of **hypovolemia.** Administration to patients who have inadequate blood volume results in decreased cardiac output and hypotension.

b. Decreased intracranial compliance is a relative contraindication to the use of the direct-acting vasodilators. If possible, they should be used in conjunction with ICP monitoring. The ability of some drugs to reduce MAP and increase ICP can markedly decrease CPP.

c. A relative contraindication to the use of the mixed arterial and venous vasodilators may be the excessive quantity of **infused volume** required to keep the preload at optimal levels. This is a consideration in patients who have renal failure and increased pulmonary or brain water.

d. Cyanide toxicity is a potential complication of administration of sodium nitroprusside; if it develops the drug must be discontinued.

C. Positive inotropic and chronotropic drugs

1. Mechanism of action. For the most part, drugs that have positive inotropic effects are beta-1 adrenergic agonists. The more beta-1 activity, the more positive the inotropic effect. Drugs that exert their positive inotropic effect by beta-1 stimulation include epinephrine, ephedrine, dopamine, dobutamine, and isoproterenol. Calcium and the digitalis glycosides are positive inotropic compounds that work directly on the heart. A comparison of pharmacologic characteristics is listed in Table 6-5.

2. **Hemodynamic effect.** As with the other vasoactive drugs, the hemodynamic effects of each positive inotropic drug depend on the particular drug, its dosage, and the clinical setting (cardiovascular status). Sympathomimetic drugs that have nearly pure beta-1 effects (isoproterenol and dobutamine) increase myocardial contractility, heart rate, and cardiac output. Atrioventricular conduction is enhanced, as is automaticity of pacemaker cells (see Table 6-1). They also, through beta-2 effects, cause weak vasodilatation and decrease systemic vascular resistance and blood pressure. The drugs that have mixed alpha and beta activity tend to increase contractility, cardiac output, and systemic resistance. Changes in heart rate are variable, but are usually increased as is blood pressure. The onset and duration of action of all the sympathomimetic amines are rapid and short-lived.

Calcium and digitalis are both nonadrenergically mediated positive inotropic drugs that increase cardiac output and slightly decrease systemic vascular resistance. The positive inotropic effects of calcium occur within 1 minute, whereas it takes 10 to 30 minutes to achieve the inotropic effects of digoxin. Therefore, if a nonadrenergic effect is needed to increase contractility rapidly, calcium is the more effective drug since its onset is faster than digoxin. Digoxin is more appropriate for long-term positive inotropic support. All inotropic drugs shift the ventricular function curves to the left, as illustrated in Figure 6-5; therefore, cardiac output is augmented at a lower filling pressure, and cardiac work is more efficient.

3. **Cerebral effects.** In addition to alpha receptors, cerebral arteries also possess dopaminergic receptors and beta receptors. Beta receptors react as beta-1 receptors rather than as beta-2 receptors. (Beta-2 receptors are usually found outside the heart.) When used to treat hypotension from low cardiac output, the positive inotropic drugs can restore cerebral perfusion pressure with an improvement in CBF. Their effects on the cerebral circulation have not been clearly established when administered in the presence of a normal cardiac output. As with the alpha-adrenergic agonists, the positive inotropic agents will increase CBF either if autoregulation is absent or if the upper limits of autoregulation are exceeded.

The effect of dopamine on the cerebral circulation is dose-

Table 6-5. Comparison of pharmacologic characteristics of positive inotropic drugs

| Generic name | Trade name | Receptor activity | | | Adult dose (IV) | Comments |
| | | Vascular | | Cardiac | | |
		Alpha	Beta-2	Beta-1		
Epinephrine	Adrenalin	+ + + +	+	+ +	0.05–0.15 µg/kg/min infusion	Relative alpha and beta activity is dose-related (beta in low doses and alpha in higher doses)
Dopamine*	Intropin	+ +	+	+ +	1–10 µg/kg/min infusion	Relative alpha and beta effects are dose-related (like epinephrine), but splanchnic and renal vasoconstriction is spared. Used in patients with compromised renal function
Ephedrine	Ephedrine	+ + +	0	+ +	5–10 mg bolus	Beta effects are primarily secondary to release of norepinephrine. Lasts 5–10 min after bolus injection. Tachyphylaxis may occur
Dobutamine	Dobutrex	+	+	+ + +	1–10 µg/kg/min infusion	Theoretically, primarily beta-1 effects on myocardial contractility and little other beta-1 cardiac effect. Given by infusion

Drug	Trade name				Dose	Comments
Isoproterenol	Isuprel	0	++++	++++	0.025–0.05 µg/kg/min infusion	Pure beta effects. High doses cause ventricular irritability.
Calcium chloride	Calcium	0	0	0	1–10 mg/kg bolus	Rapid-acting positive inotropic drug with effects that persist for 5–10 min. Mechanism of action is direct and not beta adrenergic. Useful in patients on propranolol to increase contractility
Digoxin	Lanoxin	0	0	0	0.125–0.25 mg bolus	Has delayed onset of inotropic action and low therapeutic safety ratio which makes acute use inappropriate in most cases. Mechanism of action does not involve beta system

Note: The number of + denotes increasing activity or time; 0 = no activity.
* Dopamine also stimulates dopaminergic receptors, which causes mild renal and splanchnic arterial dilatation.

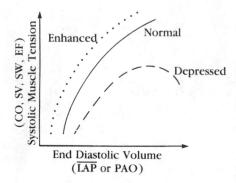

Fig. 6-5. Frank-Starling force-length relationship. Systolic muscle tension is plotted against end diastolic volume. The solid line describes the normal Frank-Starling force-length relationship, the dashed line represents cardiac function with a diseased or depressed ventricle, and the dotted line demonstrates the enhanced force-length relationship of a heart that is stimulated with a positive inotropic drug (e.g., calcium or epinephrine). CO = cardiac output; SV = stroke volume; SW = stroke work; EF = ejection fraction; $\overline{LAP}$ = mean left atrial pressure; PAO = pulmonary artery occluded pressure.

dependent. When low-dose (<2 μg/kg/min) dopamine was administered intravenously to dogs, CBF was either slightly decreased or unchanged (Von Essen, 1980). The administration of moderate doses (2–6 μg/kg/min) resulted in an increase in CBF, whereas high-dose (7–20 μg/kg/min) dopamine caused a decrease in CBF. The latter effect can be blocked by either the alpha antagonist phentolamine or the serotonin receptor antagonist methysergide; the increase in CBF caused by moderate-dose dopamine can be blocked by the dopamine receptor antagonist haloperidol. Epinephrine, which crosses the blood-brain barrier, has been shown to increase CBF, whereas norepinephrine and metaraminol have, in some models, caused a mild reduction in CBF (Michenfelder, 1980).

4. Indications

a. Positive inotropic drugs are used in patients who have **chronically decreased cardiac output** or **failing left ventricular function.** However, positive inotropic drugs are not a substitute for appropriate volume replacement, afterload reduction, or heart rate. The specific drug used depends on the clinical condition. Dopamine or epinephrine is useful when a positive inotropic effect is needed, as in a patient who has low systemic vascular resistance and poor renal perfusion (low urine output). In the presence of increased systemic vascular resistance, normal heart rate, and low cardiac output, dobutamine or isoproterenol is indicated.

b. Calcium and ephedrine will increase contractility during **brief periods of myocardial dysfunction.** Whenever cardiac output is depressed for prolonged periods, infusions of catecholamines, mechanical assist devices, or both are required to aid the failing heart.

c. Positive inotropic agents that have primarily beta or dopaminergic effect (e.g., isoproterenol or dopamine) have been used in the treatment of **cerebral vasospasm.**

5. **Contraindications**

   a. Particular drugs should not be used when their primary hemodynamic effects will aggravate the clinical situation. For example, isoproterenol and perhaps dobutamine and dopamine may exacerbate **tachyarrhythmias.** Isoproterenol will increase myocardial oxygen demand and diminish supply; therefore, it is usually contraindicated in patients who have **ischemic heart disease.**

   b. High doses of norepinephrine and epinephrine are likely to decrease nutrient flow to many tissue beds (because of alpha-adrenergic–mediated vasoconstriction) and may contribute to **renal failure** and the state known as "irreversible shock" in patients who have low cardiac output and high systemic vascular resistance.

   c. Digoxin must be used cautiously in previously **digitalized** or **hypokalemic patients** and patients in **renal failure** because of the potential for development of digitalis toxicity and associated arrhythmias.

   d. Although seemingly benign, prolonged or excessive administration of calcium can cause toxicity. If continued inotropic support is warranted, it is prudent to switch to a catecholamine or digoxin rather than to give repeated doses of calcium.

D. **Negative inotropic and chronotropic drugs**

   1. **Mechanisms of action.** Propranolol and metoprolol are negative inotropic and negative chronotropic drugs. Both are beta-1 adrenergic blocking drugs of approximately equal potency. Propranolol is also a beta-2 blocker. The major differences between propranolol and metoprolol are in the greater cardioselective (beta-1) effects of metoprolol and greater mem-

brane stabilizing activity of propranolol. The clinical significance of these differences is difficult to document, and, indeed, when high dosages of metoprolol are used, some beta-2 blockade occurs. A comparison of pharmacologic characteristics of negative inotropic and chronotropic drugs is shown in Table 6-6.

Calcium channel–blocking drugs (verapamil, nifedipine) inhibit calcium conductance of the slow calcium channel of the sarcolemma and affect the electrical and mechanical function of the heart. They exert a negative inotropic effect on the heart by interfering with calcium-mediated excitation contraction. Their primary hemodynamic effect, however, is vasodilatation.

2. **Hemodynamic effect.** Propranolol given intravenously in incremental dosages of 0.25 to 0.5 mg up to 0.1 mg/kg decreases (in a dose-related fashion) heart rate, blood pressure, and cardiac output. With moderate doses, the negative chronotropic effects are more pronounced than the negative inotropic effects. Verapamil causes a dose-related decrease in blood pressure owing to decreased systemic vascular resistance and a variable (usually increased) effect on heart rate and cardiac output. The negative inotropic effect of verapamil (and most calcium channel–blocking drugs) is relatively unimportant clinically and is counteracted by reflex increases in heart rate and, presumably, contractility secondary to its pronounced vasodilatory action.

3. **Cerebral effect.** The negative inotropic drugs apparently do not affect the cerebral circulation significantly. Calcium channel–blocking drugs cause cerebral vasodilatation.

4. **Indications**

   a. The primary indication for negative inotropic and chronotropic drugs is to **reduce myocardial oxygen consumption** associated with increases in myocardial contractility and heart rate, particularly in patients who have ischemic heart disease.

   b. Propranolol and verapamil are additionally useful in treating **supraventricular arrhythmias.**

   c. In the neurologic ICU, beta-adrenergic blocking drugs are useful adjuncts to the treatment of **hypertension.**

   d. Calcium channel–blocking drugs (e.g., nimodipine) are effective in treating **cerebral vasospasm.**

Table 6-6. Comparison of pharmacologic characteristics of negative inotropic and chronotropic drugs

Generic name	Trade name	Negative inotropic effect	Negative chronotropic effect	Mechanism of action	Adult dose	Comments
Halothane	Fluothane	+ +	0	Direct	0.5–1.0 vol% (inhalation)	
Enflurane	Ethrane	+ + +	0	Direct	1–1.5 vol% (inhalation)	
Propranolol	Inderal	+ +	+ + + +	Beta-1 adrenergic blockade	0.25–0.5 mg (IV)	Used primarily to decrease HR and treat arrhythmias
Metoprolol	Lopressor	+ +	+ + + +	Beta-1 adrenergic blockade	50–100 mg (PO)	Used primarily for medical therapy of hypertension. Not given parenterally now
Verapamil	Isoptin	+	0	Ca^{2+} antagonism	0.1 mg/kg (IV)	Used primarily for supraventricular arrhythmias

The number of + denotes increasing activity; 0 = no activity; IV = intravenous administration; PO = oral administration.

5. Contraindications

a. **Low cardiac output** is a relative contraindication to the use of negative inotropic and chronotropic drugs. An obvious exception is the patient whose low cardiac output is secondary to an arrhythmia that can be treated with propranolol or verapamil.

b. Since there is a significant beta-2 blockade effect of propranolol, it should be given cautiously in patients who have **bronchospastic pulmonary disease.**

III. Management of cardiovascular complications of neurologic disorders

A. **Cerebral arterial spasm.** The management of patients who have subarachnoid hemorrhage (SAH) from ruptured intracranial aneurysms may be complicated by cerebral arterial spasm and infarction. The incidence of radiographic vasospasm after aneurysmal rupture ranges from 30% to 50%, while 40% to 65% of patients undergoing cerebral aneurysm surgery will demonstrate vasospasm postoperatively. Vasospasm may also complicate craniocerebral trauma, particularly when subarachnoid hemorrhage is present.

1. **Pathophysiology.** Vasospasm has two phases. The early phase is probably due to the hemorrhage itself that either mechanically causes vasoconstriction or precipitates release of catecholamines from sympathetic nerve endings. This early phase is a transient phenomenon. The second or delayed phase of vasospasm probably results from the breakdown of the subarachnoid blood and/or the gradual release of serotonin and vasoactive amines from platelets and other blood elements. Prostaglandins may also play a role. Vasospasm decreases CBF to the affected vessels. If CBF is reduced below critical levels, ischemic damage may occur.

2. **Prevention.** Aneurysm surgery is frequently delayed for 10 to 14 days after SAH to allow time for resolution of vasospasm. However, delay increases the risk of rebleeding from the aneurysm, maximal at 7 to 14 days. Reserpine and kanamycin have been used to deplete the platelets of serotonin and reduce serotonin blood levels. These drugs, as well as nifedipine and other calcium-channel blockers, have been shown to be effective in the prevention and treatment of experimental vasospasm (Wilkins, 1980).

3. Treatment

a. The circulating blood volume should be increased with balanced salt solutions, blood transfusions, and albumin.

b. The pharmacologic therapy of vasospasm is based in part on the assumption that autoregulation in the involved vessels is probably not intact. Therefore, CBF will vary directly with the CPP. Drugs that raise the blood pressure, cardiac output, or both have been used alone or in combination with drugs that promote cerebrovasodilatation, either by direct action, inhibition of phosphodiesterase, or increase in cAMP. Combination therapies include isoproterenol (125 μg/hr) and aminophylline (125 mg/hr). However, these drugs increase myocardial oxygen consumption through increased heart rate and contractility. Myocardial ischemia, irritability, or both may be produced, which has prompted the addition of lidocaine (1–4 mg/min) to these regimens to prevent serious ventricular arrhythmias.

Other drugs being investigated in the treatment of this disorder include the calcium antagonists, verapamil and nifedipine, which have been shown to relax isolated constricted cerebral arteries (Hayashi, 1977). The cerebral arterial vasodilatation by calcium-channel blockers may be greater than systemic arterial dilatation. If these drugs prove effective in human beings, their less hazardous cardiac effects could make them useful in the treatment of cerebral arterial spasm.

B. Hypotension after head injury

1. Pathophysiology. Hypotension after head injury results from either the cerebral injury or hypovolemia secondary to systemic trauma. When head injury is complicated by shock, the mortality is significantly higher. Hypotension in the presence of increased ICP markedly reduces cerebral perfusion pressure and increases the likelihood of irreversible damage.

2. Treatment

a. The intravascular volume should be expanded rapidly with balanced salt solutions, blood, and albumin. The use of albumin is controversial; it may leak into cerebral tissue if the blood-brain barrier is disrupted. Avoiding volume overload is essential. Measurement of cardiac filling pressures with a right atrial or pulmonary artery catheter is helpful. The goal, however, is not to achieve a specific filling pressure but rather to maintain organ perfusion as monitored by physical examination and measurement of blood pressure, pulse, and urine output and specific gravity (which may be misleading when osmotic or loop diuretics are used). Direct measurement of cardiac output and calculation of systemic vascular resistance may be necessary if left ventricular dysfunction is suspected. Overzealous fluid administration may promote cerebral edema as well.

b. Postive inotropic agents or vasoconstrictors are indicated, depending on the systemic vascular resistance (see Tables 6-2 and 6-5 for drugs and dosages), if cardiac output remains low despite adequate cardiac filling pressures.

c. In a patient who is brain-dead, hypotension warrants treatment if organs are to be donated. Therapy includes vigorous fluid administration and infusion of dopamine. Dopamine increases renal perfusion at doses below 8 μg/kg/min.

C. Autonomic hypotension

1. Pathophysiology. Hypotension may either accompany spinal cord injury or be a preterminal event in the head-injured patient. Hypotension results from loss of sympathetic influence on the heart and systemic circulation, which causes a decrease in cardiac output and systemic vascular resistance.

2. Treatment

a. Raising the legs will augment preload, increase venous return, and enhance cardiac output.

b. Judicious management of fluids is necessary to avoid over-transfusion and congestive heart failure. These patients may be unable to increase heart rate in response to either hypovolemia or hypervolemia.

c. Vasopressors or positive inotropic drugs are required if hemodynamic performance is not improved by replacement of intravascular volume (see Tables 6-2 and 6-5 for drugs and dosages).

d. If the decreased sympathetic nervous system activity causes bradycardia, *atropine* (0.6–0.8 mg IV) is indicated.

D. Hypotension after carotid endarterectomy

1. Pathophysiology. Patients who have carotid artery disease are usually elderly and may have marked cardiovascular dysfunction and reduced carotid sinus baroreceptor function. These factors predispose them to hypotension as well as hypertension in the perioperative period. Hypotension can decrease perfusion of both brain and heart and also cause thrombosis of the operated vessel. The blood pressure should be maintained within the preoperative range.

2. **Treatment**

   a. Intravascular volume is augmented by administering fluids, recognizing that these patients may have left ventricular dysfunction.

   b. If hypotension is accompanied by bradycardia, atropine (0.6–0.8 mg IV) should be administered.

   c. Vasoconstrictors (see Table 6-2), such as phenylephrine, given by continuous infusion are indicated if perfusion pressure is not restored by increasing heart rate and intravascular volume. Monitoring for myocardial ischemia and renal hypoperfusion is imperative.

   d. If phenylephrine is not tolerated or is ineffective, then a mixed alpha- and beta-adrenergic drug such as dopamine is an alternate choice (see Table 6-5 for drugs and dosages).

E. **Hypertension**

   1. **Pathophysiology.** There are many causes of hypertension. Present in approximately 20% of the adult population in the United States, hypertension is an incremental risk factor in the development of cerebrovascular accidents as well as cardiac disease. Patients admitted to the neurologic ICU frequently have hypertension because of their pre-existing disease, head injury, or surgical procedure (especially exploration of the posterior fossa).

   2. **Treatment.** Treatment of hypertension in the patient who has intracranial pathology risks intolerable reductions in cerebral perfusion pressure. The chronically hypertensive patient requires a higher than normal blood pressure for preservation of autoregulation. Left untreated, hypertension may increase CBF, cerebral blood volume, and ICP, induce hemorrhage into the brain, and promote formation of cerebral edema. There is recent evidence that cerebral ischemia is better tolerated in the treated hypertensive patient than in the untreated patient. Vasodilators (see Table 6-3) and other antihypertensive drugs, such as alpha methyldopa, are useful in controlling chronic hypertension. The goal of treatment in the neurologic ICU is to reestablish blood pressure control with the drugs that the patient took before the acute episode.

F. Hypertension after head injury

1. Pathophysiology. Cerebral perfusion pressure (CPP) is dependent on the difference between MAP and ICP. Therefore, reduction of MAP without a concomitant reduction in ICP may compromise cerebral perfusion. Hypertension often occurs when ICP is elevated (Cushing reflex). Therefore, there may be reluctance to treat hypertension in the head-injured patient for fear of compromising cerebral perfusion. However, ICP monitoring has demonstrated that the systemic arterial pressure is not a reliable indicator of ICP since the Cushing reflex does not occur universally in the presence of intracranial hypertension. Other patients may have hypertension despite normal ICP.

2. Treatment

a. Careful assessment of the hypertensive head-injured patient is necessary. Hypercapnia, distended bladder, pain, anxiety, and other causes should be treated before vasodilator therapy is initiated.

b. Our policy is to keep the systolic arterial pressure below 160 mmHg and the diastolic pressure below 90 mmHg with the use of vasodilators (see Table 6-3 for drugs and dosages). ICP monitoring and direct arterial blood pressure measurement have greatly facilitated the treatment of hypertension coexistent with intracranial pathology by enabling calculation of the CPP at all times.

(1) The best antihypertensive drugs for these patients are vasodilators that do not dilate cerebral vessels (see Table 6-4). Initial choice is chlorpromazine, 2.5 mg IV, titrated to a maximum dose of 15 mg. Trimethaphan, another suitable drug, lowers blood pressure without increasing ICP. Drawbacks to its use are tachyphylaxis, tachycardia, and cycloplegia. Direct cerebral toxicity of this drug has been reported, but only when MAP is less than 50 mmHg. Propranolol may be used as well.

(2) Hydralazine, diazoxide, nitroglycerin, and sodium nitroprusside are cerebrovasodilators and thus may increase ICP when intracranial compliance is decreased. The effect of sodium nitroprusside on ICP may be attenuated by hypocapnic and hyperoxic conditions as well as by administering the drug slowly. Since sodium nitroprusside and trimethaphan must be mixed in 5% dextrose in water, it may be advantageous to make a more concentrated solution to decrease the amount of hypotonic so-

Table 6-7. Concentrations of vasoactive drugs used at the University of Alabama

Drug	For bolus IV	For infusion IV (infants and children)	Adults
Calcium	1 gm/10 ml (100 mg/ml)	—	—
Dobutamine	—	250 mg/250 ml (1 mg/ml)	500 mg/250 ml (2 mg/ml)
Dopamine	—	200 mg/250 ml (0.8 mg/ml)	400 mg/250 ml (1.6 mg/ml)
Ephedrine	50 mg/10 ml (5 mg/ml)	—	—
Epinephrine	0.1 mg/10 ml (10 μg/ml)	2 mg/250 ml (8 μg/ml)	4 mg/250 ml (16 μg/ml)
Isoproterenol	—	0.5 mg/250 ml (2 μg/ml)	1.0 mg/250 ml (4 μg/ml)
Methoxamine	20 mg/10 ml (2 mg/ml)	—	—
Nitroprusside	—	50 mg/500 ml (100 μg/ml)	50 mg/250 ml (200 μg/ml)
Norepinephrine	—	2 mg/250 ml (8 μg/ml)	4 mg/250 ml (16 μg/ml)
Phenylephrine	1 mg/10 ml (100 μg/ml)	—	10 mg/250 ml (40 μg/ml)
Trimethaphan	—	—	500 mg/250 ml (2 mg/ml)

The carrier fluid is D5W; when large volumes of D5W are contraindicated, the concentrations are increased.

lution administered (Table 6-7). These drugs should only be administered through a calibrated infusion pump.

G. Postoperative hypertension

1. **Pathophysiology.** Postoperative hypertension is common in the neurosurgical patient. Multiple causes include increased ICP (Cushing response), hypothermia, emergence excitement with sympathetic discharge, hypercapnia, and distended bladder. Postoperative hypertension is usually accompanied by increased systemic vascular resistance and cardiac output.

   a. **After craniotomy.** Patients who have undergone debulking of large tumors usually show improvement in intracranial compliance; however, patients who have had a craniotomy for epidural or subdural hematoma may have severe underlying cerebral contusion and edema and therefore still have poor intracranial compliance.

b. **After carotid endarterectomy.** The combination of a labile cardiovascular system, preexisting hypertension, and altered baroreceptor function is responsible for the high incidence of postoperative hypertension. Impaired baroreceptor function is more likely to contribute to postendarterectomy hypertension if both carotid arteries have been operated. As with hypertension after head injury, controversy exists as to whether the elevated blood pressure should be treated. The argument against therapy is the potential risk of hypotension and cerebral hypoperfusion, particularly with the more potent antihypertensive agents. Patients who have carotid artery disease, however, commonly have ischemic heart disease as well. While hypertension increases the rate-pressure product, pharmacologic treatment to decrease the systolic blood pressure to acceptable levels may produce undesirable diastolic hypotension and jeopardize adequate coronary blood flow.

There is substantial evidence, however, that postendarterectomy hypertension should be treated. Uncontrolled hypertension may lead to cerebral edema (particularly if autoregulation is impaired), myocardial ischemia, or infarction. Hemorrhage from the arteriotomy site may cause a hematoma in the neck, which can impede carotid blood flow and compromise the airway by compressing and displacing the trachea and larynx. Fatal intracerebral hemorrhage within 24 hours after carotid endarterectomy is a complication of hypertension.

2. **Treatment**

a. **Hypertension after craniotomy.** Therapy and considerations are the same as for hypertension after head injury (see sec. **III.F.2**).

b. **Hypertension after extracranial surgery**

(1) **Vasodilators** (see Table 6-3) are used to treat arterial hypertension. Hydralazine, 5 to 7.5 mg IV initially supplemented by doses of 4 mg as needed, or sodium nitroprusside, 0.2 μg/kg/min up to 10 μg/kg/min, are both effective. Hypotension can be prevented by (a) using a calibrated infusion pump to deliver drugs that are given as a continuous infusion, (b) placing the infusion pump line as close as possible to the IV site to avoid the dead space in long tubing (a pediatric T connector may be useful here), (c) allowing sufficient time for evaluation of drug effect before increasing the dose, (d) basing the

end point of therapy on diastolic or mean arterial pressure rather than on systolic pressure, and (e) ensuring adequate intravascular volume.

(2) Tachycardia either before or after therapy with vasodilators should be treated with propranolol, 0.25 mg IV, in incremental doses up to 0.1 mg/kg.

IV. Drug interactions. Patients who have CNS disease usually come to the neurologic ICU with a history of having taken many drugs, some of which involve the cardiovascular system. The purpose of this section is to outline potential interactions between chronic medications and vasoactive drugs administered in the perioperative period (Table 6-8).

A. Digitalis. Digitalis and the synthetic cardiac glycosides are used in the medical treatment of patients who have heart failure and atrial fibrillation. Frequently, they are given in combination with potassium-wasting diuretics which may cause digitalis toxicity manifested as one or a combination of three dysrhythmias: (1) premature ventricular contractions, (2) paroxysmal atrial tachycardia with block, and (3) Wenckebach (Mobitz type I) atrioventricular block. Therefore, close monitoring of potassium in patients receiving digitalis is necessary, particularly if loop or osmotic diuretics are used.

B. Antihypertensive medications. Antihypertensive medications such as alpha methyldopa, hydralazine, prazosin, and clonidine should be continued up to the day of surgery. Pharmacologically controlled hypertensive patients appear to tolerate anesthesia better than partially controlled or uncontrolled patients. There actually may be some danger of rebound hypertension in patients who discontinue antihypertensive therapy (e.g., clonidine withdrawal). The one group of antihypertensive drugs that should be discontinued two weeks before surgery and replaced with others at that time are the monamine oxidase (MAO) inhibitors. (These drugs also are used as antidepressants and a partial list of them appears in Table 6-8.) MAO inhibitors alter both the function of the normal adrenergic nerve terminal and the synthesis of catecholamines and their metabolites, which may lead to unusual interactions between drugs such as catecholamines and meperidine. Severe hypertension and unpredictable adrenergic drug effects have all been encountered during the perioperative period in patients taking MAO inhibitors.

C. Diuretics. Diuretics treat hypertension by counteracting the compensatory sodium retention that accompanies antihypertensive therapy. They also improve congestive heart failure by reducing the blood volume. In high doses, these drugs may cause depletion

Table 6-8. Interactions of vasoactive drugs used in the perioperative period with patient medications

Drug group	Representative drugs	Interactive drugs	Complications	Recommendations
Beta-adrenergic blockers	Propranolol, metoprolol	Halogenated anesthetics (methoxyflurane, halothane)	Possible potentiation of myocardial depression	Taper propranolol to 80–160 mg/day as tolerated. Do not discontinue
		Beta-agonist drugs	Resistance (larger doses required for beta effects)	Use calcium or other nonbeta agonist for + inotropic effects. Use atropine for + chronotropic effect
Digitalis	Digoxin, Lanoxin (many others)	Pre-op diuretics and diuresis during operation	Digitalis toxicity manifest by arrhythmias	Discontinue on day of surgery, monitor serum K^+
Anti-hypertensive medications	Methyldopa, hydralazine, prazosin, clonidine (others)	Anesthetics or drugs that produce vasodilatation	Hypotension	Continue drug, monitor volume status, give volume or alpha-adrenergic agonist if hypotension occurs
	Monamine oxidase inhibitors (pargyline and others)	Sympathomimetic amines	Hypertension, unpredictable hemodynamic responses to vasoactive drugs	Discontinue drug 2 weeks before anesthesia
Diuretics	Chlorthiazide, hydrochlorothiazide, furosemide	Anesthetics or drugs that produce vasodilatation	Hypotension	Continue drug, monitor volume status and serum K^+
		Digitalis	Arrhythmias with hypokalemia	Monitor serum K^+
Tricyclic anti-depressants	Amitriptyline, imipramine, nortriptyline, protriptyline (others)	Sympathomimetic amines	Tachycardia, hypertension	Taper if possible, administer adrenergic drugs cautiously

of extracellular fluid volume, which, combined with vasodilator therapy, can result in postoperative hypotension. Postoperative hypotension is also a problem in patients whose intracranial hypertension is treated with fluid restriction or patients who have hypertension and coronary artery disease and a reduction in plasma volume.

D. Tricyclic antidepressants. Patients are often treated with tricyclic antidepressants because of depression associated with neurologic and major cardiac disease. These drugs have three principal actions: sedation, peripheral and central anticholinergic effects, and inhibition of the amine pump responsible for norepinephrine reuptake at the adrenergic nerve terminal. It is the last action that probably accounts for the antidepressant activity of these drugs. The anticholinergic and adrenergic effects are also responsible for the undesirable cardiovascular sequelae and perioperative drug interaction problems. The anticholinergic effects of tricyclic therapy cause a sustained increase in heart rate and a transient decrease in atrio-

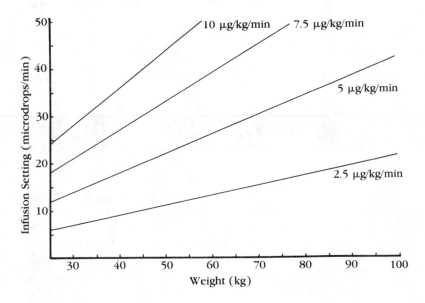

Fig. 6-6. Nomogram for the administration of dopamine (160 mg/250 ml) in patients ranging in weight from 25 kg to 100 kg. The drug infusion in microdrops/min is shown on the vertical axis and the dose from 2.5 µg/kg/min to 10 µg/kg/min is plotted as isobars above the weight of the patient. To calculate the correct infusion setting for a patient in whom the desired dosage is 5 µg/kg/min, a vertical line is drawn from the patient's weight to intersect the 5 µg/kg/min line and then drawn horizontally to intersect the infusion setting line. Nomograms for commonly used drugs given by infusion should be constructed to facilitate the accurate administration of vasoactive drugs.

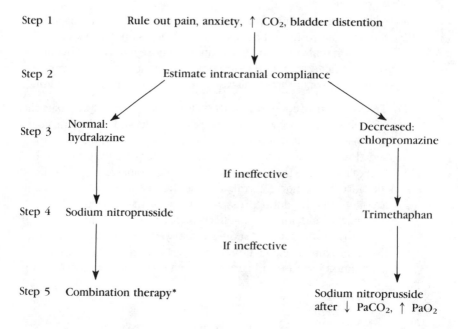

Fig. 6-7. A stepwise protocol for the evaluation and treatment of arterial hypertension in the neurosurgical intensive care patient. If tachycardia is either present initially or develops with therapy, propranolol is the treatment of choice.
*Combination therapy is the use of two or more vasodilators.

ventricular conduction. Myocardial depression is also a transient feature after initiation of tricyclic antidepressant therapy.

Potential problems from drug interactions include the tachycardia that occurs after the administration of sympathomimetic amines such as epinephrine, norepinephrine, and ephedrine. Patients who require tricyclic antidepressants for the treatment of psychiatric depression should continue taking them, but ideally the drugs should be tapered or discontinued before surgery in all other patients. The use of the combination of halothane and pancuronium is avoided during anesthesia for patients taking tricyclic antidepressants. Tricyclic antidepressants may be reinstituted during the postoperative hospital course for appropriate psychiatric indications.

V. Decision-making. The decision to intervene or, perhaps more importantly, not to intervene in the treatment of cardiovascular lability is crucial to appropriate management. Administration of all drugs entails risks and requires thorough consideration of the indications and contraindications.

To make correct decisions all the time is difficult under ideal conditions and impossible in less than optimal circumstances. The most favorable conditions exist when the physician knows the pertinent physiologic data (no more, no less) and the probability of success using a particular intervention in a given circumstance. Calm, efficient management of threatened circulatory failure is best achieved by combining thorough understanding of the clinical pathophysiology with knowledge of the pharmacodynamics of vasoactive drugs. Decision schemes or "protocols" are extremely valuable in organizing therapeutic approaches. The protocols are based on well-defined physiologic and pharmacologic principles, which aid in the selection of appropriate therapy. It is also helpful to have nomograms for infusion of vasoactive drugs to facilitate rapid and accurate selection of infusion rate (Fig. 6-6) and standardized, institution-wide drug concentrations (see Table 6-7).

An example of a logical progression in decision making is presented in the steps for treating high blood pressure (Fig. 6-7). Generally, the interventions with the least risk and/or highest probability of success are made first, and interventions with greater risk and lesser probability of success made later.

References

1. Ahlquist, R. P.   Adrenergic receptors and others. *Anesth. Analg.* (Cleve.) 58:510, 1979.
2. Allen, G. S.   Cerebral arterial spasm. Part 8: The treatment of delayed cerebral arterial spasm in human beings. *Surg. Neurol.* 6:71, 1976.
3. Britton, M., de Faire, V., and Helmers, C.   Hazards of therapy for excessive hypertension in acute stroke. *Acta Med. Scand.* 207:253, 1980.
4. Bronshvag, M. M.   Cerebral pathophysiology in hemorrhagic shock. Nuclide scan data, fluorescence microscopy, and anatomic correlations. *Stroke* 11:50, 1980.
5. Caplan, L. R., Skillman, J., Ojemann, R., et al.   Intracerebral hemorrhage following carotid endarterectomy: A hypertensive complication? *Stroke* 9:457, 1978.
6. Cohn, J. N., and Franciosa, J. A.   Vasodilator therapy of cardiac failure. *N. Engl. J. Med.* 297:27, 1977.
7. Cottrell, J. E., Gupta, B., and Turndorf, H.   Induced hypotension. In J. E. Cottrell and H. Turndorf (Eds.), *Anesthesia and Neurosurgery.* St Louis: Mosby, 1980.
8. Davies, M. J., and Cronin, K. D.   Post-carotid endarterectomy hypertension. *Anaesth. Intensive Care* 8:190, 1980.
9. Doherty, J. E., and Kane, J. J.   Digitalis glycosides: Recent advances in clinical pharmacology and treatment. *South. Med. J.* 70:470, 1977.
10. Fleischer, A. S., and Tindall, G. T.   Cerebral vasospasm following aneurysm rupture: A protocol for therapy and prophylaxis. *J. Neurosurg.* 52:149, 1980.
11. Frishman, W.   Clinical pharmacology of the new beta-adrenergic blocking drugs. Part I. Pharmacodynamic and pharmacokinetic properties. *Am. Heart J.* 97:663, 1979.
12. Graham, R. M., and Pettinger, W. A.   Drug therapy. Prazosin. *N. Engl. J. Med.* 300:232, 1979.
13. Gregory, P. C., McGeorge, A. P., Fitch, W., et al.   Effects of hemorrhagic hypotension on the cerebral circulation. II. Electrocortical function. *Stroke* 10:719, 1979.
14. Halsey, J. H., Jr., O'Brien, M., and Strong, E. R.   Amelioration of cerebral ischemia by prior treatment of hypertension. *Stroke* 11:235, 1980.
15. Hayashi, S., and Toda, N.   Inhibition by Ca^{2+}, verapamil and papaverine of Ca^{2+}-

induced contractions in isolated cerebral and peripheral arteries of the dog. *Br. J. Pharmacol.* 60:35, 1977.

16. Koch-Weser, J.   Drug therapy. Metoprolol. *N. Engl. J. Med.* 301:698, 1979.
17. Kones, R. J.   The catecholamines: Reappraisal of their use for acute myocardial infarction and the low cardiac output syndromes. *Crit. Care Med.* 1:203, 1973.
18. MacKawa, T., McDowall, D. G., and Okuda, Y.   Brain-surface oxygen tension and cerebral cortical blood flow during hemorrhagic and drug-induced hypotension in the cat. *Anesthesiology* 51:313, 1979.
19. Mackenzie, E. T., Farrar, J. K., Fitch, W., et al.   Effects of hemorrhagic hypotension on the cerebral circulation. I. Cerebral blood flow and pial arteriolar caliber. *Stroke* 10:711, 1979.
20. Marsh, M. L., Aidinis, S. J., Naughton, K. V. H., et al.   The technique of nitroprusside administration modifies the intracranial pressure response. *Anesthesiology* 51:538, 1979.
21. Marsh, M. L., Marshall, L. F., and Shapiro, H. M.   Neurosurgical intensive care. *Anesthesiology* 47:149, 1977.
22. Marsh, M. L., Shapiro, H. M., Smith, R. W., et al.   Changes in neurologic status and intracranial pressure associated with sodium nitroprusside administration. *Anesthesiology* 51:336, 1979.
23. Michenfelder, J. D.   The cerebral circulation. In C. Prys-Roberts (Ed.), *The Circulation in Anaesthesia*. Oxford: Blackwell, 1980.
24. Michenfelder, J. D., and Theye, R. A.   Canine systemic and cerebral effects of hypotension induced by hemorrhage, trimethaphan, halothane, or nitroprusside. *Anesthesiology* 46:188, 1977.
25. Miletich, D. J., Gil, K. S. L., Albrecht, R. F., et al.   Intracerebral blood flow distribution during hypotensive anesthesia in the goat. *Anesthesiology* 53:210, 1980.
26. Morawetz, R. B., De Girolami, V., Ojemann, R. G., et al.   Cerebral blood flow determined by hydrogen clearance during middle cerebral artery occlusion in unanesthetized monkeys. *Stroke* 9:143, 1978.
27. Reves, J. G., Sheppard, L. C., Wallach, R., and Lell, W. A.   Therapeutic uses of sodium nitroprusside and an automated method of administration. *Int. Anesthesiol. Clin.* 16:51, 1978.
28. Satiani, B., Vasko, J. S., and Evans, W. E.   Hypertension following carotid endarterectomy. *Surg. Neurol.* 11:357, 1979.
29. Shapiro, H. M.   Cerebral blood flow, cerebral metabolism, and the electroencephalogram in anesthesia. In Miller, R. D. (Ed.), *Anesthesia*. New York: Livingstone, 1981. Pp. 795–824.
30. Sonnenblick, E. H., Frishman, W. H., and LeJemtel, T. H.   Drug therapy. Dobutamine: A new synthetic cardioactive sympathetic amine. *N. Engl. J. Med.* 300:17, 1979.
31. Sundt, T. M., Jr., Szurszewski, J., and Sharbrough, F. W.   Physiological considerations important for the management of vasospasm. *Surg. Neurol.* 7:259, 1977.
32. Von Essen, C., Zervas, N. T., Brown, D. R., et al.   Local cerebral blood flow in the dog during intravenous infusion of dopamine. *Surg. Neurol.* 13:181, 1980.
33. Wilkins, R. H.   Attempted prevention and treatment of intracranial arterial spasm: A survey. *Neurosurgery* 6:198, 1980.

7. Fluid Management

Neal H. Cohen

An important consideration in the perioperative care of the neurosurgical patient is the maintenance of circulatory (cardiovascular) stability and fluid and electrolyte balance. Attempts to maintain normal intravascular volume and electrolyte homeostasis often interfere with preservation of adequate cerebral perfusion pressure (CPP = mean arterial pressure minus intracranial pressure) and contribute to the formation of cerebral edema. This chapter will review the normal body composition of fluids and electrolytes and maintenance fluid requirements in neurosurgical patients. Special fluid and electrolyte problems that arise in patients who have neurologic dysfunction will be discussed, providing a background on which to develop a rational approach to fluid management in the neurosurgical patient.

I. Basic principles of fluid management

A. Normal body composition

1. **Body water distribution.** Body water normally averages 45% to 75% of body weight. The highest concentration of water is in the most metabolically active cells (e.g., muscle, viscera); the lowest concentration is in relatively inactive tissues (e.g., bone, fat). The proportion of body water is highest in the neonate (about 75%) and declines to about 65% of body weight by one year of age. During childhood, the proportion of body water remains relatively constant. As fat stores increase, the percentage of water decreases. Total body water in the adult male is about 60% of body weight. Since the female has a larger percentage of fat as compared to skeletal muscle, total body water in the normal female averages 50% of body weight. Total body water decreases steadily with advancing age, falling to about 45% of body weight in the older female, 50% in the older male.

   Total body water is distributed in two major compartments: extracellular fluid (ECF) and intracellular fluid (ICF). Extracellular water constitutes approximately 20% of body weight. The distribution of extracellular water is summarized in Table 7-1. Extracellular fluid contains sodium, chloride, and bicarbonate. Interstitial fluids and plasma have similar electrolyte composition (Fig. 7-1). Plasma contains more protein, primarily albumin. The protein produces a high colloid osmotic pressure in plasma that maintains a normal fluid distribution between the intravascular and interstitial compartments. Intact capillary endothelial membranes are freely permeable to water and electrolytes, but not to protein, which accounts for the similarity in the electrolyte composition of the intravascular and interstitial fluids.

   Intracellular fluid constitutes 30% to 40% of body weight. The predominant electrolytes are potassium and phosphate. Intracellular fluid has a high protein content.

Table 7-1. Distribution of extracellular fluid

Fluid	% Body weight
Plasma	4.5
Interstitial	16.0
Lymph	2.0
"Transcellular water" (water component of extracellular solids, tendons, fascia, etc.)	1–2

2. **Regulation of intravascular volume.** Although certain ions are not readily diffusible, water as well as urea can move freely between fluid compartments. Transport is controlled by hydrostatic and oncotic pressure gradients. Glucose, which is freely movable through extracellular compartments, enters cells only by active transport mechanisms.

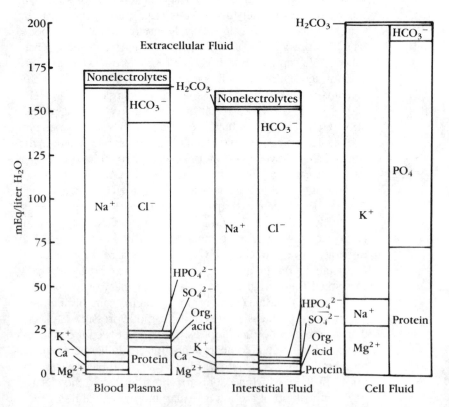

Fig. 7-1. Electrolyte composition of human body fluids (mEq/L of water). HPO_4^{2-} = phosphate; H_2CO_3 = carbonic acid; HCO_3^- = bicarbonate; SO_4 = sulfate.

The total solute concentration (osmolality) of the fluid compartments is maintained within a narrow range by the kidneys. The kidneys regulate water excretion in response to secretion of antidiuretic hormone (vasopressin) and filter and reabsorb sodium to match intake and excretion. In a normal adult, the kidneys can compensate for wide variations in salt and water intake and excrete a daily solute load of 0.5 to 17.0 liters each day. Renal control of body osmolality allows the kidneys to excrete urine with an osmolality of 50 mOsm/L to 1400 mOsm/L to maintain plasma osmolality within a narrow range (285–295 mOsm/L).

3. **Blood volume.** Normal blood volume is estimated as follows:

Adult	70–75 ml/kg
Child	80–85 ml/kg
Neonate	90–100 ml/kg

The normal distribution of body water for a 70-kg male is summarized in Figure 7-2. The blood volume is approximately 5 liters, which includes 2 liters of red blood cells and 3 liters of plasma. Within the vasculature, the majority of the blood volume is in the capacitance (venous) circulation. Any change in capacitance, as may occur with anesthetic drugs or change in position, can have a marked effect on distribution of intravascular volume, venous pressure, and, in the neurosurgical patient who has altered intracranial compliance, intracranial pressure (ICP).

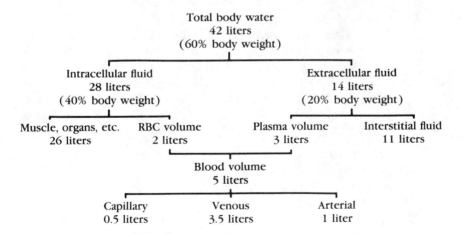

Fig. 7-2. Normal body water distribution (70-kg man).

B. Maintenance requirements

1. **Fluids.** Exogenous fluids are required to preserve the careful balance between intake and losses. In the patient taking a normal diet, ingested fluids and solid foods account for about 1800 to 2000 ml water each day. With chronic disease states, endogenous water of oxidation, normally minimal, increases to as much as 500 to 1500 ml/day: 700 ml/kg from cell water, 150 ml/kg from oxidation of protein, and 1080 ml/kg from oxidation of fat.

   In the patient who has a neurologic disorder, fluid intake may be markedly diminished owing to obtundation, inability to swallow, loss of thirst response from a hypothalamic lesion, loss of appetite, or nausea and vomiting as a result of increased ICP. Fluid intake by the patient who has evidence of intracranial hypertension will be deliberately (iatrogenically) restricted to prevent increases in cerebral extravasation of intravascular fluid and exacerbation of cerebral edema.

   Fluid and electrolyte losses occur from urine (1000–1500 ml/day), the gastrointestinal tract (primarily feces, 100–200 ml/day), and insensible losses (averaging 500–1000 ml/day). Insensible losses are variable and unpredictable, particularly in the patient who is hyperventilating or hypermetabolic. The patient who has centrally mediated hyperventilation may have a significant increase in insensible water loss. Insensible losses also increase by about 10% for every 1° above 37°C and similarly decrease with hypothermia. Any impairment in temperature regulation will therefore alter basal fluid requirements.

   Normally, fluid replacement is managed both by replacing water deficits with water to maintain intravascular volume and by administering electrolytes to replete electrolyte losses. Insensible losses are essentially water and can be replaced with free water. Urinary losses should be replaced with 0.45% normal saline and gastrointestinal losses with isotonic solutions (saline or Ringer's lactate solution). Replacing the sum of these losses with 0.45% saline will balance most of the usual basal fluid and electrolyte losses in the adult. In the child, the maintenance replacement fluid should be 0.2% saline.

2. **Electrolytes.** Sodium is the principal extracellular cation responsible for maintaining the normal osmolality of the extracellular fluid compartment. Excretion of sodium is primarily urinary, amounting to about 70 to 75 mEq/L. Replacement with 75 mEq sodium per day prevents a negative sodium balance. Under normal circumstances, the body is capable of conserving sodium if losses begin to exceed replacement. This adaptation, however, may take 4 to 7 days to occur.

Most of the body potassium is intracellular. Only about 2% of potassium is extracellular. In the 70-kg person, total body potassium is about 3200 mEq. The majority of the potassium is readily exchangeable; only the 5% to 10% of potassium that is within red blood cells is slowly exchanged.

The normal daily oral intake of potassium averages 100 mEq/day (40–120 mEq/day). The obligatory daily loss in a patient who has normal renal function is approximately 25 to 30 mEq in urine and 12 mEq in stool. Parenteral replacement of potassium should be at least 40 mEq/day in the patient who has no oral intake.

Other electrolytes do not normally need intravenous replacement in the patient who requires parenteral fluids for only a short time. Calcium is readily mobilized from bone in adults, so replacement is not usually necessary. Children, however, may need calcium replacement (calcium gluconate 200–300 mEq/kg/day in divided doses) if they are not taking oral feedings. Magnesium deficiency is rare, although 10 mEq magnesium are lost each day in the urine. Zinc deficiency is also unusual in the previously normal patient who receives intravenous fluids for a short time. Replacing these electrolytes and trace minerals is important in the patient who has received parenteral fluids for 5 to 7 days.

3. **Caloric requirements.** Glucose is generally the source of maintenance caloric intake, although hyperalimentation with amino acids and fats is becoming more common in the perioperative and long-term management of the neurologically impaired patient. When fasting, the 70-kg adult loses about 80 gm of protein each day. Administration of glucose, 100 gm (2 liters of 5% dextrose solution daily), reduces this loss by about one half. Glucose reduces the utilization of the body's protein, prevents depletion of liver glycogen and starvation ketosis, and prevents mobilization of fatty acids. The glucose in 2 liters of 5% dextrose solution can supply part or all of the daily caloric needs, as well as provide endogenous water (i.e., water of oxidation) to replace some of the insensible water losses. The osmolar load may help maintain an osmotic diuresis.

II. Surgical considerations

A. Preoperative assessment

1. **Volume status.** The patient undergoing an elective neurosurgical procedure who has no evidence of increased ICP is usually in normal fluid and electrolyte balance preoperatively. The pri-

mary perioperative consideration is the fluid restriction imposed for 8 or more hours before surgery. This deficit should be replaced intraoperatively. Half of the fluid deficit is replaced in the first hour of the surgical procedure; the remaining deficit is replaced during the rest of the procedure along with intraoperative fluid and blood product requirements.

Neurosurgical patients who have evidence of altered intracranial compliance pose a challenge both in assessing intravascular volume status and managing fluids perioperatively. Inappropriate fluid therapy in these patients, particularly preoperatively, may cause or exacerbate brain swelling, increase ICP, and decrease CPP. An accurate assessment of intravascular volume in these patients is critical, although difficult.

2. **Assessment of intravascular volume.** Preoperative volume status is generally determined clinically. Skin turgor should be reasonable, mucous membranes should be moist, and urine output should be 0.5 to 1.0 ml/kg/hr. In elderly patients, heart rate will increase and systemic blood pressure will fall gradually as intravascular volume decreases. Children and young adults will maintain blood pressure by increasing their systemic vascular resistance. Heart rate will increase only minimally until intravascular volume falls markedly.

Clinical evidence of dehydration may not be apparent until intravascular volume falls 5% to 10%. Since many patients who have increased ICP have received osmotic and loop diuretics and have had their fluids restricted to prevent further brain edema, intravascular volume may be severely diminished but clinical evidence of dehydration may not be apparent. For example, if maintained with osmotherapy, the urine output becomes a poor guide to adequacy of intravascular volume.

The "tilt test" has been used to assess fluid deficits in adults. The patient who has had an intravascular fluid loss of 1000 ml will develop tachycardia when placed in the reverse Trendelenburg position. If the loss approximates 1500 ml, the patient will become hypotensive with tilting. Losses in excess of 1500 ml cause hypotension in the supine position.

Patients who have head trauma requiring surgical intervention (depressed skull fracture, epidural or subdural hematoma) often have associated peripheral injuries. The extent of blood loss and intravascular fluid deficit is often difficult to assess before inducing anesthesia. Closed wounds can mask significant blood loss; femoral fractures or retroperitoneal bleeding may cause sequestrations of 500 to 1500 ml of blood. Blood and fluid losses from open wounds can be more easily assessed, although underestimating these losses is common. The "hand" or "fist" rule can be a useful guide to acute blood loss. Each hand required to cover a wound or each fist required to fill a wound represents about a 10% loss of blood volume.

3. **Electrolyte imbalance.** Serum electrolytes are helpful in assessing intravascular volume status. Low serum sodium most often results from excess free water rather than from true sodium depletion. Water intoxication causes increased ICP and seizures. Hypertension and bradycardia may occur as a result of the increase in ICP. Exogenous water overload must be differentiated from the syndrome of inappropriate antidiuretic hormone secretion (SIADH; see section **III.C**) and from the hyponatremia that can result from prolonged mannitol-induced diuresis without adequate sodium replacement.

Hypernatremia may be a reflection of preoperative intravascular water deficit. This deficit must be differentiated from hypernatremia that results from rapid administration of solutions containing sodium salts and from diabetes insipidus that often accompanies head trauma. Urine and serum electrolytes and osmolalities are useful in differentiating the etiology of hypernatremia.

4. **Effect of underlying diseases.** Despite the utility of these guides to volume status before induction of anesthesia, many patients also have associated or underlying diseases that influence preoperative fluid and electrolyte balance. For example, the hypertensive patient may be intravascularly volume depleted despite abnormally high systemic blood pressure. Such patients also have altered autoregulation of cerebral blood flow (CBF), with higher upper and lower limits (i.e., the autoregulatory curve is displaced to the right, see Fig. 6-1). These patients will tolerate high arterial pressure better than normotensive patients, but they will not tolerate the low perfusion pressures that may follow induction of anesthesia when hypovolemia is present.

Patients who have impaired myocardial function have altered fluid requirements and less tolerance for rapid fluid administration. Volume status both preoperatively and intraoperatively is best assessed by measuring cardiac filling pressures. Monitoring the central venous pressure (CVP) is a useful guide to right ventricular function. Normal CVP is 4 to 8 mmHg. Pulmonary artery catheterization and measurement of pulmonary capillary wedge pressure (PCWP), normally 8 to 12 mmHg, provide a better guide to left atrial and left ventricular function. The triple lumen pulmonary artery catheter allows measurement of cardiac output and calculation of systemic vascular resistance (SVR) and pulmonary vascular resistance (PVR).* This knowledge of overall myocardial function in patients who have neurologic disease and impaired intracranial compliance facilitates more controlled manipulation of parameters that influence cerebral perfusion pressure through the use of a rational combination of fluids, osmotic diuretics, vasodilators, and vasopressors.

B. Intraoperative management

1. **Fluid management.** Fluid management during neurosurgical procedures requires replacement of preoperative deficits and intraoperative losses without increasing cerebral edema, compromising cerebral perfusion pressure, or causing rupture of an aneurysm or AVM. Dextrose solutions in combination with free water rapidly equilibrate throughout all fluid compartments. If the brain becomes hyperosmolar relative to the blood, it will accumulate water, exacerbating cerebral edema. With an open skull, brain edema interferes with the surgical exposure. Administering isotonic intravenous fluids (5% dextrose in Ringer's lactate solution) is preferred to 5% dextrose in water. In most clinical situations, fluids are administered in a volume that maintains peripheral perfusion without causing overhydration. For the patient who has underlying cardiac, vascular, or renal disease, careful monitoring of intravascular volume and myocardial filling pressure is necessary.

During major surgical procedures or trauma, patients have a marked reduction in functional extracellular fluid as a result of internal redistribution of fluids ("third space" losses; Fig. 7-3). The loss of intravascular volume is directly proportional to the degree of tissue trauma. The extracellular fluid losses originate initially from the plasma compartment, but quickly equilibrate with the interstitial fluid. The body attempts to compensate for the sequestered losses of extracellular fluid by renal conservation of sodium and water. After major tissue manipulation, a large volume of fluid is sequestered in both traumatized and other tissue spaces. Although the degree of tissue manipulation in neurosurgical patients is generally small, the third space fluid

$$*SVR = \frac{MAP - CVP}{cardiac\ output} \times 80$$

normal $= 800\text{--}1200$ dynes-sec-cm^{-5}

$$PVR = \frac{mean\ pulmonary\ artery\ pressure - PCWP}{cardiac\ output} \times 80$$

normal $= 50\text{--}150$ dynes-sec-cm^{-5}
(MAP = mean arterial pressure.)

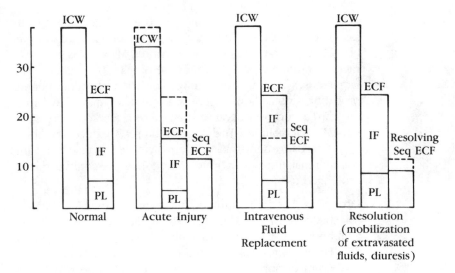

Fig. 7-3. Redistribution of fluid after injury. ICW = intracellular water; ECF = extracellular fluid; IF = interstitial fluid; PL = plasma; Seq ECF = sequestered extracellular fluid.

loss can be significant and result in decreased intravascular volume, impaired peripheral perfusion, and impaired renal function. The sequestered extracellular fluid can be replaced with isotonic fluids although care is necessary to prevent overhydration. Urine output should be 0.5 to 1.0 ml/kg/hr, and cardiac filling pressures should be maintained in the low normal range (CVP 4 to 6 mmHg, PCWP 6 to 8 mmHg).

2. **Hyperosmotic agents.** The intraoperative management of patients who have increased ICP and cerebral edema often includes intravenous administration of hyperosmotic agents. Mannitol, urea, and glycerol decrease edema by inducing an osmotic gradient between plasma and the brain and drawing water from the brain's interstitium into the intravascular compartment across intact areas of the blood-brain barrier. The osmotic diuretics may also lower cerebrospinal fluid (CSF) pressure by reducing the rate of CSF production. Because these drugs can cause an initial increase in cerebral blood volume and ICP, they must be given in conjunction with other maneuvers to decrease intracranial volume (such as steroids, hyperventilation, CSF drainage). The hyperosmotic drugs are not effective in the patient whose blood-brain barrier is disrupted because the desired osmotic gradient may not be established. Instead, the brain will become hyperosmolar relative to the intravascular space, and the brain edema will increase.

Mannitol, the most commonly used osmotic agent, is relatively safe. Urea may cause a rebound increase in ICP, venous thrombosis, and tissue necrosis if it extravasates. Mannitol is given as a rapid intravenous infusion in a dose of 0.25 to 1.5 gm/kg. The larger doses may provide a longer duration of action, but are probably of no additional benefit. Large doses may even impair myocardial function because they cause a marked increase in intravascular volume. The osmotic diuresis induced by these agents leads to dehydration, electrolyte disturbances, and impaired renal function. Careful monitoring is required during prolonged use.

3. **Diuretics.** The loop diuretics, furosemide and ethacrynic acid, have been shown to reduce ICP. The induced diuresis decreases total body water, but the drugs may also diminish formation of CSF. Furosemide causes a rapid reduction in ICP without altering serum osmolality. The diuretics appear to be particularly effective in patients who have evidence of left ventricular dysfunction and interstitial pulmonary edema. Diuresis may also improve gas exchange and indirectly lower ICP. The efficacy of loop diuretics in the management of chronically increased ICP has not been established.

C. Postoperative management

1. **Management of fluid administration.** Fluid management in the postoperative period is an extension of care in the operating room. Despite the extravasation of extracellular fluid that occurs after tissue manipulation and decreases functional intravascular volume, neurosurgical patients are treated with moderate restriction of fluid intake postoperatively. This restriction prevents increases in brain edema and potential neurologic deterioration. Intravenous fluids should be administered at a rate of about one-half to two-thirds of maintenance requirements for both children and adults. This amount will usually maintain adequate intravascular volume, urine output, and peripheral perfusion without increasing edema at the surgical site. Patients are observed closely for the development of clinical signs of spinal cord or cerebral edema. Monitoring of ICP, when available, will provide evidence of postoperative edema or hematoma that might compromise neurologic outcome. Peripheral pulses, color, and temperature are good indicators of the adequacy of peripheral perfusion. If diuretics or osmotherapy is not used, urine output should be maintained at 0.5 to 1.0 ml/kg/hr in the first 24 to 48 hours after surgery. When diuresis is induced, satisfactory urine volume may be misinterpreted as a sign of adequate intravascular volume despite other evidence of dehy-

dration. Intake and output should therefore be carefully measured during the postoperative period, both to monitor intravascular volume and to observe for complications of neurologic dysfunction (e.g., diabetes insipidus or SIADH). Fluctuation in daily weight is also a useful guide to volume status, particularly when compared to the patient's preoperative weight.

Measurement of myocardial filling pressures is the most reliable guide to adequacy of intravascular volume. As is true intraoperatively, CVP and PCWP should be maintained in the low normal range to ensure adequate perfusion. Increasing fluid intake to maintain CVP or PCWP at high levels carries the risk of increasing brain edema or rupturing an unsecured aneurysm. If cardiac output, peripheral perfusion, or urine output remains inadequate, or if the patient develops a metabolic (lactic) acidosis despite adequate volume replacement, vasopressors such as dopamine or dobutamine should be administered to improve perfusion.

2. **Crystalloid versus colloid solutions.** Crystalloid solutions (Ringer's lactate solution, normal saline) are preferred in the intraoperataive and postoperative periods. Volume expansion with colloid solutions has been suggested for maintaining intravascular volume in the postoperative patient. In the patient who has altered integrity of the blood-brain barrier or vasogenic cerebral edema, protein-containing solutions will extravasate into the brain to the same extent as crystalloid solutions creating an osmotic gradient and increasing regional edema. As the patient stabilizes postoperatively, the crystalloid solution will be more readily mobilized and the edema will more rapidly resolve.

3. **Resolution phase after fluid extravasation.** During the clearing of third-space fluid accumulation (see Fig. 7-3), administration of intravenous fluid should be minimized. As the extravasated fluid is mobilized and returned to the intravascular compartment, cardiac filling pressures often increase. This excess intravascular volume is then spontaneously excreted, usually approximately 48 to 72 hours after the tissue trauma. Administering diuretics is usually not necessary if renal function is normal; diuretics will often speed elimination of fluid mobilized into the intravascular compartment, but their use may deplete intravascular volume if it is not carefully monitored.

4. **Special considerations in the neurosurgical patient.** During the immediate postoperative period, patients who have increased ICP are often treated with mannitol. The indications and

management are the same as those for the use of osmotherapy intraoperatively. In the postoperative period, prolonged administration of mannitol may lead to dehydration, hyperosmolality, and electrolyte disturbances. Urine and serum electrolytes and osmolality must be monitored closely. In general, if serum osmolality exceeds 320 mOsm/L, mannitol should be withheld. Some of the patients whose intracranial hypertension is unresponsive to other therapies (hyperventilation, fluid restriction, steroids) will respond to mannitol, even when the serum osmolality is greater than 320 mOsm/L at the time of administration.

Patients who receive barbiturates for cerebral protection or elevated ICP in the postoperative period often require large volumes of intravenous fluid to maintain adequate intravascular volume. Barbiturates in doses sufficient to induce coma are myocardial depressants and may cause capillary endothelial disruption and extravasation of fluids. A pulmonary artery catheter is necessary in these patients to monitor myocardial filling pressures in conjunction with measurement of ICP. Central venous pressure and PCWP are maintained in the low normal range; vasopressors should be given as necessary to ensure adequate cardiac output and peripheral perfusion. As the barbiturates are tapered, these patients will mobilize the extravasated fluids. Diuretics may be of value to improve urine output and prevent development of pulmonary edema.

Patients who develop clinical or angiographic evidence of cerebral vasospasm, either after subarachnoid hemorrhage or craniotomy for aneurysm clip-ligation, present a particular problem of fluid management. Hypotension has been implicated as an exacerbating event in the development of regional vasospasm. These patients tolerate dehydration poorly: the vasospasm worsens when intravascular volume is low. Patients who have evidence of vasospasm should be treated with aggressive volume replacement with blood and albumin. Mean arterial pressure should be maintained in the high normal range, and cardiac output should be augmented with isoproterenol or dopamine. Aminophylline and calcium channel–blocking drugs have also been used to dilate the cerebral vasculature and maintain cerebral blood flow.

III. Special fluid and electrolyte problems in the neurosurgical patient

A. **Neurogenic pulmonary edema.** Patients who have a variety of central nervous system disorders occasionally develop acute pulmonary edema (neurogenic pulmonary edema) in the absence of cardiopulmonary disease or other apparent etiologies. Neurogenic pulmonary edema has been reported after head trauma, intracranial tumors, ruptured aneurysms, intraventricular hemorrhage, stroke, seizures, Guillain-Barré syndrome, and hypothalamic lesions. Although the etiology is unclear, neurogenic pulmonary edema may be related to the massive alpha-adrenergic discharge associated with the neurologic disorder. As a result, systemic and pulmonary vascular resistances increase. This transiently increases left atrial and pulmonary capillary wedge pressures, and pulmonary capillary endothelial disruption occurs. The altered pulmonary capillary permeability causes the accumulation of pulmonary edema fluid, which has a high protein content. The vascular injury also accounts for the pulmonary hemorrhage seen both clinically and pathologically in neurogenic pulmonary edema. Other mechanisms for development of neurogenic pulmonary edema have also been proposed.

The treatment of neurogenic pulmonary edema is similar to the treatment of adult respiratory distress syndrome (ARDS) from any cause (see Chap. 5). In addition to ventilatory support with positive pressure ventilation (PPV) and positive end-expiratory pressure (PEEP), fluid management is of the utmost importance. Fluid intake in the form of crystalloid solution, rather than protein-containing solution, should be minimal. If PCWP is being monitored, the PCWP should be kept low (5–7 mmHg) to prevent further extravasation of proteinaceous fluid. If mean arterial pressure or perfusion is inadequate, vasopressors (dopamine, dobutamine) should be used to maintain cerebral and peripheral tissue perfusion. If systemic or pulmonary vascular resistance is elevated, vasodilators, such as sodium nitroprusside, can be used to dilate pulmonary and peripheral vascular beds and lower vascular resistance.

B. **Diabetes insipidus.** Diabetes insipidus is a common sequela of intracranial trauma, skull fractures, and neurosurgical procedures. The disease process results from decreased secretion of antidiuretic hormone (ADH) from the posterior pituitary gland. Polyuria, progressive dehyration, and hypernatremia occur subsequently. Urine output may be greater than 3 liters per day; the urine is dilute but the serum osmolality may be 320 to 330 mOsm/L.

The diagnosis of diabetes insipidus is often difficult in the neurosurgical patient who may have a concomitant solute diuresis induced by vigorous intravenous fluid administration. Diabetes insipidus is present when the urine output is excessive, the urine osmolality is inappropriately low (60–200 mOsm) relative to serum osmolality, and the urine specific gravity is 1.001 to 1.005. The patient who has diabetes insipidus is unable to concentrate urine or reduce urine volume in response to fluid restriction. Parenteral administration of aqueous vasopressin should reduce the urine volume and confirm the diagnosis.

Management of diabetes insipidus requires careful balancing of intake and output. Serum and urine electrolytes and osmolality, urine specific gravity, BUN, creatinine, and weight must be closely monitored. Hypotonic solutions (5% dextrose in 0.2% saline plus supplemental potassium) are administered to replace the hourly urine output plus estimated insensible losses. If the urine output remains excessive (greater than 200–250 ml/hr), or if maintaining fluid balance is difficult, aqueous vasopressin (5–10 IU, IM or SC) should be administered to reduce urine output. As output decreases, intravenous or oral fluid intake will have to be tapered. Since the duration of diabetes insipidus is variable, further treatment with vasopressin is dictated by recurrence of polyuria. If long-term therapy is required, desmopressin nasal spray (1-desamino-8-D-argininevasopressin; DDAVP) can be administered intranasally as needed to control urine output.

C. **Syndrome of inappropriate antidiuretic hormone secretion (SIADH).** A wide variety of central nervous system disorders are associated with inappropriate secretion of ADH, including head trauma, tumor, subarachnoid hemorrhage, and brain abscess. SIADH may develop 3 to 15 days after trauma or surgical intervention. It is self-limited, usually resolving in less than 7 days. The excessive ADH secretion causes continued renal excretion of sodium despite hyponatremia and associated hypo-osmolality. Urine osmolality is therefore high relative to serum osmolality. The patient who has SIADH has no clinical evidence of dehydration; renal and adrenal function are normal. The clinical manifestations of SIADH are variable, depending on how hyponatremic the patient becomes and how quickly the hyponatremia develops. If the serum sodium falls slowly, even to as low as 120 mEq/L, symptoms are mild. If the hyponatremia occurs more quickly, symptoms include anorexia, nausea, vomiting, irritability, and hyperreflexia, which may progress to seizures, stupor, and coma.

The mainstay of treatment for SIADH is water restriction (500 ml/ day). If the hyponatremia is severe (serum sodium less than 110 mEq/L), hypertonic (3%–5%) saline should be administered. Hypertonic saline must be used with extreme caution and careful monitoring to avoid development of acute pulmonary edema.

In patients who have increased ADH and decreased red blood cell volume, water should be restricted and intravascular volume expanded with blood.

D. **Nonketotic hyperglycemic hyperosmolar coma.** Nonketotic hyperglycemic hyperosmolar coma (NHHC) has occurred in a vari-

ety of neurosurgical conditions, including intracerebral hemorrhage, head trauma, brain tumor, and cerebral infarction. About
two thirds of patients who have NHHC have no history of diabetes
mellitus. Many have intercurrent infections, are taking drugs that
alter glucose tolerance (e.g., steroids, phenytoin, thiazides), or are
dehydrated owing to inadequate fluid intake, hyperosmolar tube
feedings, and prolonged osmotherapy.

The diagnosis of NHHC includes hyperglycemia (blood sugar
400–2500 mg/100 ml), glycosuria, and plasma osmolality greater
than 330 mOsm/L in the absence of ketosis. Patients who have
NHHC are dehydrated and often potassium depleted because of the
osmotic diuresis. They may also have evidence of prerenal azotemia
that, if untreated, can progress to acute renal failure.

Treatment is directed primarily at correction of dehydration and
hypertonicity. Normal saline is used for volume replacement, in
conjunction with careful monitoring of serum and urine electrolytes and osmolality. In patients who have underlying cardiac disease, myocardial function should be evaluated by the use of the
thermodilution pulmonary artery catheter for measuring cardiac
filling pressures and cardiac output during volume repletion. After
sodium deficits are corrected with normal saline, 0.2% or 0.45%
saline should be used to replace water deficits.

Hyperglycemia is usually responsive to insulin. Small doses of
insulin (1–10 U/hr) given as a continuous hourly infusion will often
correct hyperglycemia. Rapid lowering of the blood sugar may be
harmful, producing hypoglycemia and cerebral edema and reducing plasma volume before sodium and water deficits have been
restored.

References

1. Bartter, F. C., and Schwartz, W. B.   The syndrome of inappropriate secretion of
   antidiuretic hormone. *Am. J. Med.* 42:790, 1967.
2. Cottrell, J. E., Robustelli, A., Post, K., et al.   Furosemide- and mannitol-induced
   changes in intracranial pressure and serum osmolality and electrolytes. *Anesthesiology* 47:28, 1977.
3. Domer, F. R.   Effects of diuretics on cerebrospinal fluid formation and potassium
   movement. *Exp. Neurol.* 24:54, 1969.
4. Fox, J. L., Falik, J. L., and Salhaub, R. J.   Neurosurgical hyponatremia: The role of
   inappropriate antidiuresis. *J. Neurosurg.* 34:506, 1971.
5. Katzman, R., and Pappius, H. M.   *Brain Electrolytes and Fluid Metabolism.* Baltimore: Williams & Wilkins, 1973.
6. Lucas, C. E.   The renal response to acute injury and sepsis. *Surg. Clin. North Am.*
   56:953, 1976.
7. Miller, J. D., and Leech, P.   Effects of mannitol and steroid therapy on intracranial
   volume-pressure relationships in patients. *J. Neurosurg.* 42:274, 1975.
8. Park, B. E., Meacham, W. F., and Netsky, M. G.   Nonketotic hyperglycemic hy-

perosmolar coma: Report of neurosurgical cases with a review of mechanisms and treatment. *J. Neurosurg.* 44:409, 1976.

9. Pitts, R. F.   *Physiology of the Kidney and Body Fluids* (3rd ed.). Chicago: Year Book, 1974.

10. Randall, H. T.   Fluid, electrolyte, and acid-base balance. *Surg. Clin. North Am.* 56:1019, 1976.

11. Revlen, H. J.   Vasogenic brain oedema. *Br. J. Anaesth.* 48:741, 1976.

12. Shenkin, H. A., Bezier, H. S., and Bouzarth, W. F.   Restricted fluid intake. *J. Neurosurg.* 45:432, 1976.

13. Shires, T.   Fluid and electrolyte therapy. In J. M. Kinney (Ed.), *Manual of Preoperative and Postoperative Care* (2nd ed.). Philadelphia: Saunders, 1971.

14. Shucart, W. A., and Jackson, I.   Management of diabetes insipidus in neurosurgical patients. *J. Neurosurg.* 44:65, 1976.

15. Theodore, J., and Robin, E. D.   Speculation on neurogenic pulmonary edema (NPE). *Am. Rev. Respir. Dis.* 113:405, 1976.

III. Anesthetic Management

8. Intracranial Aneurysms

Neurosurgery

S. J. Peerless

Since 1931, when Dott (1932) first operated on an intracranial aneurysm, great progress has been made in surgical and anesthetic technique, instrumentation, and results of treatment. Although the application of a clip across the base of an aneurysm remains the procedure of choice, several novel options are available for unclippable lesions. The surgeon may elect to strengthen the wall of the aneurysm through the use of gauze or plastic compounds or to induce intraluminal thrombosis by proximal ligation of feeding vessels.

The first use of the surgical microscope for aneurysm surgery by Lougheed in 1960 was a turning point in the operative treatment of intracranial aneurysms. The perfect coaxial light and magnification added immensely to the surgeon's precision. The use of the microscope brought with it a new generation of fine instruments and new techniques for exposing the vessels at the base of the brain and dissecting with safety around these complex branching structures.

The details made visible by high magnification have become extremely important for accurate surgical treatment of aneurysms. With the aid of the microscope, the surgeon is able to dissect the neck more precisely and to avoid injury to the tiny branching arteries in the area.

I. **Incidence and classification.** The incidence of subarachnoid hemorrhage (SAH) from ruptured intracranial aneurysms has been estimated to be approximately 15 to 20 per 100,000 population (Kurtzke, 1969); the incidence of asymptomatic aneurysms is as high as 4%.

In North America, there are approximately 30,000 new cases of SAH secondary to aneurysm rupture each year (Kurtzke, 1969; Locksley, 1965). These figures may actually be underestimated since accurate population studies have been difficult to obtain. Of the 30,000 patients diagnosed as having SAH, 12,000 will die or become significantly disabled: 4000 will be seriously and rapidly brain-injured without warning at the time of the first subarachnoid hemorrhage and 8000 will suffer recurrent hemorrhage after the initial bleed had been ignored or misdiagnosed. Of the remaining 18,000 patients available for treatment, 9000 will die or be disabled as a result of rebleeding, cerebral ischemia secondary to vasospasm, and other medical or surgical complications. Therefore, there will be only 9000 functional survivors. In view of these gloomy figures, contemporary research and therapy of intracranial aneurysms must focus on early, accurate diagnosis of SAH, recognition of aneurysms before they rupture, and elimination of the two most lethal complications: rebleeding and vasospasm.

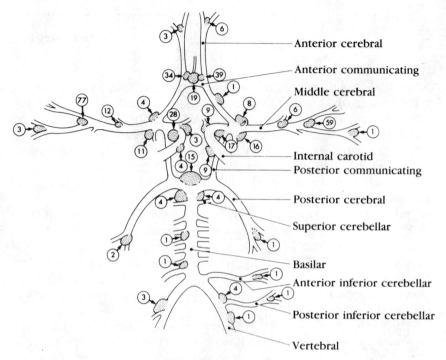

Fig. 8-1. Location of 407 aneurysms in 300 consecutive patients classified by size and location. Numbers in circles reflect the incidence.

Aneurysms are most common in the 40- to 60-year age group; 60% of all aneurysms occur in women. Aneurysms are usually classified according to location and size. The location is specified by the vessel of origin and the nearest branch vessel. Aneurysms virtually always arise at a branch or bifurcation and usually at the point where the major vessel makes a turn, changing the axial flow of blood. An aneurysm arising from the carotid artery in the crotch distal to the origin of the posterior communicating artery is called a carotid-posterior communicating aneurysm; the next most distal carotid aneurysm is labelled a carotid-choroidal aneurysm (Fig. 8-1).

After SAH, patients suffering from a ruptured intracranial aneurysm are assigned a clinical grade, depending on the presence of signs of meningeal reaction, level of consciousness, and evidence of focal neurologic dysfunction. Either Botterell's (1956) original classification or the modification proposed by Hunt (1968) is used by neurosurgeons to provide a means of estimating surgical risk and outcome (Table 8-1). Generally, direct surgical repair of an intracranial aneurysm in a Grade I patient can be accomplished with a low mortality. In contrast, virtually all Grade V patients will perish.

Table 8-1. Classification of patients with intracranial aneurysms according to surgical risk

Grade[a]	Criteria	Perioperative mortality rates (%)[b]
I	Asymptomatic, or minimal headache and slight nuchal rigidity	0–5
II	Moderate to severe headache, nuchal rigidity, no neurologic deficit other than cranial nerve palsy	2–10
III	Drowsiness, confusion, or mild focal deficit	10–15
IV	Stupor, moderate to severe hemiparesis, possibly early decerebrate rigidity and vegetative disturbances	60–70
V	Deep coma, decerebrate rigidity, moribund appearance	70–100

[a]The original classification has been revised to include Grade 0 for patients who have unruptured aneurysms and Grade Ia for patients who have a stable, residual neurologic deficit who are past the period of acute cerebral reaction.
[b]Surgical mortality varies among institutions.
Note: Serious systemic disease such as hypertension, diabetes, severe arteriosclerosis, chronic pulmonary disease, and severe vasospasm seen on arteriography result in placement of the patient in the next less favorable category.

II. Signs and symptoms of subarachnoid hemorrhage

A. **Results of initial rupture.** The signs and symptoms of SAH result from the eruption of blood into the subarachnoid space under arterial pressure. There is an abrupt, marked rise in the intracranial pressure (ICP), which reaches or momentarily exceeds the systemic arterial pressure. This intracranial pressure wave accounts for the acute onset of a severe and excruciating headache with or without loss of consciousness. Minor hemorrhages without coma ("warning leaks") occur in about 50% of patients and may be ignored or misdiagnosed as "flu" or migraine. As the irritant blood floods through the subarachnoid pathways, a meningeal reaction occurs causing photophobia, fever, nuchal rigidity, and persistent headache. After a less severe hemorrhage, normal consciousness is rapidly regained; the patient is usually alert and oriented within 24 hours and has no focal neurologic signs. With more severe bleeds, consciousness may be impaired for days or weeks. Focal or hemispheric signs immediately after the hemorrhage are most often secondary to an intracerebral hematoma. Frequently, the sudden expansion of the aneurysm or the jet of blood will impact on an adjacent cranial nerve, resulting in a focal sign. The most common example is an oculomotor nerve palsy seen in association with a carotid-posterior communicating aneurysm.

B. **Focal neurologic dysfunction.** Focal neurologic dysfunction most often occurs 5 to 9 days after the hemorrhage owing to cerebral ischemia and infarction secondary to arterial vasospasm. These clinical signs occur in 15% to 20% of patients after a major SAH and frequently may cause permanent hemiparesis, impaired consciousness, intellectual deterioration, or death.

C. **Hydrocephalus.** Hydrocephalus is also common after SAH owing to impaired CSF circulation through the basal cisterns. Hydrocephalus is best treated after the aneurysm has been secured because reducing the intracranial pressure increases the risk of rebleeding significantly. During surgery hydrocephalus is handled by lumbar subarachnoid drainage. The removal of excess fluid provides intracranial relaxation and improves access to the aneurysm. Only rarely is it necessary to insert a permanent shunting device to treat persistent hydrocephalus.

D. **Complications of subarachnoid hemorrhage.** The sudden rise of ICP in association with aneurysm rupture and the reaction of the meninges and cerebral vasculature to the subarachnoid blood will commonly cause a variety of medical complications. These complications include systemic hypertension, arrhythmias, electrolyte and water disturbances, gastric erosion, and, with coma, aspiration pneumonia.

E. **Diagnosis.** Positive confirmation of SAH should be made by lumbar puncture, taking care to centrifuge the sample immediately and examine the supernatant for xanthochromia to differentiate between true SAH and traumatic hemorrhage caused by the spinal needle.

   The noninvasive computed tomographic (CT) scan may be used in place of or in conjunction with the lumbar puncture. The CT scan may not only provide confirmation of subarachnoid blood but also information about the site and source of bleeding. Aneurysms greater than 1 cm in diameter may be located through CT scanning. Moreover, the early visualization of clot in the subarachnoid cisterns appears to be a reliable way of predicting the subsequent development of vasospasm. After confirmation of SAH, angiography is performed, using a transfemoral catheter approach, selectively injecting both carotid and vertebral arteries, and obtaining lateral, AP, and often oblique projections. The studies are used to locate the source of bleeding precisely and to rule out other causes of SAH such as arteriovenous malformation (AVM) or neoplasm.

III. **Preoperative care after subarachnoid hemorrhage.** The goals of preoperative care are to help the brain recover from the effects of SAH and to prevent recurrent hemorrhage. One must strive to maintain normal cerebral perfusion while minimizing the chance of exceeding the bursting pressure of the aneurysm. The patient should be nursed in a quiet, darkened room and given analgesics and sedation to allow sufficient sleep and rest. Phenothiazine derivatives are inadvisable as sedatives because of their variable and uncontrolled hypotensive effect. Analgesic drugs such as codeine or meperidene may be given to alleviate head and neck pain. Phenytoin is used to prevent seizures. One thousand to fifteen hundred calories per day, excluding caffeine, should be given in a soft form to conscious patients at rest in the recumbent position. Cimetidene is used in patients who have impaired consciousness to prevent gastric erosion and hemorrhage. Patients can be fed intravenously for up to three weeks, but after this time a feeding jejunostomy should be used. Straining at stool should be avoided and therefore softening agents and suppositories are given routinely. Fluid balance is carefully monitored.

A. **Complications: Rebleeding.** The complications of subarachnoid hemorrhage and surgical treatment of aneurysms include a lengthy list of potential problems that may cause progressive neurologic deterioration (Table 8-2). The most important of these are rebleeding and vasospasm.

Recurrent hemorrhage from an aneurysm is the most devastating complication and carries with it a high morbidity and mortality. Rebleeding from an aneurysm results when the bursting pressure within exceeds the tensile strength of either the clot or the wall of the sac. The bursting pressure is a function of the intra-arterial pressure and the surrounding ICP. Mild elevations in systemic blood pressure are common after SAH and usually respond to bed rest and sedation. If persistent elevation of blood pressure is a problem, we tend to restrict fluid intake modestly, giving 1500 to

Table 8-2. Complications of subarachnoid hemorrhage resulting in progressive neurologic deterioration in 420 patients

Complication	%
Vasospasm	33
Hyponatremia (ADH)	19
Hydrocephalus	14
Aseptic meningitis	9
Vascular occlusion	8
Surgery	6
Recurrent hemorrhage	6
Other	9

2000 ml over 24 hours as a simple means of controlling blood pressure. The net loss of fluid must, however, be known and replaced in the intraoperative and immediate postoperative period. Significant hypertension is controlled with loop diuretics (furosemide) and hydralazine as necessary (if the ICP is normal).

The prevention of rebleeding using antifibrinolytic agents (ϵ-aminocaproic acid [Amicar] or tranexamic acid) has been impressive but far from complete. In our experience, the rate of rebleeding has been reduced from about 20% to less than 6%. This dramatic result is not universally accepted and remains controversial. We have found that continuous infusion of ϵ-aminocaproic acid, using a calibrated pump, in a dose of 36 gm/24 hr is necessary to achieve the result. Smaller doses or oral administration is not as effective in preventing the lysis of clot in the dome of the aneurysm and rebleeding. It is important to maintain the intravenous administration of ϵ-aminocaproic acid continuously until the patient's aneurysm has been surgically secured in the operating room. We have not noted an increase in hydrocephalus or thrombotic complications with the use of ϵ-aminocaproic acid. However, ϵ-aminocaproic acid is hyperosmolar and will produce a net loss of fluid, which should be monitored and replaced.

Fundamentally, the goal of the preoperative therapy is to keep the blood pressure within the aneurysm below the bursting pressure of the sac. As noted, carefully controlling the systemic pressure and the ICP and preventing the lysis of the friable clot by sealing the rent in the aneurysm wall are critical in achieving this end. Using this regimen, we have limited the rate of rebleeding to less than 6%. Recurrent rebleeding, when it occurs, is usually attributable to imperfect control of either blood pressure of ICP or to the premature discontinuation of ϵ-aminocaproic acid.

Should rebleeding occur, the most important initial step is to control the ICP since it is the sudden explosive rise in ICP that is often so damaging. An immediate twist drill ventriculostomy and the rapid intravenous administration of mannitol (1 gm/kg) may be life-saving. The risk of further hemorrhage is increased after recurrent hemorrhage. A second bleed that occurs during the preoperative period in a patient in less than ideal condition is often considered an indication for immediate surgery.

B. Complications: Vasospasm. Reactive narrowing of the cerebral arterial tree after SAH occurs in approximately 30% of patients. This narrowing, identifiable angiographically, is associated with neurologic deterioration in about half of these patients. Although the angiogram shows narrowing only in the major conducting vessels at the base of the brain and in the sylvian fissure, it is now clear from cerebral blood flow studies that cerebral perfusion is diminished and cerebral autoregulation is often lost, suggesting that the process extends to the resistance vessels as well. Focal and generalized impairment of perfusion results in cerebral ischemia and, if untreated, may progress to infarction.

Attempts at producing vasodilatation have proven ineffective; no reliable technique or pharmacologic agent appears to exist for reversing the narrowing of arteries and arterioles. This failure may be due to the fact that vasospasm may not be simply a spastic contraction or failure of relaxation of the smooth muscle cells in the media of the vessel, but rather a structural alteration in the vessel wall involving all layers. Moreover, attempts to produce cerebral vasodilatation in the presence of a fixed narrowing of the major conduction vessels may have a paradoxical effect, resulting in decreased blood flow to the ischemic areas. The vessels proximal to the ischemic region are narrowed and cannot dilate, whereas the vessels within the ischemic zone may be already maximally dilated owing to accumulation of acid metabolites. Cerebrovasodilator drugs (aminophylline, isoproterenol, nitroprusside) may dilate arteries in normal areas of the brain, reducing local perfusion pressure and shunting blood from ischemic to normal regions: the intracerebral steal effect. Furthermore, most of the attempts to dilate cerebral vessels run the significant risk of dilating extracerebral vessels and thereby further reducing systemic arterial pressure and cerebral perfusion pressure to below critical levels. Calcium channel–blocking drugs are currently being used experimentally to counteract vasospasm.

The regimen that we have found most effective in dealing with neurologic deterioration secondary to vasospasm consists of rapidly expanding the intravascular volume with colloid and crystalloid infusion to a pulmonary capillary wedge pressure of 18 mmHg or a central venous pressure of 12 mmHg. The vasodepressor response is blocked with atropine, and pitressin is administered to diminish renal diuresis. Administration of digoxin may be necessary to ensure an optimum cardiac output. If the patient does not show signs of immediate improvement on this regimen, the systemic arterial pressure is raised in increments of 10 mmHg using dopamine or dobutamine until the neurologic deficits subside or reverse. It has been found that arterial pressure can be sustained at elevated levels for prolonged intervals using this routine.

Expanding the intravascular volume and elevating systemic arterial pressure in states of cerebrovascular insufficiency secondary to vasospasm have proved to be safe and effective providing meticulous attention is paid to the physiologic, biochemical, and hematological parameters. Volume expansion and induced hypertension are, however, clearly a hazardous regimen in the presence of an untreated or unruptured aneurysm. In a series of 36 patients, neurologic deterioration was reversed and permanent improvement achieved in 31. Improvement was only transiently maintained in five patients; in these five, the complications included rebleeding from the aneurysm, pulmonary edema, and myocardial infarction. These results are superior to any other previously attempted form of vasospasm therapy to date.

IV. **Surgery.** Hemorrhage from an intracranial aneurysm is a dramatic and often devastating event. If the patient survives the first hemorrhage, then the aim of treatment is to prevent recurrent hemorrhage. There is little doubt now that recurrent hemorrhage is best controlled by surgical obliteration of the sac.

A. **Timing of surgery**

1. **Advantages of delayed surgery.** Although surgery within 3 days of SAH was advocated by many surgeons in the past, a delay of 7 to 10 days has become common practice in the United States. Postponing surgery must be balanced, however, by the predictable increase in mortality (40%) from patients who rebleed during this period.

It is our practice to delay until the patient is in optimum condition and all evidence of vasospasm has disappeared. Delay in surgical approach often allows symptoms secondary to vasospasm to subside and seems to prevent delayed ischemic complications. In addition to antifibrinolytic agents, more precise control of blood pressure and fluid balance has appreciably diminished the wastage from rebleeding and vasospasm during the delay period while providing the surgeon with optimal conditions under which to dissect, isolate, and clip the aneurysm.

An additional advantage to delaying surgery is the almost universal finding of a slack brain that is easy to manipulate during the exposure of the aneurysm. The dissection of the aneurysmal sac also seems easier and safer after much of the blood in the subarachnoid space has been reabsorbed. The aneurysms are firmer, tougher, and less likely to rupture during dissection. Practical reasons for delay include the opportunity to diagnose or treat coexisting cardiopulmonary disease and the ability to obtain detailed and careful preoperative radiologic studies. It is important to have sufficient flexibility in operating room scheduling to provide the surgeon, the anesthetist, and the operating room team with optimal conditions for what is frequently a demanding technical exercise. Finally, our results of an operative morbidity and mortality of less than 8% in more than 2000 aneurysms of all sizes and grades, including 800 arising from the posterior circulation, compels us to continue with our practice of delay.

2. **Advantages of early surgery.** Nevertheless, in recent years there has been a growing interest once again in early operation. This interest has come as a result of major technical advances in aneurysm surgery including the microscope, removable clips, microinstruments, and developments in neurosurgical anesthesia that now almost guarantee a slack brain and the safe induction of controlled hypotension.

Theoretically, the factors in favor of early surgery are attractive. The most impressive, of course, is the prevention of early rebleeding, which is virtually assured when the neck of the aneurysm is secured. There is also some suggestion that, by operating early and removing blood in the subarachnoid space, the incidence of vasospasm may be reduced. Perhaps a more important consideration is that once the aneurysm is secured, the current treatment of vasospasm (volume expansion and deliberate systemic hypertension to improve cerebral perfusion pressure) can be carried out with relative safety in the knowledge that the aneurysm is clipped and is not likely to rebleed during the manipulations of blood pressure and intravascular volume.

Other factors of possible significance include the reduction of medical complications (e.g., pneumonia, deep vein thrombosis, pulmonary embolus, and fluid and electrolyte abnormalities) as a result of a short stay in bed and a diminished pharmacologic assault. The stress on the patient and family during the tense and anxious period of preoperative delay and the effect of prolonged hospitalization are psychologic and social factors that cannot be ignored.

There have been a few small uncontrolled series from Japan and North America suggesting that early surgery using modern techniques is the optimal method of treatment. These studies, however, lack adequate controls and numbers to be certain of their validity. A larger study from Japan consisting of Grades I and II patients who had surgery within 48 hours of SAH demonstrated a mortality rate of 56.8%, which differs markedly from the more optimistic reports of the smaller series. The controversy regarding early aneurysm surgery is now undergoing evaluation in an international cooperative study from which it is hoped that data will be obtained that will help resolve the difficult issue of timing. As stated, we continue to favor delay, operating on day 10 following SAH, providing spasm has resolved.

B. Operative choices

1. **Clipping.** The best and most effective method of surgical treatment of an aneurysm is complete dissection and clipping of the neck of the sac while sparing the parent vessel and any small perforating arteries or branches in the region. Clipping involves the placement of a removable spring clip across the neck of the aneurysm as close to the feeder artery as possible. If the clip is placed too distally on the neck of the sac, there is a high probability that a new aneurysm will form between the artery and the clip.

   Experience, detailed knowledge of the anatomy of the parent vessel, its branches, and the aneurysm, and familiarity with modern microsurgical techniques are all necessary to make the direct operative attack on an aneurysm feasible and safe. It is our opinion that these lesions are best handled by surgeons who operate on many aneurysms a year.

2. **Trapping.** In cases in which the application of a clip is impossible owing to the size of the neck of the aneurysm, consideration can be given to "trapping." Trapping is accomplished by permanently occluding the vessels proximal and distal to the aneurysm and can only be attempted if there is sufficient collateral flow to the affected area of the brain beyond the occluded vessel. Again, trapping is not an alternative if important branch or perforating vessels arise from the segment to be trapped.

3. **Hunterian proximal ligation.** Occasionally it may be necessary or desirable to ligate the feeder artery to an aneurysm. In some large or otherwise inoperable carotid aneurysms, carotid ligation has been a mainstay of treatment for many years. Reducing the pressure within, or restricting the flow through, the aneurysm decreases the chance of further enlargement and rupture and may induce thrombosis and obliteration of the sac. Such a procedure may be carried out gradually, while the patient is awake, using a graduated screw device such as the Selverstone clamp. Recently this principle of hunterian ligation has also been applied with some success to middle cerebral, posterior cerebral, and anterior communicating aneurysms, as well as to vertebrobasilar aneurysms. With these more distally located aneurysms, the risk of ischemia and infarction in the territory of the occluded vessel may be reduced by preliminary extracranial to intracranial arterial bypass.

4. **Reinforcement.** In aneurysms in which the aforementioned techniques are impossible because of size or location, reinforcement of the aneurysmal wall using gauze, gelfoam, or plastic

materials may be attempted with the hope of preventing progressive enlargement and rupture of the aneurysm. These techniques are necessarily less than perfect, because it is difficult to eradicate the sac completely. Wrapping also does nothing to reduce the bulk of a large or giant aneurysm, which may cause focal deficit by compression.

   5. **Embolization.** Some inoperable ophthalmic artery or cavernous sinus aneurysms can be embolized by introducing balloon catheters or embolic material by way of the feeder artery to promote thrombosis. Thrombotic material such as muscle, horsehair, iron filings, acrylic, and silicone have been introduced at surgery as a last resort. Obliteration as a primary technique uses insertion of iron into the aneurysmal sac by stereotactic methods.

V. **Postoperative care.** Immediate reestablishment of normal blood volume and electrolyte balance is necessary postoperatively to compensate for preoperative fluid restriction, negative nitrogen balance, blood loss, and diuresis during surgery. Normal blood pressure, temperature, and cardiopulmonary status should be maintained. Elastic stockings used intraoperatively and postoperatively improve venous circulation and may reduce the incidence of pulmonary embolism. A postoperative angiogram is performed to evaluate the success of the operation. Phenytoin should be continued for three months postoperatively. Corticosteroids are given immediately preoperatively and tapered in the week after the operation. Prophylactic antibiotics are not used.

VI. **Operative results.** Based on these methods for diagnosing and treating patients who have suffered a ruptured intracranial aneurysm, the operative mortality and morbidity in Grades I and II patients should be less than 5% in the hands of an experienced surgeon.

   Treatment of unruptured aneurysms that do not act as mass lesions results in low morbidity and mortality, often reported to be under 1%. As aneurysms increase in size, both mortality and major morbidity increase proportionately.

Anesthesia
Peter S. Colley

I. **Basic considerations.** The major concern in the anesthetic management of patients undergoing craniotomy for surgical treatment of a cerebral aneurysm is the potential for intraoperative rupture of the aneurysm, either during induction of anesthesia or during the surgical procedure itself. Anesthetic management of patients who have cerebral aneurysms is made even more hazardous if cerebral vasospasm, raised intracranial pressure (ICP), or both are present. These complications limit the safety of all anesthetic techniques designed to lessen the risk of aneurysm rupture by lowering the systemic blood pressure.

A. Intraoperative aneurysm rupture

1. Aneurysm rupture **during induction** of anesthesia has been reported to occur in less than 1% (Sundt, 1982) to 4% (Nornes, 1979) of patients undergoing cerebral aneurysm surgery; the mortality is up to 50% (Sundt, 1982). When the skull is intact, aneurysmal rupture causes a marked increase in ICP and a decrease in cerebral perfusion pressure (CPP).

2. Incidence of aneurysm rupture **during surgery** ranges from 5% (Dahlgren, 1970) to 19% (Krayenbühl, 1972), although rates as high as 65% (Pertuiset, 1974) have occasionally been reported. Increased morbidity and mortality in these patients result from greater retraction pressure, surgical trauma that results from attempts to operate in a restricted and obscured surgical field, and permanent or temporary occlusion of major cerebral vessels to control hemorrhage. Rarely, the ruptured aneurysm may be so difficult to locate that control becomes impossible and the patient exsanguinates. Rupture may occur

   a. During dissection of the aneurysm

   b. As the clip is placed around the neck of the aneurysm

   c. During removal of the clip holder from the aneurysm clip

   d. Less commonly, when the dura is incised and ICP decreases to atmospheric levels

   e. When excessive brain retraction causes reflex systemic hypertension

3. The main goal during induction and maintenance of anesthesia is to **avoid increasing transmural pressure** in the aneurysm. Transmural pressure is defined as the difference between the mean arterial pressure (MAP) and the ICP (Fig. 8-2). The relationship between the transmural pressure and wall stress or tension of the aneurysm is linear (Ferguson, 1972) (Fig. 8-3). Either an increase in the MAP (e.g., by light anesthesia) or a fall in the ICP (e.g., by ventricular drainage or hyperventilation) will increase the transmural pressure, the wall stress, and the risk of aneurysm rupture.

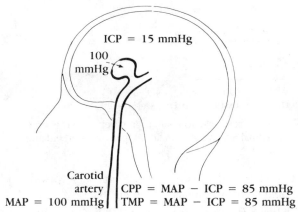

Fig. 8-2. The transmural pressure (TMP) of the aneurysm. TMP is the same as the cerebral perfusion pressure (CPP) and is equal to the difference between mean arterial pressure (MAP) and intracranial pressure (ICP). (Redrawn from Ferguson, 1972.)

4. **MAP should be maintained.** The CPP also equals the difference between MAP and ICP. If, while attempting to maintain a low aneurysm transmural pressure, the anesthesiologist allows the CPP to fall below the lower limit of autoregulation (i.e., 50 mmHg in the normal brain), a reduction in cerebral blood flow (CBF) will occur (Fig. 8-4). Prolonged reductions in CBF to less than 50% of normal will lead to EEG evidence of cerebral malfunction (Trojaborg, 1973). MAP, therefore, needs to be maintained within the range of 50 to 90 mmHg. The presence of cerebral vasospasm and raised ICP further narrows this range of "safe" blood pressure.

B. **Cerebral vasospasm.** After subarachnoid hemorrhage (SAH), a significant number of patients develop vasospasm, which decreases cerebral blood flow and impairs cerebral autoregulation (Farrar, 1981). CBF thus tends to follow changes in systemic blood pressure

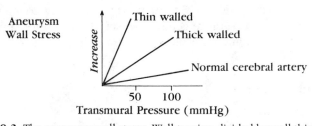

Fig. 8-3. The aneurysm wall stress. Wall tension divided by wall thickness equals aneurysm wall stress. The relationship between transmural pressure (TMP) and wall stress is linear: the thinner the wall, the greater the wall stress at any given pressure. (Redrawn from Ferguson, 1972.)

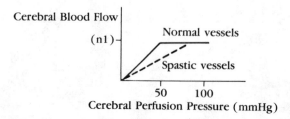

Fig. 8-4. Cerebral blood flow (CBF) response to changes in cerebral perfusion pressure (CPP) in the presence of normal autoregulation and impaired autoregulation due to cerebral vasospasm.

passively, increasing the risk of cerebral ischemia after episodes of inadvertent or deliberate hypotension (see Fig. 8-4).

When anesthetizing patients who have cerebral vasospasm, it is important to maximize oxygen delivery to the brain by maintaining blood volume, blood oxygenation, and blood pressure (keeping CPP at higher levels than would be necessary in the absence of cerebral vasospasm). Intraoperative hypotension is avoided whenever possible. The anesthesiologist may also reduce cerebral oxygen requirements by the liberal use of barbiturates and low-grade hypothermia.

C. **Increased intracranial pressure.** Most patients coming to surgery for clip ligation of a cerebral aneurysm will have normal ICP but may have decreased intracranial compliance. Patients who have depressed levels of consciousness may have raised ICP owing to the presence of cerebral vasodilatation, cerebral edema, hematoma, or hydrocephalus. About 5% of patients who have a ruptured cerebral aneurysm will have severe intracranial hypertension and will require emergency operation for evacuation of an intracranial hematoma (Skultety, 1966).

In patients who have intracranial hypertension, it is preferable to avoid inhalation anesthetics until after craniotomy because their vasodilating properties increase the potential for further elevation of ICP. If inhalation agents are required to control systemic blood pressure, moderate hyperventilation should precede their introduction, lowering the $PaCO_2$ to 25 to 30 mmHg, and thereby counteracting their tendency to dilate cerebral vessels. Hypertension, hypercapnia, and coughing are avoided to prevent further increases in ICP.

II. Preoperative evaluation

A. General status

1. A brief neurologic examination should be performed and the patient's **clinical grade** noted. The clinical grade is determined

according to the system of Hunt (1968) or Botterell (1956). Higher grades (clinically more impaired) tend to be associated with the presence of cerebral vasospasm, increased ICP, and increased surgical mortality. Approximately 55% of patients present in Hunt's Grades I and II, 30% in Grade III, 10% in Grade IV, and 5% in Grade V (see Table 8-1).

2. Any association between a **decrease in blood pressure** and the appearance of **neurologic deterioration** or deficit should be noted. Occasionally a critical level of blood pressure below which neurologic deficits occur may be observed. Blood pressures below this level should be avoided intraoperatively. Previous blood pressure measurements should be reviewed and the preoperative blood pressure determined in both arms to establish a normal value for the patient.

3. Fluid restriction, diuretics, and steroids used in the preoperative management of subarachnoid hemorrhage and intracranial hypertension may cause **dehydration** and **electrolyte abnormalities.** Hyponatremia and hypokalemia occur occasionally and may require correction before surgery.

4. A 1 to 2°C **increase in body temperature** is frequently present in patients who have ruptured aneurysms. This increase is possibly a reaction to blood in the subarachnoid space and should be treated before surgery because an elevated temperature causes an increase in cerebral oxygen requirement.

5. The anesthesiologist should **evaluate** the patient's **CT scan** for the presence of cerebral edema, midline shift, ventricular distortion, hydrocephalus, and hematoma to assess the presence and severity of intracranial hypertension.

6. Note the **location** of the aneurysm; this will determine the surgical approach and the patient's position intraoperatively (see section **III.C**).

B. **Electrocardiographic abnormalities.** Electrocardiographic (ECG) abnormalities occur preoperatively in 60% of patients who have SAH (Galloon, 1972). The ECG alterations are most likely due to increased vagal and sympathetic neural output secondary to SAH. The changes consist most frequently of T wave inversion or flattening, S–T segment depression or elevation, U waves, and Q–T interval prolongation. Arrhythmias are also common and usually appear within 48 hours of SAH. Sinus bradycardia is present in 66% of patients, and premature ventricular contractions or episodes of ventricular tachycardia appear in 20% of patients (Vidal, 1979). The

majority of ECGs return to normal within 10 days of the hemorrhage.

Unless the patient has a history of ischemic heart disease, the ECG
abnormalities are not necessarily indicative of myocardial damage
or a contraindication to either surgery or the use of controlled
hypotension (Galloon, 1972). In several studies, postmortem examination of hearts in patients who had ECG abnormalities has revealed little evidence of significant coronary artery or myocardial
disease (Galloon, 1972; Srivastava, 1964). Other studies, however,
have reported histologic evidence of focal myocardial necrosis
(Doshi, 1977). A cardiac consultation and determination of serum
myoglobin and CPK isoenzymes (Rudehill, 1982) may be necessary
to evaluate these patients.

C. **Informed consent.** Some patients can tolerate a fuller explanation of the risks involved in this operation than can others. A di-
lemma exists, however, because the physician wishes to avoid causing the patient anxiety and associated increases in blood pressure,
but also wishes to comply with laws that protect the patient's right to
be informed of the anesthetic risks. It is known that rupture of the
aneurysm often occurs during periods of emotional stress. On this
basis, we recommend that information, including discussion of
risks, such as the risks of rupture during induction and intubation
and of controlled hypotension, that may lead to increased anxiety
should not be volunteered to patients who have a history of rupture
of a cerebral aneurysm. The family is apprised of all risks and
procedures.

Patients are generally less anxious if informed of what to expect
on the day of operation. The anesthesiologist should give a brief
explanation of the anesthetic procedure, the expected duration of
operation, and the nature of the anesthetic recovery period.

In all cases, the anesthesiologist should explain the procedures
and risks thoroughly to the next-of-kin in a tactful manner. The
risks, including rupture of the aneurysm from intraoperative hypertension and brain damage from induced or unintentional hypotension, are discussed. Documentation of discussions with the patient
and relatives is entered in the patient's record.

D. **Premedication.** Patients in (Hunt) Grades I and II who appear
well tranquilized require little additional preoperative sedation. If
tranquilization is less than adequate, an increase in the dose of
drugs already in use can be ordered for the 24 hours before
surgery. Diazepam, 10 to 15 mg given orally 45 to 60 minutes preoperatively, will usually provide satisfactory sedation. Excessive sedation and narcotics such as morphine and meperidine are best withheld to prevent respiratory depression and masking of signs of

recurrent aneurysmal hemorrhage. Patients who have a decreased level of consciousness (Hunt Grades III–V) do not require preoperative sedation.

III. Anesthetic management

A. Preinduction procedures and monitoring

1. Prepare a tuberculin syringe containing **sodium nitroprusside,** 100 μg, for use during any hypertensive episodes. Apply **20% benzocaine** (Hurricaine) for topical anesthesia of the oropharynx and coat the oral airway with lidocaine ointment.

2. Place the patient in a 10- to 15-degree head-up position to reduce intracranial pressure and minimize venous bleeding.

3. Insert a large-bore (14–16 gauge) intravenous cannula in a peripheral vein for infusion of **Ringer's lactate solution.** The intravenous catheter should be equipped with a sidearm attachment that has minimal deadspace if infusion of a hypotensive drug is planned. Once an intravenous cannula is inserted, the anesthesiologist can increase sedation (i.e., intravenous diazepam in 2.5- to 5-mg increments) if the patient appears anxious. Start a second large intravenous catheter in the opposite arm after the patient is anesthetized. The presence of two intravenous catheters allows simultaneous administration of a hypotensive drug and blood in the event of intraoperative rupture of the aneurysm.

4. Make available at least 4 units of **compatible whole blood** before induction of anesthesia.

5. **Parameters monitored** during induction and maintenance of anesthesia include the following:

   a. **Cardiac rate and rhythm.** Use an ECG with a V_5 lead.

   b. **Level of neuromuscular blockade.** Use a peripheral nerve stimulator.

   c. **Arterial pressure and arterial blood gases.** Insert a 20-gauge cannula in the radial artery under local anesthesia before induction. Keep the arterial transducer at the level of the head for accurate measurement of CPP.

   d. **Central venous pressure (CVP).** Insert the central venous catheter after the patient is anesthetized via a peripheral arm vein (Cucchiara, 1980). CVP is an especially useful parameter in the event of intraoperative rupture of the aneurysm as it serves as an index of blood volume to monitor fluid replacement.

e. **End-tidal CO_2.** Monitor during both induction and maintenance of anesthesia to assure adequacy of ventilation. End-tidal CO_2 is typically 0 to 5 mmHg lower than $PaCO_2$ because of ventilation-perfusion mismatching.

f. **Heart and lung sounds, body temperature.** Place an esophageal stethoscope and temperature probe in the lower third of the esophagus after induction.

g. **Ventricular CSF pressure** (if available). These measurements are needed to diagnose and treat raised ICP.

h. **Urinary output.** Insert a urinary catheter after induction.

6. **Monitoring brain functions** during cerebral aneurysm surgery is a desirable but elusive goal. EEG techniques are limited because of the distance from scalp electrodes to surgical site (Jones, 1979). Evoked potential monitoring, however, offers promise for the future (Symon, 1979).

B. **Induction technique.** To avoid a hypertensive response, it is most important that the patient be smoothly and deeply anesthetized before laryngoscopy and intubation. We recommend thiopental and fentanyl as the primary induction drugs because thiopental rapidly produces unconsciousness. In patients who have normal or moderately elevated ICP (up to 30 mmHg), thiopental reduces the transmural pressure in the aneurysm by decreasing systemic blood pressure more than it decreases ICP (Shapiro, 1973). Fentanyl provides profound analgesia, blunting the blood pressure response to laryngoscopy and intubation (Kautto, 1982) but has relatively little effect on intracranial and mean arterial pressure in the presence of controlled ventilation and normal blood volume. The following sequence has proved to be a satisfactory technique:

1. Initially give the patient **100% oxygen** through a face mask held off to the side of the patient's face to avoid producing anxiety.

2. Administer **thiopental,** 3 to 5 mg/kg, and **fentanyl,** 50 to 100 μg, intravenously over 1 to 2 minutes to induce anesthesia. As soon as the eyelash reflex disappears, apply the mask to the face and control ventilation manually to keep the end-tidal CO_2 at approximately 30 mmHg. An oral pharyngeal airway is inserted if needed to maintain ventilation.

3. **Metocurine** (formerly called dimethyl tubocurarine), 0.3 to 0.4 mg/kg, is given intravenously. Metocurine is a good choice to produce muscle relaxation for intubation, since it appears to have the least effect on blood pressure (Savarese, 1977). Alternatively, pancuronium, 0.1 mg/kg, may be used, although pancuronium occasionally causes an increase in heart rate and blood pressure (Lebowitz, 1981). Among the choices not recommended are *d*-tubocurarine in intubating doses (0.5–0.6 mg/ kg), which may cause unpredictable and profound decreases in blood pressure, and succinylcholine, which may lead to sympathetic stimulation and hypertension and has also been reported to cause hyperkalemia in patients who have cerebral aneurysms (Iwatsuki, 1980).

4. Once ventilation is easily controlled, the inhaled gas mixture may be changed from 100% oxygen to **nitrous oxide** (N_2O) in oxygen (50:50). If the patient does not have evidence of increased ICP, add a low concentration of enflurane or isoflurane (0.5%–1.0%). For patients who have preoperative evidence of increased ICP or who develop increased ICP with induction, it is prudent to avoid using N_2O and the inhalation anesthetics during induction because these drugs may cause further increases in ICP.

5. To deepen the level of anesthesia, **fentanyl,** in 25- to 50-μg increments, is administered as the anesthesiologist monitors the fading muscle twitch. A total dose of up to 500 μg (7–10 μg/kg) or more may be used, depending on the response of the blood pressure.

6. The peripheral muscle twitch will usually disappear in about 4 minutes after injection of metocurine or pancuronium. Then give **lidocaine,** 1.5 mg/kg, intravenously in addition to **thiopental,** 100- to 200-mg.

7. Ninety seconds after administration of lidocaine and thiopental, perform **endotracheal intubation** under direct vision as gently and as expeditiously as possible. Use of a stylet is suggested to reduce the time required for intubation and hence the noxious stimulation of laryngoscopy. Fasten the endotracheal tube securely to the patient's face using tincture of benzoin and adhesive tape.

8. Insert the **esophageal stethoscope** and temperature probe so that the probe will be at the lower third of the esophagus. **Inspect the pupils** for symmetry and carefully cover the eyes.

9. Insert a **urinary catheter** and make sure the legs are wrapped from toes to groin to facilitate venous return and to prevent postoperative venous thrombosis.

C. **Positioning.** The patient is placed in one of the following positions, depending on the site of the aneurysm (Yasargil, 1975):

1. Aneurysms arising from the **anterior part of the circle of Willis:** supine position for a frontotemporal approach.

2. Aneurysms arising from the **posterior aspect of the basilic artery:** lateral position for a temporal approach.

3. Aneurysms arising from the **vertebral artery or from the lower basilic artery:** sitting or prone position for a suboccipital approach.

4. Aneurysms arising from the **anterior communicating artery** are frequently approached from the right. Aneurysms arising from the **middle cerebral and posterior communicating arteries** are approached from the side where the aneurysm is located.

D. **Maintenance of anesthesia**

1. **Control ventilation mechanically,** and adjust it to maintain an appropriate $PaCO_2$. If ICP is normal, maintain $PaCO_2$ at 35 mmHg. This relatively normal $PaCO_2$ is selected to help maintain CBF in the presence of both cerebral vasospasm and controlled hypotension. If intracranial hypertension (above 20 mmHg) is present, the anesthesiologist should lower the $PaCO_2$ to 25 to 30 mmHg by increasing ventilation, thereby reducing ICP. Arterial blood gases and pH should be measured after a stable level of ventilation has been achieved. They are repeated at hourly intervals during the procedure.

2. **Begin surface cooling** shortly after induction if moderate hypothermia is planned (see section **IV.C**).

3. **Inject bupivacaine** 0.25% (without epinephrine) subcutaneously and widely along the line of the planned incision to provide excellent prolonged local anesthesia and prevent blood pressure elevations during the early part of the procedure.

4. **Establish a deep plane of anesthesia** before the surgeon makes the scalp incision and turns the bone and dural flaps to avoid a hypertensive response. Depth of anesthesia can be increased by using additional doses of fentanyl, 25 to 50 μg, combined with isoflurane or enflurane, 0.5% to 1.5%. Isoflurane is preferable to

enflurane or halothane because it has a smaller effect on cerebral blood volume than does enflurane. It markedly decreases the cerebral metabolic rate for oxygen and confers some degree of cerebral protection (Newberg, 1982). Isoflurane's low blood-gas solubility also permits rapid elimination at the end of the surgical procedure. Isoflurane maintains cardiac output and systemic blood pressure and, unlike enflurane, does not produce spike or seizure patterns on the EEG with increasing concentration. Thiopental infusion (1–3 mg/kg/hr), in place of the volatile agents, is a technique that is also gaining popularity.

If marked intracranial hypertension is present, increase the depth of anesthesia solely by giving additional increments of fentanyl until the skull is opened. Maintain the nitrous oxide-oxygen concentration at 60:40 if isoflurane or enflurane is used and at 70:30 if only fentanyl is used, unless full hemoglobin saturation ($PaO_2 > 150$ mmHg) requires a higher concentration of oxygen.

5. **Mannitol** (1.0–1.5 gm/kg over 10–15 min) may be required to decrease the volume of the brain before the dura is opened. Do not give mannitol, however, until after the bone flap is turned to prevent premature shrinkage of the brain and tearing of the bridging veins. Mannitol begins to lower ICP within 4 to 5 minutes of infusion and produces a peak reduction in ICP in about 45 minutes (range 20–120 min). It may transiently increase blood volume and blood pressure; if so, the depth of anesthesia should be increased.

6. **Maintain anesthesia** with enflurane or isoflurane (0.5%– 1.5%) and nitrous oxide-oxygen after the dura is opened and the degree of noxious stimulation decreases and ICP falls to atmospheric levels. An occasional 25- to 50-μg increment of fentanyl may be required to adjust the depth of anesthesia. The total dose of fentanyl should be limited to less than 500 to 750 μg (10–12 μg/kg) to minimize the incidence of postoperative respiratory depression unless postoperative controlled ventilation is planned (i.e., in Grades III–IV patients).

7. **Begin infusion of the hypotensive agent** as the surgeon starts the aneurysm dissection if controlled hypotension is planned (see section **IV.B**).

8. **A unit of whole blood should be immediately available** at the beginning of the dissection of the aneurysm for infusion in case of sudden rupture of the aneurysm.

E. Intraoperative fluid management

1. **Intravenous fluid therapy.** Ringer's lactate solution is infused throughout the procedure at a rate of 3 to 4 ml/kg/hr to meet maintenance requirements and to replace fluid losses from overnight fasting and urine production. If mannitol is used to promote diuresis, only replace half the urine volume produced during the period of diuresis with additonal Ringer's lactate solution, to avoid overexpanding the intravascular volume with salt solutions. Unlike intra-abdominal or intrathoracic surgery, intracranial surgery does not entail significant third-space loss of fluid. Infusion of a large volume of salt solution is thus not needed. Although salt permeates the normal blood-brain barrier poorly, salt solutions may still cause an increase in cerebral edema if either intracerebral hemorrhage or ischemia has induced an increase in blood-brain permeability.

2. **Volume loading.** In recent years there has been a trend toward more liberal administration of blood and crystalloid solution intraoperatively in patients undergoing surgery for cerebral aneurysms. This practice evolved from the observation that expansion of blood volume frequently improved cerebral perfusion and reversed neurologic deficits in patients who had vasospasm (Pritz, 1978). The technique of volume loading with whole blood, plasma, or both received further support from the observation that patients who had cerebral aneurysms had a blood volume that was approximately 17% below normal values in the preoperative period (Maroon, 1979). We think this decrease in blood volume is due to a combination of supine diuresis, bed rest, decreased erythropoiesis, and negative nitrogen balance. Since craniotomy usually involves a blood loss of 250 to 500 ml, this additional loss, if uncorrected, would result in a 20% to 30% decrease in blood volume.

   On the basis of these observations, at least one unit of blood may be infused immediately after the aneurysm is clipped. A second unit of blood, additonal Ringer's lactate solution, or both can be administered if blood loss is greater than 500 ml to maintain the central venous pressure above 5 cmH$_2$O and a hematocrit of 30% to 35%.

F. Termination of anesthesia

1. For patients in Grades I and II who have **no intraoperative complications,** the endotracheal tube may be removed in the operating room. The primary goals at the end of surgery are to avoid coughing, straining, hypercapnia, and hypertension, which may occur during placement of the head dressing when head

movement causes movement of the endotracheal tube within the trachea and during extubation. These problems may be avoided by maintaining a deep level of anesthesia during placement of the head dressing and tracheal extubation. Before extubation and while still controlling ventilation, give neostigmine, 2.5 mg, and atropine, 1.2 mg, intravenously to reverse residual muscle relaxation. After return of the muscle twitch to normal (normal train-of-four and lack of fade on tetanic stimulation), suction the oropharynx to remove secretions. Give lidocaine, 1.5 mg/kg, intravenously; 90 seconds later extubate the trachea. The use of lidocaine in this manner has been shown to reduce hemodynamic responses to extubation.

After extubation, continue controlled ventilation with 100% oxygen by mask for several minutes to eliminate inhalation anesthetics and their respiratory depressant and cerebral vasodilator effects. Gradually decrease ventilation to allow $PaCO_2$ to rise until it stimulates spontaneous ventilation. A delay in the onset of spontaneous ventilation is usually due to the residual depressant effect of fentanyl. This may be reversed with naloxone, 1 µg/kg intravenously, repeated once if necessary. Avoid larger doses of naloxone because they cause sudden, violent awakening of the patient and marked increases in systemic blood pressure, which is especially hazardous in the patient who has multiple aneurysms.

2. Patients who have **intraoperative complications** such as occlusion of a major vessel, severe blood loss, or excessive surgical trauma and patients in Grades III to IV who have depression of consciousness preoperatively retain their endotracheal tubes and have postoperative mechanical ventilation. Tracheal extubation may be accomplished later when the patient's neurologic status is stable and an unobstructed airway and adequate ventilation can be assured.

IV. Special techniques

A. **Spinal drainage.** The purpose of spinal drainage is to produce a slack, easily retractable brain and to improve access to aneurysms situated at the base of the brain. This procedure, however, is not used by all neurosurgeons. If spinal drainage is planned, place the patient in the lateral position and insert either a subarachnoid catheter or malleable spinal needle through the lumbar 3–4 or 4–5 interspace. For a subarachnoid catheter, insert a 3½-inch 18-gauge thinwall Becton-Dickinson (BD) needle with a Crawford point using a paramedian approach, and advance a Racz epidural catheter no more than 2 cm beyond the needle tip. The Racz catheter has advantages in that supports do not need to be placed under the back and the catheter is unlikely to become obstructed or kink. Manual or mechanical withdrawal of CSF may be necessary, however, and pressure monitoring may be inaccurate because of the small lumen.

If spinal needles are used, place two malleable needles (18-gauge, 5-inch) instead of one because if one needle becomes occluded, the remaining needle may be used. An attempt should be made to avoid excessive loss of CSF when the spinal needles are first placed. Such losses decrease the ICP (increase the aneurysm transmural pressure) and promote further hemorrhage.

When the needles are placed, attach the catheters, bend the needles parallel with the back, and tape them in place. Position rolls under the back to prevent the needles from touching the table. Initially, one of the catheters attached to the needles can be attached to a venous transducer to monitor the lumbar CSF pressure. A normal or moderately elevated lumbar CSF pressure (i.e., 15–30 mmHg) provides some assurance that the aneurysm has not ruptured during induction or the initial period of surgery and provides an assessment of cerebral perfusion pressure (MAP − CSF pressure). Lumbar CSF pressure measurements are also useful in monitoring effects of the various anesthetic drugs and the level of ventilation.

Initiate spinal drainage only after the dura has been opened to prevent the development of pressure gradients across the brain that could lead to tonsillar herniation. To achieve drainage, allow CSF to flow passively through the needle-catheter system into a volume-calibrated container (i.e., Buretrol); control the rate with an adjustable clamp. Active aspiration using a syringe or mechanical pump will likely be necessary for drainage through a subarachnoid catheter. CSF should be removed at a rate no greater than 5 ml/min (approximately 1 drop/sec) to prevent reflex increases in systemic blood pressure (Barker, 1975) (Fig. 8-5). Withdraw 50 to 150 ml of

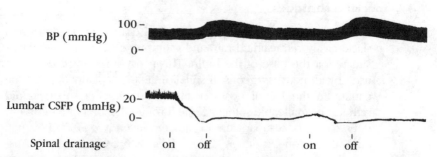

Fig. 8-5. Systemic blood pressure (BP) response to excessively rapid spinal fluid drainage. CSFP = cerebrospinal fluid pressure.

CSF as required for adequate surgical exposure. Spinal drainage is stopped when dural closure begins.

B. Controlled hypotension

1. General considerations. Although good operative results have been reported when controlled hypotension was not used, controlled hypotension has become an integral part of aneurysm surgery in many institutions. In considering the use of controlled hypotension, one should keep in mind that the blood pressure level below which CBF begins to decrease (i.e., the lower limit of cerebral autoregulation) is elevated in the more clinically ill patients (i.e., the higher clinical grades) and patients who have hypertension (Nornes, 1977).

a. Advantages of controlled hypotension

(1) The aneurysm becomes more **mobile,** facilitating dissection and placement of clips.

(2) If the aneurysm ruptures, the **slow rate of blood loss** facilitates control of bleeding.

(3) The incidence of premature rupture is "possibly" decreased by **reducing the transmural pressure.** ("Possibly" because no published studies have demonstrated a reduced incidence of intraoperative rupture with the use of hypotension.)

b. Choice of hypotensive drug

(1) Nitroprusside, a direct-acting vasodilator, has generally replaced trimethaphan and deep halothane anesthesia, and is the authors' recommended agent to produce controlled hypotension during aneurysm surgery. Whether CBF is more effectively maintained during nitroprusside-induced hypotension is controversial (Grubb, 1982; Brown, 1978; Stoyka, 1975). There is no question, however, that nitroprusside is easier to control in that it has a more rapid onset and briefer duration of action than any other currently used hypotensive agent.

Nitroprusside releases cyanide, which is normally converted to thiocyanate in the presence of endogenous thiosulfate and hepatic rhodanase. Excessive infusion of nitroprusside may overwhelm this metabolic pathway, resulting in increased blood levels of cyanide. Cyanide combines with cytochrome oxidase, which inhibits cellular uptake of oxygen. To avoid cyanide toxicity, it is recommended that infusion rates not exceed 10 μg/kg/min and that the total dose of nitroprusside not exceed 1 mg/kg.*

(2) Nitroglycerin, also a direct-acting vasodilator, would appear to have some advantages over nitroprusside. The use of nitroglycerin is associated with a lower incidence of ECG changes characteristic of myocardial ischemia than is nitroprusside (Fahmy, 1978). Nitroglycerin is essentially nontoxic and is metabolized to glyceryl dinitrate and nitrite in the presence of glutathione. Large doses (greater than 1 gm) may cause small increases in methemoglobin. However, nitroglycerin has not replaced nitroprusside because of its somewhat slower onset of action and the belief that more patients are resistant to its hypotensive effect. The drug is adsorbed on many plastics including polyvinylchloride (PVC) and should be infused using glass bottles and polyethylene tubing.

(3) Trimethaphan, in clinical use as a hypotensive drug for the past 30 years, produces hypotension primarily by ganglionic blockage, although release of histamine and direct relaxation of vascular smooth muscle may also contribute to its hypotensive effect. Its primary advantages, compared to nitroprusside and nitroglycerin, are that fewer patients (especially young adults) are resistant to its hypotensive effect. Since it is not a cerebral vasodilator, trimethaphan produces negligible changes in ICP, which may be an important consideration in the hypertensive patient before craniotomy. It is used less frequently, however, because of its relatively slow onset of action, because it may cause unreactive, dilated pupils for a variable duration postoperatively, interfering with the neurologic evaluation, and because of evidence of cerebral toxicity when MAP levels are less than 50 mmHg. Trimethaphan undergoes enzymatic hydrolysis in blood and is partly excreted unchanged by the kidney. The drug may prolong the action of succinylcholine by inhibition of plasma pseudocholinesterase (Sklar, 1977).

c. Contraindications to controlled hypotension

(1) Vascular disease of brain, heart, or kidney

---

*Treatment of cyanide toxicity includes discontinuation of nitroprusside and administration of sodium thiosulfate, 150 mg/kg IV in 5 min, and sodium nitrite, 5 mg/kg IV slowly.

Table 8-3. Hypotensive drugs

	Nitroprusside	Trimethaphan	Nitroglycerin
Preparation	0.01% 50 mg/500 ml D_5W	0.2% 500 mg/250 ml D_5W	0.04%–0.1% 0.4–1 mg/ml
Concentration	100 μg/ml	2000 μg/ml	400–1000 μg/ml
Initial dose (μg/kg/min)	0.2–0.5	20–50	0.2–0.5
Maintenance (μg/kg/min)	1–3	20–200	5–7
Maximum dose (μg/kg/min)	8–10 or 1 mg/kg total	Unknown	Unknown
Side effects	↑ ICP ↓ PaO_2 Cyanide toxicity	Histamine release Dilated pupils Cerebral toxicity (MAP < 50 mmHg)	↑ ICP ↓ PaO_2

      (2) Hypovolemia or anemia

      (3) Narrow angle glaucoma (trimethaphan)

      (4) Leber's optic atrophy*

      (5) Tobacco amblyopia*

      (6) Vitamin B_{12} deficiency*

   d. Relative contraindications to controlled hypotension

      (1) Elderly patient

      (2) Chronic hypertension

      (3) Elevated temperature

      (4) Sitting position

   e. Doses and characteristics of these hypotensive drugs appear in Table 8-3.

2. Clinical considerations

   a. Discuss the need for and timing of hypotension with the neurosurgeon before starting the procedure.

   b. Use continuous intra-arterial monitoring and oscilloscopic display of blood pressure to increase the safety of controlled hypotension.

---

*Nitroprusside is contraindicated because of impaired ability to metabolize cyanide.

c. Use a volumetric infusion pump for improved control of the rate of infusion.

d. Calculate the initial dose and set the rate of infusion before hypotension is to be started.

e. Use lower initial doses for older patients.

f. Maintain a continuous infusion of Ringer's lactate solution through the intravenous catheter to prevent pooling of the hypotensive agent.

g. Although a controversial issue, it is probably best to maintain $PaCO_2$ at levels of more than 25 mmHg to avoid causing brain ischemia during simultaneous hypocapnia and hypotension (Sullivan, 1980; Levin, 1980).

3. **Management of controlled hypotension**

   a. When the neurosurgeon is approaching the aneurysm and hypotension is needed, infuse nitroprusside at an initial rate of 0.2 µg/kg/min. Adjust the rate to reduce MAP to 50 mmHg in Grade I patients (i.e., normotensive patients who do not have evidence of cerebral vasospasm). In hypertensive patients, decrease MAP by only 30% of the preoperative value. Treat any inadvertent reduction in blood pressure to less than 50 mmHg by decreasing the infusion rate, by briefly terminating the infusion, or by administering intravenous fluid. If the blood pressure decreases to less than 30 mmHg, give ephedrine in 5-mg increments to raise the blood pressure to desired levels. An infusion of phenylephrine may be used to counteract drug-induced hypotension but, in the author's experience, this is more likely than ephedrine to produce inadvertent hypertension.

   b. Compensatory tachycardia occurring during controlled hypotension can be treated with intravenous propranolol in 0.2-mg increments up to 5.0 mg. Propranolol is contraindicated in patients who have bronchial asthma. Practolol may likewise cause bronchoconstriction but to a lesser extent.

   c. Determine arterial blood gases as soon as hypotension is established. Both nitroprusside and nitroglycerin may decrease PaO_2 by inhibiting hypoxic pulmonary vasoconstriction and increasing blood flow to poorly ventilated or atelectatic areas of the lung (Colley, 1979; Colley, 1981). An early sign of nitroprusside-induced cyanide toxicity is the appearance of metabolic acidosis. $PaCO_2$ should be maintained at levels of more than 25 mmHg.

d. Maintain hypotension until after the aneurysm is clipped. Then gradually decrease the infusion rate to avoid rebound hypertension, which, if excessive, may increase cerebral edema and interfere with hemostasis. Return blood pressure to normotensive levels before closure of the dura so the surgeon may detect and coagulate any bleeding sites and make any necessary adjustment in the position of the aneurysm clip.

C. Surgical hypothermia

1. **Moderate hypothermia.** Hypothermia reduces the cerebral metabolic requirements for oxygen ($CMRO_2$) by 5% for each degree centigrade decrease in temperature. Moderate hypothermia (i.e., 32°C) is often used during aneurysm surgery in the belief that it will decrease the risk of controlled or inadvertent hypotension and of unanticipated occlusion of a major vessel. Hypothermia in this temperature range decreases $CMRO_2$ by 25% and is not associated with cardiac arrythmias or other complications. Recently, however, the ability of low-grade hypothermia (32°C) to provide cerebral protection during hypotension has been shown to be absent in animals (Keykhah, 1982). The risks of this procedure appear negligible, however, so that hypothermia remains an adjunct to aneurysm surgery in some centers.

2. **Management.** After induction of anesthesia, circulate water at a temperature of 4°C through a thermal blanket placed above and beneath the patient until the body temperature begins to fall. Stop cooling as soon as esophageal temperature reaches 33°C; then set the water temperature control to 35° to 40°C. The body temperature will drift downward to 31° to 32°C by the time the aneurysm is clipped. Do not remove the endotracheal tube until the body temperature is 35°C or higher. An in-circuit heated humidifier for inspired gases accelerates rewarming.

3. **Deep hypothermia.** More profound levels of hypothermia were used in the late 1950s during operation for cerebral aneurysms in an attempt to provide cerebral protection and reduce the extremely high mortality rates at a time when surgical treatment frequently involved occlusion of major cerebral vessels. The risks of interference with blood clotting mechanisms, increase in operation time, possible increase in the incidence of postoperative vasospasm, cardiac arrhythmias (i.e., ventricular fibrillation), as well as the failure of published reports to show improved results, have gradually led to an avoidance of pro-

found hypothermia in many institutions. The few exceptions have been for treatment of various aneurysms that, by their location or size, are inaccessible by the usual surgical approaches and techniques and require major interruption of CBF. These aneurysms include certain giant aneurysms and aneurysms of the posterior circulation in which cardiac arrest and extracorporeal circulation are required. The development of vascular bypass techniques (i.e., superficial temporal artery to middle cerebral artery anastomosis) has further decreased the need for hypothermia in such situations.

V. Aneurysm rupture

A. Rupture during induction. An abrupt increase in blood pressure during or after induction of anesthesia may be either the result or the cause of aneurysm rupture. Increases in systemic blood pressure may be treated by administering a bolus of thiopental, 100 to 200 mg, and sodium nitroprusside, 0.5 to 1.0 μg/kg, intravenously to decrease the aneurysm transmural pressure. Marked hypotension is detrimental, however, because a decrease in systemic blood pressure coupled with an increase in ICP may severely impair CPP and reduce CBF.

B. Intraoperative aneurysm rupture

1. **Surgical attempts** to control hemorrhage from an aneurysm that has ruptured intraoperatively consist initially of placing the tip of the suction catheter over the bleeding site and, if possible, clipping the base of the aneurysm. If this is not possible, control of bleeding is achieved by placing temporary clips on the major cerebral artery proximal to the aneurysm. Some hemorrhage conditions necessitate a trapping procedure (i.e., placing clips on the involved artery both proximally and distally to the aneurysm).

2. **Anesthetic management** during rupture of the aneurysm consists of adjusting the infusion rate of nitroprusside to maintain the mean arterial pressure between 40 and 50 mmHg to decrease the rate of bleeding. If bleeding continues to be excessive, then MAP may be briefly lowered to 30 mmHg to allow the surgeon to remove blood from the field and to see the aneurysm more easily. Blood losses should be continuously replaced with infusions of whole blood to maintain blood volume. If excessive hemorrhage persists, decreasing MAP to 20 mmHg may be necessary. Alternatively, one or both carotid arteries may be compressed against the vertebral bodies for up to three minutes. Carotid compression may produce a nearly bloodless field and allow the surgeon to see the aneurysm (Botterell, 1956).

C. **Barbiturates** have been suggested to provide protection against cerebral ischemia when the risk of subsequent neurologic deficit is high. Ischemia may result from prolonged occlusion of a major cerebral artery, cerebral vasospasm, or an episode of severe hypotension. The efficacy of barbiturates in these situations is not yet supported by adequate clinical studies, but perhaps such therapy is worth attempting when the surgical outcome is otherwise likely to be one of severe morbidity or mortality. Some authors have suggested that if temporary occlusion of a major intracranial vessel or deep hypotension is required, thiopental, 3 to 5 mg/kg, be given intravenously before aneurysm clipping (Michenfelder, 1982). If prolonged barbiturate therapy is planned, use pentobarbital, 15 to 20 mg/kg, as a loading dose followed by pentobarbital, 15 mg/kg/24 hr, in divided doses for 48 hours postoperatively (Hoff, 1977).

VI. Immediate postoperative care

A. **In the intensive care unit,** place the patient in a 20- to 30-degree head-up position with the head in the midline position to prevent obstruction of the jugular veins. Assure adequate oxygenation by using supplemental oxygen delivered by face mask and heated nebulizer. Give the nurse caring for the patient a detailed account of the patient's preoperative neurologic state, anesthetic and surgical procedures, intraoperative fluid therapy, and intraoperative and any anticipated complications. Order continuous monitoring of systemic blood pressure and ECG. Maintain MAP at a level above that associated with preoperative neurologic deficits, or no lower than 80 mmHg and no higher than 120 mmHg. Because of the possibility of delayed postoperative respiratory depressant effects of fentanyl (Adams, 1978; Nilsson, 1982), if any deterioration in consciousness or respiration occurs, give naloxone, 0.1 to 0.2 mg, intravenously or instruct the nurse to notify the house staff immediately.

B. **Before leaving the intensive care unit,** be certain that the vital signs are stable and that the patient is capable of maintaining an unobstructed airway. Carry out a brief neurologic assessment of the patient's level of consciousness, pupillary symmetry and reaction to light, ability to move all extremities, and relative strength of each extremity.

References

Neurosurgery
1. Botterell, E. H., Longhead, W. M., Scott, J. W., and Vandewater, S. L.   Hypothermia and interruption of carotid or carotid and vertebral circulation in the surgical management of intracranial aneurysms. *J. Neurosurg.* 13:1, 1956.
2. Dott, N. W.   Intracranial Aneurysm: Cerebral Arterioradiography: Surgical Treat-

ment. *Transcripts of the Medical Chirurgical Society,* Edinburgh, 1932–1933. Pp. 219–234.
3. Hunt, W. E., and Hess, R. M.   Surgical risk as related to time of intervention in the repair of intracranial aneurysms. *J. Neurosurg.* 28:14, 1968.
4. Kurtzke, J. F.   *Epidemiology of Cerebrovascular Disease.* New York: Springer, 1969. P. 195.
5. Locksley, H. B.   Report on the cooperative study of intracranial aneurysms and subarachnoid hemorrhage: Natural history of subarachnoid hemorrhage, intracranial aneurysms and arteriovenous malformations. Based on 6368 cases in the Cooperative Study. *J. Neurosurg.* 22:219, 1965.

Anesthesia
1. Adams, A. P., and Pybus, D. A.   Delayed respiratory depression after use of fentanyl during anaesthesia. *Br. Med. J.* 1:278, 1978.
2. Artru, A. A.   A comparison of the effects of isoflurane, enflurane, halothane, and fentanyl on cerebral blood volume and ICP. Abstracts of Scientific Papers. *Anesthesiology* 57:A374, 1982.
3. Barker, J.   An anaesthetic technique for intracranial aneurysms. Correspondence. *Anaesthesia* 30:557, 1975.
4. Botterell, E. H., Longhead, W. M., Scott, J. W., et al.   Hypothermia and interruption of carotid or carotid and vertebral circulation in the surgical management of intracranial aneurysms. *J. Neurosurg.* 13:1, 1956.
5. Brown, F. D., Crockard, H. A., Johns, L. M., et al.   The effects of sodium nitroprusside and trimethaphan camsylate on cerebral blood flow in rhesus monkeys. *Neurosurgery* 2:31, 1978.
6. Colley, P. S., Cheney, F. W., and Hlastala, M. P.   Ventilation–perfusion and gas exchange effects of sodium nitroprusside in dogs with normal and edematous lungs. *Anesthesiology* 50:489, 1979.
7. Colley, P. S., Cheney, F. W., and Hlastala, M. P.   Pulmonary gas exchange effects of nitroglycerin in canine edematous lungs. *Anesthesiology* 55:114, 1981.
8. Cucchiara, R. F., Messick, J. M., Gronert, G. G., et al.   Time required and success rate of percutaneous right atrial catheterization: Description of a technique. *Can. Anaesth. Soc. J.* 27:572, 1980.
9. Dahlgren, B. E., Gordon, E., and Steiner, L.   Evaluation of controlled hypotension during surgery for intracranial arterial aneurysms. In *Prog. Anaesthesiology,* Excerpta Medica, 1970. P. 1232.
10. Doshi, R., and Neil-Dwyer, G.   Hypothalamic and myocardial lesions after subarachnoid haemorrhage. *J. Neurol. Neurosurg. Psychiatry* 40:821, 1977.
11. Fahmy, N. R.   Nitroglycerin as a hypotensive drug during general anesthesia. *Anesthesiology* 49:17, 1978.
12. Farrar, J. K., Gamache, F. W., Ferguson, G. G., et al.   Effects of profound hypotension on cerebral blood flow during surgery for intracranial aneurysms. *J. Neurosurg.* 55:857, 1981.
13. Ferguson, G.   Physical factors in the initiation, growth and rupture of human intracranial aneurysms. *J. Neurosurg.* 37:666, 1972.
14. Galloon, S., Rees, G. A. O., Briscoe, L. E., et al.   Prospective study of electrocardiographic changes associated with subarachnoid haemorrhage. *Br. J. Anaesth.* 44:511, 1972.
15. Grubb, R. L., and Raichle, M. E.   Effects of hemorrhagic and pharmacologic hypotension on cerebral oxygen utilization and blood flow. *Anesthesiology* 56:3, 1982.
16. Hoff, J. T., Pitts, L. H., and Spetzler, R.   Barbiturates for protection from cerebral ischemia in aneurysm surgery. *Acta Neurol. Scand.* (Suppl. 64) 56:158, 1977.

17. Hunt, W. E., and Hess, R. M. Surgical risk as related to time of intervention in the repair of intracranial aneurysms. *J. Neurosurg.* 28:14, 1968.
18. Iwatsuki, N., Kuroda, N., Amaha, K., and Iwatsuki, K. Succinylcholine-induced hyperkalemia in patients with ruptured cerebral aneurysms. *Anesthesiology* 53:64, 1980.
19. Jones, T. H., Chiappa, K. H., Young, R. R., et al. EEG monitoring for induced hypotension for surgery of intracranial aneurysms. *Stroke* 10:292, 1979.
20. Kautto, U-M. Attenuation of the circulatory response to laryngoscopy and intubation by fentanyl. *Acta Anaesthesiol. Scand.* 26:217, 1982.
21. Keykhah, M. M., Welsh, F. A., Hagerdal, M., et al. Reduction of the cerebral protective effect of hypothermia by oligemic hypotension during hypoxia in the rat. *Stroke* 13:171, 1982.
22. Krayenbühl, H., Yasargil, G., Flamm, E. S., et al. Microsurgical treatment of intracranial saccular aneurysms. *J. Neurosurg.* 37:678, 1972.
23. Lebowitz, P. W., Ramsey, F. M., Savarese, J. J., et al. Combination of pancuronium and metacurine. Neuromuscular and hemodynamic advantages over pancuronium alone. *Anesth. Analg.* 60:12, 1981.
24. Levin, R. M., Zadigian, M. E., and Hall, S. C. The combined effect of hyperventilation and hypotension on cerebral oxygenation in anaesthetized dogs. *Can. Anaesth. Soc. J.* 27:264, 1980.
25. Maroon, J. B., and Nelson, P. B. Hypovolemia in patients with subarachnoid hemorrhage: Therapeutic implications. *Neurosurgery* 4:223, 1979.
26. Michenfelder, J. D. Physiology and pharmacology of brain protection. *Annual ASA Refresher Course Lectures,* 1982. P. 242.
27. Newberg, L. A., Milde, J. H., and Michenfelder, J. D. Cerebral metabolic effects of isoflurane at and above concentrations which suppress the EEG. *Anesthesiology* 57:A334, 1982.
28. Nilsson, C., and Rosberg, B. Recurrence of respiratory depression following neurolept analgesia. *Acta Anaesthesiol. Scand.* 26:240, 1982.
29. Nornes, H., Knutzen, H. B., and Wikeby, P. Cerebral arterial blood flow and aneurysm surgery. *J. Neurosurg.* 47:819, 1977.
30. Nornes, H., and Wikeby, P. Results of microsurgical management of intracranial aneurysms. *J. Neurosurg.* 51:608, 1979.
31. Pertuiset, B., Van Effenterre, R., Goutorbe, J., et al. Management of aneurysmal rupture during surgery, using bipolar coagulation, deep hypotension, and the operating microscope. *Acta Neurochir.* 30:195, 1974.
32. Pritz, M. B., Giannotta, S. L., Kindt, G. W., et al. Treatment of patients with neurological deficits associated with cerebral vasospasm by intravascular volume expansion. *Neurosurgery* 3:364, 1978.
33. Rudehill, A., Gordon, E., Sundqvist, K., et al. A study of ECG abnormalities and myocardial specific enzymes in patients with subarachnoid haemorrhage. *Acta Anaesthesiol. Scand.* 26:344, 1982.
34. Savarese, J. J., Hassan, H. A., and Antonio, R. P. The clinical pharmacology of metacurine. *Anesthesiology* 47:277, 1977.
35. Shapiro, H. M., Galindo, A., Wyte, S. R., et al. Rapid intraoperative reduction of intracranial pressure with thiopentone. *Br. J. Anaesth.* 45:1057, 1973.
36. Sklar, G. S., and Lanks, K. W. Effects of trimethaphan and sodium nitroprusside on hydrolysis of succinylcholine in vitro. *Anesthesiology* 47:31, 1977.
37. Skultety, F. M., and Nishioka, H. The results of intracranial surgery in the treatment of aneurysms. *J. Neurosurg.* 25:683, 1966.
38. Srivastava, S. C., and Robson, A. O. Electrocardiographic abnormalities associated with subarachnoid haemorrhage. *Lancet* 2:431, 1964.
39. Stoyka, W. W., and Schultz, H. The cerebral response to sodium nitroprusside and trimethaphan controlled hypotension. *Can. Anaesth. Soc. J.* 22:275, 1975.

40. Sullivan, K. H., Keenan, R. L., Isrow, L., et al.   The critical importance of $PaCO_2$ during intracranial aneurysm surgery. *J. Neurosurg.* 52:426, 1980.
41. Sundt, T. M., Kobayashi, S., Fode, N. C., et al.   Results and complications of surgical management of 809 intracranial aneurysms in 722 cases. *J. Neurosurg.* 56:753, 1982.
42. Symon, L., Hargadine, J. R., Zawirski, M., et al.   Central conduction time as an index of ischaemia in subarachnoid haemorrhage. *J. Neurol. Sci.* 44:95, 1979.
43. Trojaborg, W., and Boysen, G.   Relation between EEG, regional cerebral blood flow and internal carotid artery pressure during carotid endarterectomy. *Electroencephalogr. Clin. Neurophysiol.* 34:61, 1973. ·
44. Vidal, B. E., Dergal, E. G., Cesarman, E., et al.   Cardiac arrythmias associated with subarachnoid hemorrhage: Prospective study. *Neurosurgery* 5:675, 1979.
45. Yasargil, M. G., and Fox, J. L.   The microsurgical approach to intracranial aneurysms. *Surg. Neurol.* 3:7, 1975.

9. Ischemic Cerebrovascular Disease

Elizabeth A. M. Frost

All anesthetic drugs and techniques influence cerebral circulation and metabolism. In patients who have cerebral ischemic disease, these changes may prove inappropriate to the brain's nutritional needs, and the consequences may be devastating. Thus, anesthetic effects must be carefully controlled to provide optimal protection and improved conditions, so that a rational choice of neuroanesthetic measures is essential.

I. Basic considerations of cerebral circulation

A. Anatomy

1. **Cerebral arterial supply** is provided by the carotid and vertebral circulations. Normally 90% of the cerebral blood flow is supplied through the carotid arteries and 10% through the vertebral arteries.

   a. **Carotid arteries.** The left carotid and left subclavian arteries are direct branches of the aortic arch. The right carotid and right subclavian arteries arise from the innominate branch of the aorta. Each common carotid artery divides at the level of the fourth cervical vertebra (C4) into the internal and external carotid arteries. The external carotid artery supplies the glands, muscles, and bones of the head and face, and the dura mater. The internal carotid artery enters the skull through the foramen lacerum and carotid canal and crosses the cavernous sinus. Ophthalmic, posterior communicating, and anterior choroidal branches are given off before the internal carotid artery terminates on the basal surface of the brain by dividing into the anterior and middle cerebral arteries.

   b. **Vertebral arteries.** The vertebral arteries are given off by the subclavian arteries. The larger left vertebral and the smaller right vertebral arteries enter the foramen transversarium of C6 on either side and ascend through the neck to C1 where they cross the dura to the anterolateral surface of the upper cervical spinal cord.

   The vertebral arteries give origin to (1) the posterior inferior cerebellar arteries and (2) the rami for the common midline anterior spinal artery that supplies the anterior two-thirds of the spinal cord before joining the midline to form the basilar artery. Paired branches of the basilar artery include the anterior inferior cerebellar arteries, the segmental perforating branches, the superior cerebellar arteries, and the terminal posterior cerebral arteries.

2. Venous drainage is through superficial and deep systems. Cortical veins drain into the veins of Trolard and Labbé laterally and inferiorly and into the superior sagittal sinus medially and superiorly. Drainage from the deep gray nuclei passes along periependymal veins to the basal veins of Rosenthal and the vein of Galen to the straight sinus and torcular and thence to the superior sagittal sinus. Lateral sinuses carry venous blood to the sigmoid sinus and to internal jugular veins that empty into the superior vena cava. From the posterior fossa, drainage is through cerebellar and basilar plexi into the sigmoid sinus.

3. Anastomotic pathways between the arterial systems, of which there are several, exist to maintain flow in cases of cerebral ischemic disease. The circle of Willis connects the left and right carotid circulations and the carotid and vertebrobasilar circulations. Retrograde flow from maxillary ophthalmic arteries can fill the internal carotid artery. Emissary channels connect scalp, bony, and dural arteries through petrotympanic branches to the internal carotid artery.

B. Physiology

1. The brain's lack of phosphorylase and glycogen means that it requires a continuous supply of glucose and oxygen to function. A relatively high blood flow is therefore mandatory and is maintained as long as autoregulatory mechanisms remain intact. The normal value for global cerebral blood flow (CBF) is 44 ml/100 gm/min. However, this figure may vary regionally from 20 to 80 ml/100 gm/min, the faster flows generally occurring through gray matter and the slower rates calculated from white matter. Values for metabolic rates for consumption of cerebral nutrients are given in Table 9-1.

2. Physiologic control of the cerebral circulation is maintained by a precise interaction of myogenic, metabolic, chemical, and neurogenic vascular responses (Table 9-2).

a. Autoregulation, or myogenic control, maintains CBF near a constant value even though the mean arterial pressure (MAP) may range between 50 and 150 mmHg. The exact mechanism for this control is not completely understood, although it is known to be dependent on changing cerebrovascular resistance. Autoregulation is not an instantaneous effect, as several minutes are required for equilibration. This myogenic response is impaired by trauma, hypoxia, anesthetic agents, seizures, chronic hypertension, diabetes, and vasospasm.

Table 9-1. Normal values for metabolic rates of consumption of cerebral nutrients

Full name	Abbreviation	Normal values and units
Cerebral blood flow	CBF	44 ml/100 gm/min
Regional cerebral blood flow	rCBF	20–80 ml/100 gm/min
Cerebral perfusion pressure*	CPP	80 mmHg
Cerebrovascular resistance	CVR	1.8 mmHg/ml/100 gm/ min
Arteriovenous oxygen content difference	$(A\text{-}V)O_2$	6.8 ml/100 ml
Cerebral metabolic rate for oxygen	$CMRO_2$	3.0 ml/100 gm/min
Cerebral metabolic rate for glucose	CMR glucose	4.5 mg/100 gm/min
Cerebral metabolic rate for lactate	CMR lactate	2.3 mg/100 gm/min
Cerebral venous oxygen tension	PvO_2	35–40 mmHg
Oxygen glucose index	OGI	90–100%
Lactate glucose index	LGI	0–10%
Cerebral blood flow equivalent	$CBF/CMRO_2$	14–15 ml blood/ml O_2

*Defined as mean arterial pressure minus mean cerebral venous pressure or mean arterial pressure minus intracranial pressure.

b. Metabolic control of CBF refers to the close association between flow and the level of oxidative metabolism in brain tissue. As the metabolic rate increases or the relative supply of oxygen within small areas of the brain decreases, release of local metabolites results in vasodilatation. An increase in hydrogen ion (H^+) concentration rather than a decrease in oxygen is considered the major metabolic factor coupling flow and metabolism. Alteration of serum calcium (Ca^{2+}) and potassium (K^+) levels and changes in carbonic anhy-

Table 9-2. Physiologic control of the cerebral circulation

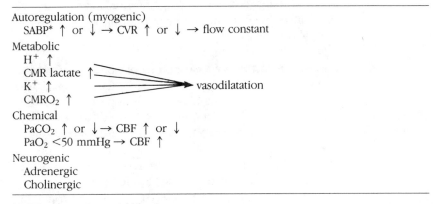

Autoregulation (myogenic)
   SABP* ↑ or ↓ → CVR ↑ or ↓ → flow constant
Metabolic
   H^+ ↑
   CMR lactate ↑
   K^+ ↑   → vasodilatation
   $CMRO_2$ ↑
Chemical
   $PaCO_2$ ↑ or ↓ → CBF ↑ or ↓
   PaO_2 <50 mmHg → CBF ↑
Neurogenic
   Adrenergic
   Cholinergic

*SABP = Systemic arterial blood pressure.

drase activity and adenosine diphosphate concentrations influence local flow.

c. **Chemical control** is mediated by alteration of arterial carbon dioxide tension ($PaCO_2$). A linear relationship exists between CBF and $PaCO_2$: there is a 4% rise in CBF for each 1 mmHg increase in $PaCO_2$ between $PaCO_2$ levels of 30 to 60 mmHg. Within the same range, $PaCO_2$ has no apparent effect on cerebral metabolic rate of oxygen consumption ($CMRO_2$). Alteration of CBF by changing $PaCO_2$ occurs almost immediately as carbon dioxide (CO_2) diffuses rapidly from blood vessels to affect the pH of extracellular fluid. If $PaCO_2$ is kept constant and only arterial H^+ or bicarbonate (HCO_3^-) altered, little immediate change is seen in CBF, since these ions enter the extracellular fluid space more slowly.

The decrease in CBF with hypocapnia is limited, and minimal flow is reached at about 15 to 20 mmHg, when cerebral tissue hypoxia may prevent further reduction in flow. Lowering arterial oxygen tension (PaO_2) when the $PaCO_2$ is normal does not affect CBF until PaO_2 falls below 50 mmHg, at which point cerebral vasodilatation occurs and CBF increases.

d. The precise role of **neurogenic control** is still debated. Both adrenergic and cholinergic nerves innervate extracranial and intracranial blood vessels. Stimulation of nerves can markedly affect the caliber of pial vessels. However, the response of these pial vessels—to hypoxia, hypercapnia, and hypertension—appears to be similar whether the nervous pathways are intact or not. The nerve plexuses on cerebral vessels are identical to these in other vascular beds, but the nerve actions are minimal or nonexistent. Neurogenic control is probably not of major significance under normal circumstances but becomes important during stress states such as hypovolemic shock.

3. Noninvasive **quantitative assessment** of CBF and metabolism may be made by monitoring washout of ^{133}Xe from small areas of the brain after the patient inhales the isotope. CBF can also be measured externally by using up to 250 scintillation counters, each of which looks at a small cylinder of brain tissue. In centers with access to a cyclotron, it is now possible to measure the metabolic rates for CO_2 generation, ammonia turnover, oxygen consumption, and local cerebral blood volume in small regions of cerebral tissue, using tomographic scanners that image positron-emitting radioisotopes.

C. **Pathophysiology.** Anesthetic management of patients who have ischemic cerebrovascular disease must be aimed at institution of conditions that will favor resolution of ischemia, protection against the development of ischemic infarction, and maintenance of normal intracranial dynamics.

   1. Development of cerebral infarction is governed by the degree to which the metabolic needs of the brain are met by the cerebral circulation. Factors that decrease substrate supply or increase metabolic demand increase the risk of infarction. Factors that augment blood flow or lower metabolism decrease the chance of infarction. How much ischemia produces a clinical deficit is unknown, but slowing of the EEG is seen when CBF is < 20 ml/ 100 gm/min.

   2. CBF is decreased by systemic hypotension and focal vascular occlusion; also sickle cell anemia and paraproteinemias increase cerebrovascular resistance and decrease CBF. Cerebral edema and hydrocephalus increase critical closing pressures and reduce CBF. Hematomas cause a mass effect and decrease perfusion pressure at the point of focal compression; reactive edema and hyperemia are present in the surrounding brain.

   3. Hypoxic ischemia from respiratory or central neurogenic disorders causes a relative shift from oxidative metabolism within mitochondria to anaerobic, largely extra-mitochondrial glycolysis with conversion of pyruvate to lactate. As lactate concentration increases, there is a decrease in the rate of production of adenosine triphosphate by oxidative phosphorylation. The blood-brain barrier, which restricts permeability, breaks down and injury to the endothelial cells of the capillaries occurs. Edema aggravates ischemia by increasing critical closing pressure. A vicious cycle of ischemia and edema may then lead to irreversible infarction.

   4. Therapy can interrupt this sequence of events at several points, and must be directed toward increasing CBF, reducing edema formation, or decreasing metabolic demand. Anesthetic techniques and drugs may be used to maintain or decrease CBF or to exert a protective effect on the brain by reducing the metabolic rate of oxygen utilization.

II. **Major cerebrovascular ischemic disease entities**

   A. **Thromboembolism** accounts for approximately 78% of new "strokes." Sources of emboli include obstructive lesions in the arterial circulation from atheromas, cardiac emboli, or ulceration of atheromatous plaques. Other causes of stroke include vasculitis and hematologic disorders.

B. Classification of ischemic disease reflects duration and severity of the clinical deficit. *Transient ischemic attacks* (TIA) are characterized by deficits that persist for less than 24 hours and resolve completely. *Reversible ischemic neurologic deficits* (RIND) persist for longer than 24 hours but resolve within a week. *Progressive stroke* (PS) is the most unstable condition and is characterized by serial worsening of the deficit. *Completed stroke* (CS) describes a persistent deficit that may range from minor to disabling.

C. Noninvasive tests to evaluate the extent of the ischemic disease include ophthalmodynamometry, assessment of flow reversal in ophthalmic-facial collaterals with directional Doppler equipment, thermography, and oculoplethysmography. Plain skull and cervical x-rays may show calcification, and computed tomographic (CT) scan with contrast enhancement may show the extent of infarction. Noninvasive arteriographic methods, including digital subtraction (or intravenous) angiography, permit visualization of arterial channels. Arterial angiography is often reserved either for symptomatic patients or for visualization of intracranial vessels.

D. Choice of **surgical technique** is determined by the site of the lesion. Severe stenosis or ulcerative plaques near the carotid bifurcation are best treated by carotid endarterectomy. Complete occlusions or inaccessible stenoses of the internal carotid or middle cerebral arteries or the posterior circulation respond best to microvascular anastomosis of an extracranial to an intracranial artery.

III. Preoperative anesthetic evaluation

A. Multisystem disease

1. **Hypertension.** The majority of patients who have cerebrovascular disease are hypertensive and pose a number of problems for the anesthetist.

   a. The hypertensive patient undergoing general anesthesia is at increased risk of **myocardial infarction.**

   b. Hypertensive patients may be particularly **unstable during the anesthetic period,** becoming hypotensive intraoperatively and further compromising an ischemic area of the brain.

   c. Postoperatively, hypertension may develop, putting atheromatous cerebral vessels at risk of rupture.

d. Control. Since patients who have untreated or inadequately treated hypertension are at greater risk during anesthesia of arterial hypotension and of associated myocardial and cerebral ischemia, it has been recommended that the arterial pressures be brought under control *before* the patient undergoes anesthesia. The risk of anesthesia can be reduced when the diastolic pressure is stable and not higher than 110 mmHg, and when close monitoring and prompt therapy avoid intraoperative and postoperative episodes of hypotension or hypertension.

2. **Carotid artery disease.** Cerebral ischemia usually does not cause neurologic deficit until carotid artery stenosis reaches about 80% or embolization of an atheromatous plaque occurs. The disease is bilateral in about 50% of cases. Abnormalities of the circle of Willis (usually hypoplastic communicating vessels) are found in the majority of cases and further decrease the ability to augment collateral flow. Thus the margin of safety is greatly reduced, and relatively small decreases in systemic blood pressure or cerebral vessel diameter may precipitate a catastrophic situation. Preoperative evaluation of patients who have carotid artery disease should include a test of neck motion to ascertain that consciousness is maintained with lateral movement.

3. **Myocardial infarction.** A history of previous myocardial infarction is obtained from 25% of patients and has been shown to correlate closely with postoperative cardiac complications regardless of the age or the severity of the infarction. If patients also have ischemic cardiac disease and require coronary artery bypass, their cerebral ischemia should be relieved before they undergo heart surgery. About 20% of patients have also had previous major vascular surgery.

4. **Diabetes mellitus** occurs in about 20% of patients who have cerebrovascular disease, and they usually require insulin for control. Coincidental use of corticosteroids in neurosurgical management to decrease cerebral edema may aggravate hyperglycemia and increase insulin needs.

5. About 40% of patients have smoked one to two packs of **cigarettes** per day for more than 20 years. Consequently bronchitis, emphysema, chronic hypoxia, or even carcinoma are frequently complicating factors.

6. Stroke victims also have altered muscular function. **Hyperkalemia** is a recognized danger in patients who have central nervous system lesions and skeletal muscle paralysis. The phe-

nomenon may occur in patients who have both upper and lower motor neuron abnormalities. Elevated serum potassium levels persist in the venous blood returning from all paralyzed muscles for several weeks after injury, indicating that the source of the potassium is the abnormal muscle distal to the neural lesion. Therefore, administration of succinylcholine to these patients may increase serum potassium levels and cause cardiac arrhythmias or even arrest. It is imperative that preoperative serum potassium levels be within normal limits. The patient is pretreated with small doses of a nondepolarizing muscle relaxant; succinylcholine is used only in minimal amounts or avoided altogether.

B. Multiple pharmacologic regimens

1. Approximately 85% of patients who have cerebrovascular insufficiency take a combination of several drugs. Most commonly, these medications include digitalis, diuretic, antihypertensive, antiarrhythmic, anticoagulant, insulin, and corticosteroid preparations.

2. Antihypertensive and antiarrhythmic drugs should be continued until the morning of surgery to minimize the risk of postoperative rebound hypertension. Rebound hypertension is most commonly seen after withdrawal from clonidine. It is important to restart hypertensive drugs as soon as possible in the postoperative period.

3. Diuretics may cause fluid and electrolyte imbalance that can result in critical intraoperative hypotension and arrhythmias. Serum electrolytes must be measured immediately before surgery. Input-output charts should be carefully balanced for 24 to 48 hours preoperatively to assess fluid status.

4. Patients receiving long-acting insulin preparations should be stabilized preoperatively on soluble compounds.

5. Aspirin, usually given for several weeks before surgery to reduce platelet adhesiveness, may decrease essential coagulation factors, especially factor X. In addition, patients who have suffered transient ischemic attacks often take coumadin preparations. These drugs must be discontinued for up to 1 week to allow clotting to revert to normal. Emergency therapy with large doses of vitamin K may prove relatively ineffective in returning prothrombin times to standard levels. A clotting profile is essential on the day of surgery.

C. Preanesthetic medication. The use of atropine is best avoided because of its unpleasant drying and tachycardiac effects. Small

doses of tranquilizers such as diazepam (5–10 mg orally) may be given about one hour before surgery. If the patient exhibits bradycardia after succinylcholine is given or after intubation, atropine may be given intravenously.

IV. Intraoperative anesthetic management

A. Carotid endarterectomy (See Table 9-3.)

1. **Cerebral perfusion pressure** (CPP) must be maintained. Normotension or slight hypertension is essential since autoregulatory mechanisms are frequently altered regionally if not globally. The long-term use of antihypertensive medications makes patients susceptible to hypotensive episodes initially. These changes may be detected immediately if an arterial line has been established before or during induction. Stabilization of blood pressure is achieved by increasing fluid administration, infusing a 0.02% phenylephrine hydrochloride solution, and using light planes of anesthesia.

2. $PaCO_2$ should be kept in the normocapnic range (35–40 mmHg), since CBF increases linearly with increase in $PaCO_2$.

   a. In cases of carotid artery stenosis, establishment of **hypercapnia** will increase collateral flow and might be beneficial. However, ischemic areas of the brain are probably already

Table 9-3. Anesthetic management of the patient undergoing carotid endarterectomy

---

Careful preoperative history
  Assessment of multisystem disease
  Optimal medical condition
  Continue cardiovascular therapeutic regimen
Maintain cerebral perfusion pressure
  Avoid hypotension and bradycardia
  Normocapnia
  Surgical shunt
Select anesthetic agent to lower $CMRO_2$ and maintain cerebral blood flow
Monitoring
  ECG
  Intra-arterial BP
  EEG
  Stump pressure
  CBF
Close postoperative observation
  Maintain normotension or slight hypertension
  Resume antihypertensive drugs
  Clear airway
  Neurologic assessment

---

maximally dilated owing to regional autoregulation, and a reduction in resistance in nonischemic areas may cause blood to flow from ischemic to normal areas of the brain, resulting in the **intracerebral steal phenomenon.** Retained CO_2 increases systemic blood pressure (which is beneficial) but causes a higher incidence of arrhythmias, especially in patients who already have generalized vascular disease. In addition, hypercapnia decreases stump pressure and increases cerebral venous pressure, both of which lower CPP.

   b. Hypocapnia has the opposite effect: it increases resistance in nonischemic areas and may direct flow to ischemic areas. However, this effect may jeopardize healthy brain tissue and increase resistance in collateral vessels supplying ischemic areas. A shift of the oxygen dissociation curve to the left in respiratory alkalosis also makes oxygen less available to tissues.

3. Precise, continuous **monitoring** is essential. Monitoring should include electrocardiogram, direct arterial blood pressure and gases (from an arterial line), and temperature. The Cerebral Function Monitor, an electroencephalographic processor giving information essentially from a single pair of parietal electrodes, provides only a gross indication of activity (see Chap. 3). Continuous, full EEG recording is preferable, especially during the period of carotid clamping. Although stump pressures above 50 mmHg are said to indicate adequate flow, the EEG may be abnormal at values even higher than this. Therefore, stump pressures are an indication of global flow at best and afford no information as to regional conditions.

4. Assessing the adequacy of cerebral circulation

   a. Assessment is most accurate when **local anesthesia** allows the patient to respond verbally. Even though carotid endarterectomy is performed successfully in many centers under cervical plexus block, local anesthesia is not always possible because of either lack of patient acceptance or surgical difficulties. In addition, this technique may cause the patient anxiety and some pain, resulting in tachycardia, hypertension, hypercapnia (from rebreathing under the drapes), and increased myocardial and brain oxygen consumption. Finally, neurologic damage does not always occur immediately after carotid artery clamping and may even be delayed for up to 30 minutes, a time when surgical attention may be directed elsewhere.

b. Under **general anesthesia,** means of assessing cerebral circulation include jugular bulb oxygen tension (an indicator of global flow), EEG monitoring (regional and global flow), stump pressure (indicating the pressure of back flow from the opposite carotid artery and vertebral arteries), and the Cerebral Function Monitor. The use of collimated scintillation crystals and measurement of ^{133}Xe washout rates after inhalation may soon be the most accurate means of measuring regional flow intraoperatively.

5. An **anesthetic agent** should be used that will lower cerebral metabolic oxygen requirements but maintain flow without myocardial depression.

    a. **Barbiturates** decrease $CMRO_2$ but they also decrease CBF. In addition, blood pressure may be difficult to maintain, and emergence is frequently delayed. A cerebral protective effect of barbiturate has been suggested but is still under considerable question (see Chap. 4).

    b. An **inhalation agent** such as isoflurane also decreases cerebral metabolic rate, but will increase total CBF (which may result in some, but not total, intracerebral steal effect). Although blood pressure may decrease initially, emergence from anesthesia is usually prompt and complete. Isoflurane may also confer some protective effect. Thus, low-dose inhalational techniques are probably preferable to barbiturates.

    c. Reliance on the mechanical effect of a **surgical shunt** to maintain flow during clamping is preferable to the assumption that the metabolic requirements of the brain have been adequately reduced pharmacologically.

6. Sudden episodes of **bradycardia and hypotension** intraoperatively are caused by surgical manipulation at the carotid bifurcation. The reflex may be blocked by intravenous atropine 0.4 mg, repeated twice, as necessary, or by local instillation of 1% lidocaine. The surgeon should be advised immediately of the response.

B. **Extracranial–intracranial anastomosis.** The technique of microvascular extracranial to intracranial anastomosis was developed to increase collateral blood flow in patients who have cerebrovascular insufficiency from atheromatous disease that is inaccessible by carotid surgery.

1. The **characteristic profile** of patients undergoing these operations is as follows:

    a. Age greater than 50 years

b. Male/female ratio of 3:1

c. Presence of cardiovascular disease and diabetes

d. Multiple drug regimen

e. Transient ischemic attacks and progressive stroke

f. Generalized low cerebral perfusion syndrome

g. Heavy smoking

2. **Surgical considerations.** Anastomosis may be performed in the anterior circulation between the superficial temporal artery and the middle cerebral artery or in the posterior circulation between the occipital artery and the posterior inferior cerebellar artery. If the occipital artery is used, surgery is performed in a sitting position and all precautions necessitated by this position must be observed (see Chap. 11).

3. **Anesthetic considerations.** The main anesthetic considerations are to maintain cerebral perfusion pressure, maintain normocapnia, decrease $CMRO_2$, reduce brain movement, and administer low-molecular-weight dextran.

   a. Maintenance of adequate CPP is essential. An arterial line must be established immediately, and systemic arterial pressure must be held as close to the patient's customary levels as possible with the use of 0.02% phenylephrine hydrochloride solution intravenously, if necessary.

   b. Normocapnia should be maintained ($PaCO_2$ of 35–40 mmHg). During bypass surgery, the brain may appear swollen and edematous and the temptation exists to use hyperventilation to reduce ICP. However, this maneuver is rarely effective since the area involved has usually lost responsiveness to changes in $PaCO_2$. Hyperventilation may be counterproductive since the resultant vasoconstriction is deleterious to the collateral blood supply and to other marginally supplied areas. During anesthesia, hyperventilation may cause cerebral damage as determined by a critical flicker fusion or reaction time test postoperatively. Hyperventilation may also adversely affect the patient who already has neurologic damage because the increased cerebral vasoconstriction that occurs as $PaCO_2$ decreases leads to a fall in cortical PO_2. Judicious use of osmotic diuretics and cerebrospinal fluid drainage is preferable to reduce brain volume.

   c. Routine monitoring should include all vital signs, input-output charting, temperature recording, and frequent blood gas determinations. The inspired oxygen concentration may require adjustment if significant lung disease exists. Blood transfusion is rarely necessary although blood should be available in the event of profuse scalp bleeding or inadvertent displacement of the arterial clamp.

d. Reduction of brain movement. The operation is performed under high magnification through a narrow exposure. Respiratory and cardiac pulsations are magnified and cause a distracting brain bounce, which may be attenuated by a head-up position, minimal head turning, lower tidal volumes with increased respiratory rate, and use of small doses of furosemide. Although not yet clinically employed, a modification of jet ventilation may lend itself to these situations.

e. Anesthetic drugs

(1) The surgical technique necessitates clamping a branch of the middle cerebral artery for approximately 1 hour. Therefore, a drug that may afford ischemic protection, such as a barbiturate, may seem to be preferable for anesthesia. However, barbiturates cause marked cerebral vasoconstriction, which could impair collateral flow to ischemic areas.

(2) Alternatively, low-dose inhalational drugs in combination with efforts to maintain normocapnia cause some cerebral vasodilatation and decrease $CMRO_2$. Thus, blood flow is maximally maintained to poorly perfused areas. In a series of 80 patients who were anesthetized with low-dose inhalation agents, no new neurologic deficits developed immediately postoperatively; this, and the ability to perform accurate neurologic assessment (since the patient awakens promptly), would indicate that the regimen is satisfactory (Table 9-4).

f. Low-molecular-weight dextran infused at a rate of 50 to 100 ml/hr has been shown to maintain flow through freshly anastomosed vessels. In about 50% of patients, however, persistent oozing of blood or increasing blood pressure results, at which point this therapy should be discontinued.

g. The surgery essentially does not invade the brain. Thus, **extremely light planes of anesthesia** can be tolerated and the patient should be awake at the end of the operation. Intravenous administration of lidocaine, 50 to 100 mg, as the head dressing is applied will prevent or greatly decrease the

Table 9-4. Postoperative condition in 80 patients undergoing extracranial-intracranial anastomosis

Condition		
Uneventful recovery	50	(62%)
Wound infection	10	(13%)
Flap necrosis	7	(9%)
Severe hypertension	6	(8%)
Urinary tract infection	5	(6.5%)
Thromboembolism	4	(5%)
Pneumonia	1	(1.5%)
Myocardial infarction (fatal)	1	(1.5%)

coughing that not only puts strain on newly anastomosed vessels but possibly causes considerable tissue damage if the pin headholder has not been removed.

V. Postoperative care

A. Carotid endarterectomy

1. **Careful monitoring** and trend recording in an intensive care unit setting are essential. Frequent evaluation of neurologic status is important to detect obstruction of the carotid artery, hematoma, or embolization that may require additional surgical exploration.

2. **Blood pressure** must be kept at or slightly above normal to prevent thrombosis. Both hypotensive and hypertensive episodes may occur in the immediate postoperative period because of reduced baroreflex function. Hypotension reduces perfusion of both the brain and the heart; hypertension increases the work and the oxygen demand of the myocardium. In both instances the end result is likely to be myocardial ischemia. The major cause of serious postoperative morbidity in patients undergoing carotid endarterectomy is myocardial infarction. In addition, hypertension may increase capillary hydrostatic pressure, especially in ischemic areas of the brain, and lead to protein leakage, edema, or hemorrhagic infarction.

   a. **Hypotension** is treated with fluid replacement, ventilation, and infusion of 0.02% phenylephrine hydrochloride solution as necessary.

   b. For **hypertensive episodes,** which occur more commonly, preoperative antihypertensive medications should be restarted as soon as possible. When mean arterial pressure rises more than 15% to 20% above baseline recordings, aggressive therapy is required. However, rapid reduction of arterial pressure by more than 25% may in itself cause cerebral ischemia. Therefore, therapy must be instituted with care, and extremely close observation of continuous arterial pressure recordings is mandatory. Useful drugs for parenteral therapy include sodium nitroprusside by slow infusion (70 μg/kg/hr), hydralazine (5–20 mg IM or IV), or diazoxide in a bolus injection of 50 mg that may be repeated twice. Propranolol 0.5 to 1.0 mg given slowly may augment the effects of hydralazine. There is some evidence to suggest that intraoperative use of propranolol (0.5–1.0 mg/hr slowly) may attenuate hypertensive responses in the postoperative period.

3. The **airway must be easily accessible;** close monitoring is necessary to detect intrinsic or extrinsic obstruction from laryngeal edema or hematoma formation. Patients frequently complain of throat pain probably related to intraoperative retraction on the trachea or esophagus. Treatment consists of reassurance and topical anesthetic lozenges.

B. Extracranial–intracranial anastomosis

1. Because these anastomoses involve only the superficial cortex of the brain, patients should be awake and their tracheas should be extubated before entry to the recovery room.

2. Close observation in the intensive care unit of all vital signs for 48 to 72 hours is necessary. Patients who have a previous history of myocardial infarction are at particular risk of postoperative cardiac complications such as ventricular arrhythmias, which usually respond to lidocaine in a bolus injection or continuous infusion. Blood pressure should be maintained as close to preoperative levels as possible (see section **A.2**). Careful, frequent neurologic assessment must be performed and charted.

3. All previous medications (with the exception of aspirin) should be restarted as quickly as possible. Patients who had been taking barbiturate preparations to control seizures should not receive full doses in the immediate postoperative period since this will interfere with emergence from anesthesia.

4. Necrosis of the flap may occur in the area of the scalp supplied by the diverted superficial temporal artery and may cause postoperative fever or sepsis.

References

1. Bentsen, N., Larsen, B., and Lassen, N. A.   Chronically impaired autoregulation of cerebral blood flow in long term diabetics. *Stroke* 6:497, 1975.
2. Cooper, E. S., West, J. W., Jaffe, M. E., et al.   The relation between cardiac function and cerebral blood flow in stroke patients. I. Effect of CO_2 inhalation. *Stroke* 1:330, 1970.
3. Fitch, W.   Anaesthesia for carotid artery surgery. *Br. J. Anaesth.* 48:791, 1976.
4. Föex, P., and Prys-Roberts, C.   Anesthesia and the hypertensive patient. *Br. J. Anaesth.* 46:575, 1974.
5. Goldman, L., and Caldera, D. L.   Risks of general anesthesia and elective operation in the hypertensive patient. *Anesthesiology* 50:285, 1979.
6. Goldman, L., Caldera, D. L., Southwick, F. S., et al.   Cardiac risk factors and complications in non-cardiac surgery. *Medicine* 57:357, 1978.
7. Harper, A. M.   The inter-relationship between $PaCO_2$ and blood pressure in the regulation of blood flow through the cerebral cortex. *Acta Neurol. Scand.* 41 (Suppl. 14):95, 1965.
8. Howe, J. R., and Kindt, G. W.   Cerebral protection during carotid endarterectomy. *Stroke* 5:340, 1974.
9. Kuschinsky, W., and Wahl, M.   Local chemical and neurogenic regulation of cerebral vascular resistance. *Physiol. Rev.* 58:656, 1978.
10. Lassen, N. A., Ingvar, D. H., and Skinhoj, E.   Brain function and blood flow. *Sci. Am.* 239:62, 1978.
11. McKay, R. D., Sundt, T. M., Michenfelder, J. E., et al.   Internal carotid artery stump pressure and cerebral blood flow during carotid endarterectomy. Modification by halothane, enflurane and Innovar. *Anesthesiology* 45:390, 1976.
12. Popp, A. J., and Chater, N.   Extracranial-to-intracranial vascular anastomosis for occlusive cerebrovascular disease. Experience in 110 patients. *Surgery* 82:648, 1977.
13. Rich, N. M., and Hobson, R. W.   Carotid endarterectomy under regional anesthesia. *Am. Surg.* 253, 1975.
14. Shapiro, H. M., Wyte, S. R., Harris, A. B., et al.   Acute intraoperative intracranial hypertension in neurosurgical patients. *Anesthesiology* 37:399, 1972.
15. Sharbrough, F. W., Messick, J. M., Jr., Sundt, T. M., Jr.   Correlation of continuous electroencephalograms with cerebral blood flow measurements during carotid endarterectomy. *Stroke* 4:674, 1973.
16. Strandgaard, S., Olesen, J., and Skinhoj, E.   Autoregulation of brain circulation in severe arterial hypertension. *Br. Med. J.* 1:507, 1973.
17. Tobey, R. E., Jacobsen, P. M., Kahle, C. T., et al.   The serum potassium response to muscle relaxants in neural injury. *Anesthesiology* 37:332, 1972.
18. Wollman, S. G., Orkin, L. R.   Postoperative human reaction time and hypocarbia during anesthesia. *Br. J. Anaesth.* 40:920, 1968.

10. Cerebrovascular Lesions and Tumors in the Pregnant Patient

Mark A. Rosen

Maternal mortality has declined during the past 35 years owing to better management of the major obstetric problems of hemorrhage, infection, and toxemia. As a result, there has been an increase in the incidence of maternal deaths from nonobstetric causes. Prominent among nonobstetric causes of maternal mortality are neurosurgical disorders, of which the most commonly encountered during pregnancy are subarachnoid hemorrhage (SAH) and intracranial tumor. SAH secondary to rupture of either a saccular aneurysm or an arteriovenous malformation (AVM) now ranks high as a cause of maternal mortality. As documented by angiography, surgery, or autopsy, SAH is reported to cause 12% to 24% of maternal deaths. Primary and metastatic intracranial tumors are uncommon during the childbearing years, but their clinical course may be aggravated by pregnancy, and surgery may be necessary before it is possible to deliver a viable infant.

This chapter will review the pathophysiology of SAH and intracranial tumors during pregnancy, and discuss an approach to the anesthetic management of these clinical situations. Although other neurosurgical disorders such as pseudotumor cerebri, cerebral cysts or abscesses, sinus thrombosis, and spinal cord diseases occur less frequently, the principles of anesthetic management discussed in this chapter are applicable to them as well.

Regardless of the neuropathology, the anesthesiologist will be involved in providing anesthesia for either the neurosurgical procedure or the vaginal or abdominal delivery. The objectives in the neuroanesthetic management of pregnant women are (1) ensuring maternal safety, (2) avoiding teratogenic drugs, (3) avoiding fetal asphyxia, and (4) preventing preterm labor. The goal of anesthesia for labor and delivery is to provide analgesia without either endangering the fetus or aggravating the maternal neurologic disorder.

I. **Intracranial tumors during pregnancy.** Although the incidence of brain tumors is not greater in pregnant women than in nonpregnant women, a tumor's clinical course is often aggravated by pregnancy. The mechanism for the exacerbation of tumor progression in pregnancy is probably the generalized water retention that occurs, which causes tumor swelling. There is no evidence that mitotic activity increases. Clinical presentation, signs, symptoms, indications for diagnostic work-up, and decisions regarding radiation therapy are not altered by pregnancy. Consideration should be given to postponing elective surgical resection until after delivery, when the maternal physiologic changes of pregnancy have returned toward normal and there is no chance to adversely affect the fetus. Craniotomy may be necessary during pregnancy, however, if the patient's clinical condition deteriorates.

II. **Subarachnoid hemorrhage during pregnancy**

A. **Etiology and incidence.** Subarachnoid hemorrhage during pregnancy is most commonly related to congenital saccular (berry) aneurysms or cerebral AVMs with approximately equal frequency. Although the precise incidence is not known, estimates from different series vary from less than 1 per 10,000 to 1 per 2500 pregnancies (Miller, 1970).

B. Pathology

1. **Saccular aneurysms** are caused by congenital defects in the muscularis of arterial walls that occur at bifurcation or branching sites at or near the circle of Willis. These aneurysms are usually less than 1 cm in diameter but can be as large as 5 cm. Autopsy specimens from women of reproductive age reveal an incidence of unruptured saccular aneurysms of 0.5% to 1.0%. With continued overstretching by the forces of blood pressure, the internal elastica undergoes degeneration.

2. **AVMs** are a network of tangled, interconnected thin-walled vessels in which arterial blood passes directly to venous drainage without intervening capillaries. The network is usually supplied by more than one artery and ranges in size from microscopic to massive. AVMs commonly extend from the surface of the brain into the parenchyma and can occur in the spinal cord.

C. Etiology of rupture.
Although distention leading to rupture of an AVM or saccular aneurysm often occurs at rest, the most clearly related predisposing factor appears to be an episode of increased blood pressure, which may occur with coughing, straining, coitus, defecation, lifting, or emotional stress.

D. Relation of pregnancy to rupture.
A clear correlation between pregnancy and rupture of saccular aneurysms or AVMs has not been established. Although some conclude that the association is merely coincidental, there is an increased incidence of rupture of saccular aneurysms in the thirtieth to fortieth gestational week and of AVMs during the second trimester, shortly before labor, during delivery, and in the early puerperium. Rupture of either aneurysms or AVMs can occur, however, at any time during gestation, labor, or delivery. Several physiologic factors may cause rupture during pregnancy. The cardiovascular stresses of increased cardiac output and increased blood volume and the hormonal changes affecting the connective tissue integrity of the vessel walls may all play contributory roles, but none has been proven or directly implicated.

E. Pathophysiology.
With rupture of AVMs or aneurysms, the sudden high-pressure leakage of blood raises the intracranial pressure (ICP) and can cause rapid brain displacement and death, coma, drowsiness, or merely headache, depending on the severity of the hemorrhage. The hemorrhage may remain subarachnoid or blood

may dissect into brain parenchyma, resulting in focal neurologic deficits. Parenchymal involvement is more common with AVMs than aneurysms. The blood and its breakdown products are irritants to meninges, blood vessels, and brain parenchyma. Meningeal irritation causes headache and sterile meningitis, which can lead to subacute or chronic communicating hydrocephalus. Brain irritation can evoke adverse descending autonomic discharges, causing hypertension or cardiac arrhythmias. Vasospasm, at least partially caused by the breakdown products of extravasated blood, can lead to ischemia or infarction with resulting neurologic deficits 5 to 7 days after the initial hemorrhage.

F. Prognosis. The prognosis after rupture of either a saccular aneurysm or AVM in pregnancy is comparable to nonpregnant patients. There is a high incidence of recurrent hemorrhage within the first few weeks, especially within the first 48 hours after the initial bleed. The overall mortality is higher in hemorrhages from saccular aneurysms than from AVMs, although there is increased neurologic disability among survivors of AVMs because of their location and tendency to bleed into brain tissue.

G. Diagnosis. The diagnosis of AVM (more often than aneurysm) can sometimes be made before rupture by history of severe headaches, seizures, bruits, cranial nerve palsies, or focal neurologic deficits. The presentation, however, is almost invariably SAH. The initial symptoms are abrupt onset of severe headache (usually described as bursting or explosive), photophobia, nuchal rigidity, diplopia, nausea, vomiting, disturbance of consciousness ranging from drowsiness or confusion to coma, seizures, migraines, bruits, and possibly focal or lateralizing neurologic signs.

  The diagnosis of SAH is made by history and physical examination and confirmed by computed tomographic (CT) scanning and grossly bloody or xanthochromic CSF (if sufficient time has elapsed for the blood to hemolyze after the rupture) at lumbar puncture. If there are lateralizing neurologic deficits or suspicion of increased ICP, the lumbar puncture should be deferred. The specific etiology is confirmed by angiography. Protective radiographic shielding for the fetus is important and should be used.

H. Differential diagnosis. The principal differential diagnosis is either fulminant toxemia of pregnancy, with or without intracerebral hemorrhage, or a cerebrovascular accident secondary to chronic hypertension. In fact, many patients with SAH are erroneously diagnosed and treated as toxemics. Hypertension, proteinuria, and either convulsions or coma can occur with both toxemia and SAH. Severe hypertension, generalized edema, and severe proteinuria are more often associated with toxemia, however. The headache of toxemia is usually frontal and boring or throbbing rather than explosive, and the epigastric pain sometimes seen with toxemia is not a symptom of SAH. Although unusually high blood pressure occurs more frequently with toxemia, the hemorrhage of a ruptured aneurysm or AVM may raise ICP, causing a reflex increase in blood pressure. Because of these similarities, early neurosurgical consultation is advised whenever toxemics present with unusual findings.

I. **Treatment.** Successful outcome requires aggressive and prompt investigation and treatment. The neurologic management of SAH in pregnancy is the same as that for the nonpregnant patient. The goals of treatment are (1) to preserve life, (2) to reduce disability, and (3) to prevent recurrent hemorrhage.

1. **Medical treatment.** The initial treatment is conservative.

   a. Avoid increase in blood pressure by the following measures:

      (1) Antihypertensives for hypertension caused by preexisting disease or secondary to the irritation from subarachnoid blood

      (2) Absolute bed rest in a dark, quiet room to avoid emotional excitement

      (3) Cautious use of sedatives to prevent excitement

      (4) Cautious use of analgesics

      (5) Stool softeners to avoid straining and Valsalva maneuver

   b. Administer steroids to reduce edema

   c. Administer antifibrinolytic agents (ϵ-aminocaproic acid) to inhibit lysis of the clot formed at the bleeding site to prevent rebleeding (see Chap. 8)

2. **Surgical treatment.** The decision to operate, as well as the timing of operation, are based on the site and surgical accessibility of the lesion, the patient's clinical condition, and the presence of vasospasm. These decisions should rarely, if ever, be influenced by pregnancy. Surgery reduces the mortality and incidence of recurrent hemorrhage from saccular aneurysms. The advantages of surgical resection and ligation of the feeding arteries of AVMs depend on the size and location. Alternative interventional therapy includes particulate embolization, obliteration with intravascular glue, and proton-beam irradiation.

III. **Physiologic changes of pregnancy and their anesthetic implications.** The particular hazards of anesthesia during pregnancy are related to the physiologic changes in the mother and to the possible adverse effects on the fetus. Hormonal secretions from the corpus leuteum and the placenta and mechanical effects of the gravid uterus induce major changes in practically every organ system. Familiarity with these alterations and their implications for anesthetic management is essential for the safest possible administration of anesthesia to the pregnant woman.

A. **Pulmonary changes**

   1. **Decreased functional residual capacity (FRC).** FRC is decreased 10% at 16 weeks' gestation and 20% at term, owing to an increase in tidal volume and a decrease in expiratory reserve volume in the face of unchanged total lung capacity.

   2. **Increased ventilation.** Alveolar ventilation is increased 25% at 16 weeks' gestation and 70% at term because of an increase in tidal volume with only small increases in respiratory rate. With this increased ventilation, normal $PaCO_2$ is decreased to 32 mmHg. Compensatory metabolic acidosis (bicarbonate reduced to 22 mEq/L) keeps maternal pH close to 7.4 units.

   3. **Increased oxygen consumption.** Oxygen consumption increases 20% from the development of the fetus, placenta, and uterus.

B. **Anesthetic implications of pulmonary changes**

   1. **Rapid inhalation induction.** With a decreased FRC and increased alveolar ventilation, the rapidity of induction with inhalation anesthetics is increased. This effect is partially balanced by an increase in cardiac output.

   2. **Decreased oxygen reserve.** A decreased FRC combined with increased oxygen consumption makes pregnant women more likely to become hypoxic in the face of respiratory obstruction or difficult intubation during the period of apnea. Rapid development of hypoxia is avoided by administering 100% oxygen before induction and intubation. Even during rapid intubation with only 30 seconds of apnea, PaO_2 can fall to 50 mmHg if preoxygenation is not performed.

C. **Cardiovascular changes**

   1. **Increased cardiac output.** Cardiac output increases 30% to 40% during the first trimester and remains elevated throughout

gestation. It increases even more during labor with painful uterine contractions and reaches its greatest increase (80% elevation) immediately after delivery. Despite this increase in cardiac output, there is normally no increase in blood pressure, indicating a decrease in peripheral vascular resistance.

2. **Increased blood volume.** Increases in maternal blood volume begin in the first trimester. The increase in plasma volume is greater than the increase in red blood cell (RBC) volume. This accounts for the relative anemia of pregnancy. At term, the RBC volume is increased about 20% and the plasma volume is increased about 40%.

3. **Supine hypotension.** When lying supine, pregnant women in the second and third trimesters may develop hypotension from aortocaval compression by the gravid uterus. Caval compression impedes venous return to the heart, which decreases cardiac output. Uterine blood flow decreases both from increased uterine venous pressure and, occasionally (in 10% of parturients), from uterine arterial hypotension. Direct compression of the aorta by the gravid uterus will directly decrease uterine blood flow. Anesthesia may augment these detrimental changes by mechanisms such as the vasodilatation produced by halothane and thiopental or the sympathectomy from regional epidural anesthesia, both of which reduce venous return to the heart. Therefore, it is important to avoid the supine position. For uterine displacement off the great vessels to prevent supine hypotension and uterine hypoperfusion, left lateral tilt should be employed during all anesthetic procedures.

D. **Gastrointestinal changes**

1. **Increased gastric acid production.** The hormone gastrin is produced by the placenta. Gastrin levels are elevated throughout pregnancy, with especially high levels occurring in the second and third trimesters. This hormone stimulates gastric acid and enzyme production.

2. **Gastroesophageal sphincter incompetence.** During pregnancy there is a shift in the position of the stomach due to the enlarging uterus, which changes the angle of the gastroesophageal junction and may permit passive regurgitation.

E. **Anesthetic implications of gastrointestinal changes.** With increased gastric acid production and compromise of the cardiac sphincter, the pregnant woman, when anesthetized, is more susceptible than her nonpregnant counterpart to regurgitation and aspiration of acidic gastric contents. Although the precise time in gestation when she is at greater risk is unknown, the gastric emptying time is significantly increased in pregnant women beyond 34 weeks gestation.

All pregnant women should receive 15 ml of 0.3 M sodium citrate before undergoing anesthesia. The safety and effectiveness of other drugs, such as metoclopramide and cimetidine, for reducing gastric volume and acidity are currently being investigated.

Airway protection using cuffed endotracheal tubes and rapid intubation with preoxygenation and cricoid pressure should be employed for women in the second half of pregnancy or anytime during pregnancy if the woman has symptoms of reflux esophagitis.

F. **Neurologic changes**

1. **Decreased inhalation anesthetic requirement.** The minimum alveolar concentration (MAC) of pregnant women is reduced 25% to 40%, which is possibly related to elevated endorphin levels.

2. **Decreased size of epidural and subarachnoid spaces.** With the increase in femoral venous and intra-abdominal pressures, the epidural veins are enlarged, decreasing the epidural space. This increased epidural pressure is transmitted to the subarachnoid space, decreasing the volume of CSF in the vertebral column. The CSF pressure is not elevated.

G. **Anesthetic implications of neurologic changes**

1. **Increased likelihood of inhalation anesthesia overdose.** With the decreased MAC, pregnant women are more sensitive to inhalation anesthetics. Concentrations that would otherwise be safe may produce overdose and cardiovascular depression.

2. **Decrease in epidural anesthetic requirements.** With the decrease in epidural space and CSF volume, there is a 30% decrease in the amount of local anesthetic required to produce a given level of epidural or subarachnoid block in parturients during the period from midpregnancy to term as compared to the nonpregnant patient.

H. **Renal and hepatic changes.** During pregnancy there is an increase in the renal plasma flow, glomerular filtration rate, and tubular reabsorption of water and electrolytes, with an increased creatinine clearance. Therefore, the normal BUN is 8–9 mg/100 ml, and the normal creatinine is 0.6 mg/100 ml, but electrolytes are unchanged.

Many liver enzymes are normally elevated during pregnancy, including SGOT, LDH, and alkaline phosphatase, although bilirubin levels and hepatic blood flow remain unchanged. There is a decrease in total protein and the albumin-globulin ratio. Serum cholinesterase is also decreased, which is usually clinically insignificant but may prolong the neuromuscular blockade of succinyl-choline.

I. Uterine blood flow. Uterine blood flow at term is about 700 ml/min, which is 10% of the maternal cardiac output. About 70% to 90% of the uterine blood flow perfuses the placenta and the rest supplies the myometrium. The uterine vascular bed, almost maximally dilated under normal conditions, has little capacity to dilate further. It is not autoregulated, so the uterine blood flow is proportional to the mean perfusion pressure. The uterine vessels are, however, capable of marked vasoconstriction.

J. Anesthetic implications of uterine blood flow. Reductions in uterine blood flow can cause serious fetal hypoxia with disasterous results. Uterine blood flow is significantly decreased by several factors relevant to the anesthesiologist.

    1. Hypotension

        a. Sympathetic blockade

        b. Hypovolemic shock

        c. Supine-hypotension syndrome

        d. Iatrogenic: Nitroprusside-induced hypotension or deep halothane anesthesia

    2. Vasoconstriction (increased uterine vascular resistance)

        a. Endogenous sympathetic discharge

        b. Essential hypertension

        c. Toxemia

        d. Exogenous alpha-adrenergic drugs (e.g., phenylephrine)

    3. Uterine contractions or hypertonus

    4. Excessive positive pressure ventilation (by decreasing venous return and cardiac output)

IV. Anesthesia for craniotomy during pregnancy. Anesthetic management of patients undergoing neurosurgical procedures is modified during pregnancy to protect the fetus (by avoiding asphyxia, teratogenicity, and preterm labor) and the mother.

A. Fetal considerations

1. **Avoidance of fetal asphyxia.** Fetal oxygenation is dependent on maternal arterial oxygen content and placental blood flow. Induced hypotension and hypocapnia are commonly employed during neurosurgery, but these techniques may affect the fetus adversely. Intrauterine fetal asphyxia is avoided by maintaining normal maternal PaO_2, $PaCO_2$, and uterine blood flow.

   The causes of maternal hypoxia during general anesthesia do not differ from those for any ventilated patient. Elevated maternal oxygen tensions that commonly occur during anesthesia are safe for the fetus. A rise of maternal PaO_2 even to 600 mmHg seldom produces a fetal PaO_2 above 45 mmHg and never above 60 mmHg. Thus, premature closure of the ductus arteriosus or retrolental fibroplasia cannot be produced in utero with normobaric maternal hyperoxia.

   Fetal $PaCO_2$ is directly related to maternal $PaCO_2$. Maternal hypercapnia will cause fetal respiratory acidosis. Maternal hypocapnia produced by excessive positive pressure ventilation may increase mean intrathoracic pressure, decrease venous return, and hence decrease cardiac output. This causes a fall in the uterine blood flow, which is deleterious to the fetus. Also, maternal alkalosis reduces umbilical blood flow by direct vasoconstriction, and shifts the oxyhemoglobin dissociation curve to the left. This shift increases the affinity of maternal hemoglobin for oxygen and decreases the release of oxygen to the fetus at the placenta. Thus, fetal hypoxia and acidosis can result from maternal hyperventilation.

   As uterine arterial blood flow is directly dependent on maternal blood pressure, maternal hypotension will cause a fall in uterine blood flow and may lead to asphyxia. A small fall in blood pressure with low concentrations of halothane is not associated with significant reduction of uterine blood flow because of the concomitant decrease in uterine vascular resistance. Deep halothane anesthesia that results in maternal hypotension (30% decrease from control) will, however, produce fetal asphyxia. Significant maternal hypotension should therefore be avoided or corrected promptly by administering fluids, reducing anesthetic concentration or, if necessary, administering an appropriate vasopressor (ephedrine).

2. **Avoidance of teratogenic drugs.** Teratogenicity may be induced at any stage of gestation by exogenous agents and detected at birth, or later. To produce a defect, the teratogenic agent must be given in an appropriate dose, during a particular

developmental stage of the embryo or fetus, in a species or individual who has a particular genetic susceptibility. Each organ and each system undergoes a critical stage of differentiation during which vulnerability to teratogens is greatest and specific malformations can be produced. In humans, the first trimester appears to be the most vulnerable period.

Almost all commonly used anesthetic and premedicant drugs have been shown to be teratogenic in some animal species. Also, in the experimental animal, hyperbaric oxygenation, hypoxia, and hypercapnia may be teratogenic. In several surveys of women who received anesthesia for operations during pregnancy, including the vulnerable first trimester, no drug has been shown to be safer than another, and no specific agent has been implicated as a teratogen. (Shnider and Webster, 1965; Smith, 1963.) These studies in humans are too small, however, to support a categorical statement that anesthetic drugs are *not* teratogenic. At this time, the choice of specific anesthetic agents for pregnant women undergoing neurosurgical procedures is not influenced by concerns of teratogenicity.

3. **Prevention of preterm labor.** There have been suggestions that abdominal operations during pregnancy may cause preterm labor during the postoperative period, and that anesthesia and surgery during pregnancy are associated with an increased risk of first and second trimester spontaneous abortions. Despite this, there is no association between neurosurgical procedures and preterm labor. It is unknown whether anesthetics can stimulate or inhibit preterm labor, but it is unlikely that preterm labor would begin during the neurosurgical intraoperative period. Patients should be monitored for uterine contractions intraoperatively and postoperatively for at least 24 hours. Early detection of preterm labor is important because effective drugs are available to inhibit labor and avoid premature delivery.

   Drugs that increase uterine tone such as alpha-adrenergic vasopressors should be avoided as should rapid intravenous administration of anticholinesterase drugs.

4. **Possible fetal complications of adjuvants to lower intracranial pressure.** Osmotic diuresis, controlled hypotension, hypothermia, and hypocapnia are commonly employed during neurosurgery. These adjuvants may, however, have adverse effects on the fetus. Special consideration must be given to the fetus in relation to the use of these techniques and adjuncts during the anesthetic course. Their use depends on the seriousness of the maternal impairment, and whether that im-

pairment will result in more severe fetal morbidity than the
morbidity associated with the therapy.

a. Osmotic diuretics. Osmotic diuretics (mannitol, urea)
used to reduce cerebral water content, have been shown to
traverse the placenta, raise the fetal plasma osmotic pressure,
and cause a net flow of water from the fetus to the mother.
This decreases fetal blood volume, total body water, and
extracellular fluid volume. Such fluid exchange can cause
severe fetal dehydration. Therefore, these drugs should only
be used when absolutely necessary during pregnancy.

b. Induced hypotension. Induced hypotension reduces cerebral bleeding and the likelihood of rupture of a saccular
aneurysm during surgical manipulation, but it can cause fetal
asphyxia with disastrous effects on the newborn. Although
there have been several successful cases reported using hypotensive techniques for craniotomies during pregnancy
(Wilson, 1959; Minielly, 1979), there have also been reports
of fetal demise or distress (based on fetal heart rate monitoring) (Robinson, 1972; Pevehouse, 1960). Further, the "success" reported has often been a living fetus or live birth with
neither follow-up nor assessment of neurologic status.

(1) Fetal asphyxia. The hazard to the fetus depends on the
severity and duration of maternal hypotension. Fetal risk
is directly related to uterine blood flow, which varies
directly with maternal blood pressure. When uterine
blood flow is reduced sufficiently, fetal asphyxia results.
Fetal asphyxia is most damaging to the central nervous
system, heart, and lungs. In experimental fetal monkeys
who sustained fetal asphyxia of intermediate severity
and duration with consequent acidosis, permanent brain
injury occurred, with lesions similar to those of human
cerebral palsy (Brann, 1975). Severe asphyxia produces
fetal death from myocardial failure.

(2) Hypotensive drugs. The drugs commonly used to induce hypotension are halothane, nitroprusside, nitroglycerin, and trimethaphan. Regardless of which drugs
are used, the reduced maternal blood pressure may lead
to fetal asphyxia.

(a)   Halothane. Light halothane anesthesia is not associated with significant reductions in uterine
blood flow because of concomitant decreases in

uterine vascular resistance. High concentrations of halothane anesthesia that depress myocardial contractility and produce significant hypotension cause a fall in uterine blood flow and, consequently, fetal asphyxia.

(b) Nitroprusside. Nitroprusside, the most widely used drug for inducing hypotension, carries the potential hazard of fetal toxicity. The placenta is readily permeable to nitroprusside. It is degraded to cyanide, which is transformed to thiocyanate by the liver enzyme rhodonase. In experimental animals, peak fetal arterial cyanide levels have been shown to be significantly higher than maternal levels. This may be due to either more rapid formation of cyanide or a slower rate of detoxification and excretion by the fetus. Although several patients have received nitroprusside for acute treatment of systemic and pulmonary hypertension without adverse effects on the fetus, nitroprusside administration should be limited to small doses for short periods of time.

(c) Nitroglycerin. Although there have been recent case reports involving the use of nitroglycerin during pregnancy, no studies of its placental transfer or the fetal effects are available. However, no adverse fetal or neonatal effects have been observed in the few cases reported to date.

(d) Trimethaphan. Pregnant women have a greater reaction to ganglionic blockade, as with trimethaphan, than nonpregnant women. The hypotensive effect of autonomic blockade in supine pregnant women depends mainly upon venous pooling of blood with decreased return to the heart and a consequent diminution of cardiac output. Autonomic blockade prevents the increased neurogenic tone of the capacitance vessels that ordinarily compensates for the interference with venous return from uterine compression.

(3) Monitoring. When it is necessary to induce hypotension, blood pressure reduction should be limited in depth and duration to the minimum required, based on clinical judgment, and fetal heart rate should be closely monitored. Fetal tolerance will depend on fetoplacental reserve. Maternal arterial pH should be measured frequently to avoid potentially severe fetal toxicity.

c. **Hypocapnia.** Extreme maternal hyperventilation may result in a reduction of uterine blood flow, a fall in placental oxygen transfer, a fall in fetal PO_2, anaerobic metabolism, and fetal metabolic acidosis. In theory, hyperventilation should therefore be avoided. Mild hyperventilation is probably safe, however, especially if the fetal heart rate is monitored for adverse effects. Some fetuses that have good reserve will not become acidotic because of anaerobic metabolism. Fetuses in borderline or in precarious situations, however, may react adversely to even mild degrees of maternal hyperventilation. The normal $PaCO_2$ in pregnant women is 32 mmHg, with a pH of 7.4 units. Hyperventilation to decrease $PaCO_2$ to 20 mmHg is most likely safe and easily reversible if fetal tachycardia or bradycardia indicates fetal intolerance. As with induced hypotension, the use of hyperventilation should be limited in extent and duration to the minimum required, based on clinical judgment.

d. **Hypothermia.** Moderate hypothermia (temperatures of 28–32°C), properly used, decreases cerebral oxygen demand and reduces blood flow to the brain. If maternal respiratory acidosis is prevented, the gas and acid-base contents of fetal blood will parallel those of the mother. Although uterine vascular resistance increases and uteroplacental blood flow falls during hypothermia, oxygen transfer is unaffected. Since the fetus also becomes hypothermic, its metabolic needs are proportionately decreased. Hypothermia as an ancillary aid to intracranial surgery does not increase fetal morbidity, which is substantiated by many case reports (Kamrin, 1965).

5. **Monitoring during craniotomy.** Besides the usual monitors for major neurosurgical procedures (intra-arterial catheter, Doppler air-embolism monitor, and right atrial catheter), the fetus and uterus should be monitored when a pregnant woman undergoes craniotomy. After the sixteenth week of pregnancy, the external Doppler fetal heart rate monitor should be employed. Monitoring fetal heart rate provides an indication of abnormalities in maternal ventilation or uterine perfusion, as well as fetal well-being. Careful observation of the maternal blood pressure and prompt correction of hypotension and hypoxia are mandatory if the fetus is to have the best chance of survival with an intact nervous system.

Anesthetics that readily traverse the placenta diminish the

normal beat-to-beat variability of the fetal heart rate. During induced hypothermia, the fall in fetal heart rate parallels the decrease in maternal heart rate. Patterns of bradycardia are, however, associated predominantly with maternal hypotension or hypoxia and, as such, are valuable for diagnosis. The relationship between maternal hypotension and fetal bradycardia is well known in obstetrics. A maternal systolic blood pressure of less than 100 mmHg may be associated with pathologic fetal bradycardia, which begins a few minutes after the onset of the hypotension, and is sometimes preceded by mild fetal tachycardia. Fetal tachycardia has also been recognized as an early sign of maternal hypoxia in the third trimester of pregnancy and of fetal distress in the full-term infant.

Additionally, an external tocodynamometer to monitor uterine tone is indicated if the uterine fundus is above the level of the umbilicus.

B. Preanesthetic visit. The preanesthetic visit, an essential part of each patient's preparation and assessment before operation, includes attention to physical examination, history, laboratory findings, and consultants' reports. Special efforts should be made to decrease the patient's apprehension by providing reassurance and emotional support. Maternal stress and anxiety are associated with increased release of endogenous catecholamines, which decreases uterine blood flow. These women are concerned not only for their own welfare, but for that of their unborn child. The anesthesiologist should convey optimism about both maternal and fetal prognosis and reassure the mother that the welfare of the baby will be considered at all times.

C. Premedication. Heavy sedation is contraindicated because of possible respiratory depression, potential exacerbation of depressed consciousness, and delayed postoperative recovery of consciousness. Preoperative sedation may be omitted in most cases with increased safety for the patient. If some sedation is necessary, pentobarbital, 50 to 100 mg IM, is preferred to benzodiazepines, phenothiazines, or narcotics. All patients should receive an oral antacid 30 to 60 minutes before induction to reduce gastric acidity.

D. Transport and positioning. Beginning in the second trimester, women must not be transported or positioned on the surgical table in a supine or prone position. They should either be placed in a sitting or lateral decubitus position. Proper positioning will minimize the risk of obstruction of the vena cava by displacing the gravid uterus off the great vessels. The legs should be wrapped in elastic bandages and placed at the level of the heart to facilitate venous return from the lower extremities. The eyes should be protected with a small amount of protective eye ointment, tape, and patches.

E. Induction and intubation. Induction of anesthesia with intravenous drugs, followed by immediate endotracheal intubation, is performed with standard rapid-sequence technique to establish an airway and protect the patient from possible regurgitation and aspiration. This is essential for pregnant women whose gestation is greater than 20 weeks and for all women who have a history of gastric reflux.

The rapid-sequence intravenous induction and endotracheal intubation, commonly performed for women undergoing cesarean section, is acceptable for the neurosurgical patient provided she is adequately anesthetized before laryngoscopy. Succinylcholine after pretreatment with a nondepolarizing drug will not itself raise the ICP. Laryngoscopy and intubation in a lightly anesthetized patient will cause hypertension, but a large dose of thiopental ameliorates this response. Additionally, the use of nitroprusside to achieve a stable, modest blood pressure reduction (15%–20%) during the few minutes prior to induction will blunt the hypertensive response from the rapid-sequence intravenous induction. The technique is as follows:

1. Induce a stable, modest blood pressure reduction (15%–20%) with nitroprusside, using an infusion pump and direct arterial pressure monitoring.

2. Administer 100% oxygen for at least 3 minutes to avoid maternal hypoxia during intubation.

3. Administer *d*-tubocurarine, 3 mg IV, to prevent fasciculations and the rise in intragastric pressure associated with succinylcholine. Reassure the patient that she and the fetus are both doing well. Wait 3 to 5 minutes, continuing preoxygenation.

4. Apply pressure over cricoid cartilage to occlude the esophagus and prevent passive regurgitation (Sellick maneuver). This pressure should be applied by an assistant until the trachea is successfully intubated and the endotracheal tube cuff is inflated.

5. Administer thiopental, 4 to 5 mg/kg IV, to conscious patients (less thiopental required for patients with altered states of consciousness) *and* administer succinylcholine, 100 mg IV, followed by a 60- to 90-second pause, during which positive pressure ventilation by mask is avoided.

6. Intubate the trachea with a cuffed endotracheal tube, using a stylet.

7. Inflate the cuff immediately after the trachea is intubated.

8. Control the ventilation, and undertake maneuvers to ensure correct endotracheal tube placement.

9. Stop the nitroprusside infusion.

F. **Maintenance of anesthesia.** Fifty percent nitrous oxide with 50% oxygen supplemented by intravenous thiopental, narcotics, and neuromuscular blocking drugs will be adequate for positioning and placement of the pin headholder. Once adequate hyperventilation has been assured by blood gas determination, anesthesia can be supplemented by the addition of low concentrations of halothane, enflurane, or isoflurane.

G. **Postoperative management.** The postoperative management of a pregnant woman after craniotomy involves only a few modifications from that of her nonpregnant counterpart.

1. **Extubation.** Although smooth emergence and extubation are ideal, extubation should be delayed until the patient is sufficiently awake to protect her airway from regurgitation and aspiration of gastric contents.

2. **Position.** Maintenance of left uterine displacement is important to avoid supine hypotension from compression of the great vessels by the gravid uterus. The patient should be maintained in a lateral position, with the head slightly elevated, during the entire postoperative period (including transport from the operating room to the recovery area).

3. **Monitoring.** The fetal heart rate and uterine tone should be monitored for at least 24 hours, or until the mother's condition is stable. Maternal hypotension, hypertension, or respiratory depression may have adverse effects on the fetus as well as the mother. Efforts should be made to avoid these complications. If they do occur, they should be promptly investigated, diagnosed, and aggressively treated.

V. **Obstetric management and anesthesia for vaginal delivery or cesarean section.** For the patient who has a documented saccular aneurysm or AVM, whether ruptured or unruptured, surgically or conservatively treated, elective cesarean section is not necessarily warranted since it affords no advantage over vaginal delivery in protecting against intracerebral hemorrhage. Cesarean section should be performed only for accepted obstetric indications. If labor supervenes after SAH, vaginal or even abdominal delivery should be considered before neurosurgical intervention. This decision is affected by the severity of the maternal clinical condition, the feasibility of stopping preterm labor, and the maturity of the fetus.

Management of labor and delivery in women who have documented aneurysms, AVMs, or intracranial tumors (especially tumors that have not been surgically treated) includes avoidance of hypertension and increased ICP. The second stage of labor should be shortened and maternal straining should be avoided. Maternal straining with the Valsalva maneuver raises both the intracranial and CSF pressures. After the Valsalva maneuver, there is an immediate reduction in CSF pressure but an increase in cardiac output and blood pressure owing to increased venous return to the heart. The net effect on transmural pressure of cerebral vessels from the Valsalva maneuver is not precisely known. Until cerebral hemodynamics during labor are better understood, it is best to avoid Valsalva maneuvers in women who have increased ICP or cerebrovascular disease to reduce the possibility of herniation of the brain or rupture of tenuous cerebral vessels.

Shortening the second stage of labor and avoiding maternal straining can be best achieved by segmental lumbar epidural or caudal anesthesia and the elective application of outlet forceps for delivery. A properly administered epidural block for labor will (1) decrease pain and prevent the increased blood pressure and cardiac output from painful contractions, (2) avoid the Valsalva maneuver by blocking the reflex urge to bear down, and (3) allow painless and easy application of forceps. There is an obvious risk of lumbar epidural techniques in these women because of inadvertent dural puncture. A sudden leakage of CSF can result in cerebral herniation. Consequently, this technique should only be performed by a skilled anesthesiologist. There is a somewhat reduced likelihood of dural puncture with the caudal approach to the epidural space.

Alternate forms of analgesia include paracervical and pudendal blocks, inhalation analgesia and systemic narcotics. These techniques are not as effective as epidural anesthesia. Also, administration of narcotics and inhalation agents during spontaneous ventilation may raise $PaCO_2$, increase cerebral blood flow, raise ICP, and induce maternal respiratory acidosis. If general anesthesia is necessary for either vaginal delivery or manual removal of the placenta, the anesthetic considerations and techniques for induction and intubation discussed in section **V** should be employed.

Low spinal anesthesia is contraindicated in patients who have intracranial hypertension. For women who have aneurysms or AVMs, a reduction in CSF pressure might increase the transmural pressure (MAP-ICP) in the aneurysm and the risk of aneurysm rupture (see Chap. 8).

Should a cesarean section be required, epidural anesthesia with a sensory level of T4 is recommended. However, if general anesthesia is indicated, the considerations and techniques discussed in section **V** are applicable.

After successful surgical occlusion of an aneurysm or AVM, there appears to be no need for specialized management of labor and delivery. Even elective induction of labor employing an oxytocic agent is not contraindicated. Considering that the reported incidence of aneurysms is 0.5% to 1%, a large number of women who have this vascular anomaly must go through labor and delivery without undue difficulty.

References

1. Brann, A. W., and Myers, R. E. Central nervous system findings in the newborn monkey following severe in utero partial asphyxia. *Neurology* 25:329, 1975.
2. Bruns, P. D., Linder, R. O., Drose, V. E., and Battaglia, F. The placental transfer of water from fetus to mother following the intravenous infusion of hypertonic mannitol to the maternal rabbit. *Am. J. Obstet. Gynecol.* 86:160, 1963.
3. Hehre, F. W. Hypothermia for operations during pregnancy. *Anesth. Analg.* (Cleve.) 44:424, 1965.
4. Hunt, H. B., Schifrin, B. S., and Suzuki, K. Ruptured berry aneurysms and pregnancy. *Obstet. Gynecol.* 43:827, 1974.
5. Kamrin, R. P., and Masland, W. Intracranial surgery under hypothermia during pregnancy. *Arch. Neurol.* 13:70, 1965.
6. Miller, H. J., and Hinkley, C. M. Berry aneurysms in pregnancy: A ten year report. *South Med. J.* 63:279, 1970.
7. Minielly, R., Yuzpe, A. A., and Drake, C. G. Subarachnoid hemorrhage secondary to ruptured cerebral aneurysm in pregnancy. *Obstet. Gynecol.* 53:64, 1979.
8. Naulty, J., Cefalo, R. C., and Lewis, P. E. Fetal toxicity of nitroprusside in the pregnant ewe. *Am. J. Obstet. Gynecol.* 139:708, 1981.
9. Pevehouse, B. C., and Boldrey, E. Hypothermia and hypotension for intracranial surgery during pregnancy. *Am. J. Surg.* 100:633, 1960.
10. Ring, G., Krames, E., Shnider, S. M., and Levinson, G. Comparison of nitroprusside and hydralazine in hypertensive pregnant ewes. *Obstet. Gynecol.* 50:598, 1977.
11. Robinson, J. L., Chir, B., Hall, C. J., and Sedzimir, C. B. Subarachnoid hemorrhage in pregnancy. *J. Neurosurg.* 36:27, 1972.
12. Shnider, S. M., and Levinson, G. Anesthesia for operations during pregnancy. In S. M. Shnider and G. Levinson (eds.), *Anesthesia for Obstetrics.* Baltimore: Williams & Wilkins, 1979. Pp. 312–330.
13. Shnider, S. M., and Webster, G. M. Maternal and fetal hazards of surgery during pregnancy. *Am. J. Obstet. Gynecol.* 92:891, 1965.
14. Smith, B. E. Fetal prognosis after anesthesia during gestation. *Anesth. Analg.* (Cleve.) 42:521, 1963.
15. Vandewater, S. L., and Paul, W. M. Observations on the foetus during experimental hypothermia. *Can. Anaesth. Soc. J.* 7:44, 1960.
16. Wilson, F., and Sedzimir, C. B. Hypothermia and hypotension during craniotomy in the pregnant woman. *Lancet* 2:947, 1959.

11. Posterior Fossa Procedures

Robert F. Bedford

I. Physiologic considerations

A. Brainstem considerations

1. Within the posterior fossa, the pons and medulla contain the major motor and sensory pathways, the primary respiratory and cardiovascular centers, and the lower cranial nerve nuclei. Because of the posterior fossa's small size, a localized lesion or a small amount of edema may have profound neurologic effects.

2. Patients who have posterior fossa lesions have decreased levels of consciousness, increased sensitivity to sedative medications, depressed respiration, and impaired airway protective reflexes, all of which must be carefully considered throughout the perioperative period.

3. Posterior fossa operations are complicated by fluctuations in heart rate and blood pressure. Meticulous cardiovascular monitoring is therefore required during operation and in the postoperative period.

B. Obstructive hydrocephalus and increased intracranial pressure.
Exploration of the posterior fossa is frequently performed in the presence of obstruction of cerebrospinal fluid (CSF) outflow at the level of the fourth ventricle from compression by tumor or cyst. Continued production of CSF by the choroid plexus of the lateral ventricles causes intracranial hypertension. When intracranial pressure (ICP) is increased further by volatile anesthetics or arterial hypertension, herniation of brain contents may result, causing potentially fatal brainstem compression. Signs of increased ICP must be sought constantly and techniques for prompt decompression must be available.

II. Preoperative evaluation

A. Patient history

1. Headache, vomiting, and lethargy are indicative of **intracranial hypertension** and often subside after corticosteroid therapy. If signs of intracranial hypertension persist, a ventriculostomy drainage tube or ICP monitor should be placed preoperatively under local anesthesia before general anesthesia is induced.

2. A history of a recent preoperative **air-contrast study** should be sought, since residual air may take up to a week to reabsorb. Nitrous oxide (N_2O) inhalation will expand the volume of residual intracranial air and thus increase ICP.

3. The patient's **sensitivity to general anesthetics** can be estimated from his reponse to sedative medications if they were used for preoperative neuroradiologic procedures. Prolonged somnolence after sedatives usually indicates a decrease in intraoperative anesthetic requirement.

B. **Physical examination**

1. **Intravascular volume depletion** often occurs during an extensive period of neurologic diagnosis. Somnolence may limit fluid intake, bed rest causes supine diuresis, and these patients often develop vomiting. Flat neck veins and poor tissue turgor indicate the need for vigorous preoperative volume replacement.

2. **Vascular sites** for monitoring catheters require evaluation. Allen's test for ulnar-artery collateral blood flow to the hand should be performed before radial artery cannulation, and suitable sites for peripheral and central venous catheters must be sought. Increased ICP from head-down positioning and decreased cerebral venous outflow can be avoided if antecubital veins are used instead of the jugular or subclavian route.

3. **Preoperative papilledema** confirms the diagnosis of increased ICP and limited intracranial compliance. If papilledema disappears after corticosteroid therapy, improved intracranial compliance can be anticipated.

4. Preoperative **pulmonary function** should be evaluated. Impaired consciousness and protective reflexes may have allowed "silent" aspiration to occur. Previously undiagnosed pulmonary dysfunction may present as intraoperative hypoxia and may be life-threatening if combined with uncontrolled hemorrhage during surgery.

5. Evaluation of **concurrent cardiovascular disease** is important. Patients who have limited myocardial reserve or cerebrovascular insufficiency should be considered for operation in the prone or lateral decubitus position rather than risking cardiovascular instability in the seated position.

C. **Medications.** High-potency corticosteroids reduce edema around brain tumors and frequently cause marked preoperative neurologic improvement. The potential complications of hyperglycemia and electrolyte disturbances must be evaluated, and plans for continued perioperative steroid and diuretic therapy formulated.

III. Intraoperative considerations

A. Choice of anesthetic

1. The use of **nitrous oxide and oxygen in combination with narcotic and muscle relaxant** has minimal effect on cerebral blood flow and ICP, yet it allows maximal cardiovascular stability during postural changes. This technique is preferred for most patients who have space-occupying lesions undergoing operations in the seated position.

2. **Volatile drugs** may be used in patients who have normal intracranial dynamics for nerve root section, microvascular decompression, or electrode implantation. Patients who have obstructive pulmonary disease or coronary artery disease may require volatile anesthetics. An ICP monitor should be placed before induction of anesthesia to facilitate titration of volatile drugs; cerebral perfusion pressure (CPP) can be maintained through hyperventilation and other measures to control ICP.

B. Monitoring

1. **Direct arterial pressure monitoring** is extremely useful during posterior fossa exploration in the seated position. An estimate of CPP can be obtained by placing the pressure transducer at head level, and sudden cardiovascular changes can be observed on a beat-to-beat basis. Furthermore, correlation of pulse-pressure waveforms with electrocardiogram (ECG) patterns allows instant recognition of the hemodynamic impact of arrhythmias caused by brainstem or cranial nerve stimulation.

2. **Right atrial and pulmonary artery pressure monitoring** afford means for diagnosis and recovery of intravenous air and also reflect cardiac preload. Although insertion of flow-directed balloon-tip catheters requires added time and effort, several centers now use them routinely. However, most institutions still prefer right atrial catheterization with ECG or x-ray confirmation of the position of the tip.

3. **Precordial Doppler monitoring** is virtually mandatory. The probe is affixed along the right sternal border between the third and sixth intercostal spaces. Proper positioning over the right atrium is confirmed by eliciting a change in Doppler signal when a 10-ml bolus of saline is injected rapidly into the right atrial catheter.

4. **End-tidal CO_2 analysis** complements the capabilities of the Doppler device, since small, hemodynamically insignificant air

emboli heard with the Doppler device can be differentiated from emboli that may produce arterial hypotension. Capnography is almost as sensitive as pulmonary artery pressure monitoring but has the added advantage of being noninvasive. Initial cost, however, ranges from $2000 to $7000.

5. **Neuromuscular transmission** requires monitoring during posterior fossa surgery, particularly if there is a possibility that the patient will cough or strain during the light levels of anesthesia occasionally required for the seated position to prevent cardiovascular instability.

6. Knowledge of **urinary output** is necessary as an indicator of perioperative fluid balance. During craniotomy the initial diuresis is frequently augmented by osmotic or loop diuretics. Urine output, however, may be reduced by either hypovolemia or release of antidiuretic hormone (ADH).

C. Position

1. **The seated position** affords access to the apex of the posterior fossa and facilitates exploration and dissection because blood and CSF drain away from the surgical site. In addition, it is possible to observe the airway and to note the response to cranial nerve stimulation.

2. **Cardiovascular instability** is the primary disadvantage of the seated position. General anesthesia and positive pressure breathing reduce blood pressure mainly by reducing cardiac output. These effects are augmented as patients are placed in the seated position since venous return is impeded. Vigorous volume replacement with balanced salt solutions, wrapping the legs with ace bandages, and keeping the knees flexed at heart level are all techniques that promote venous return and maintain cardiac output (Fig. 11-1). Although blood pressure at the level of the heart may be normal, it is crucial to remember that mean arterial pressure (MAP) at the level of the head is significantly lower in the seated position.

3. **Positional complications**

   a. Hyperflexion of the neck causes **jugular venous obstruction,** which can result in increased ICP and a "tight" posterior fossa. Swelling of the face and tongue will also occur. Excessive neck flexion may cause **quadraplegia** from ischemia of the cervical spine (Hitselberger, 1980). Placing two fingers between the chin and suprasternal notch while the patient's head is being fixed in position in the headholder is

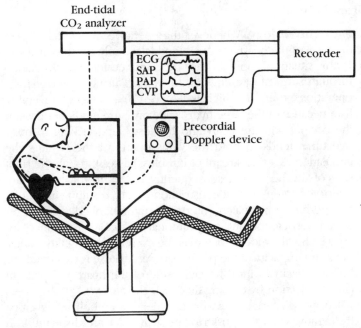

Fig. 11-1. Diagrammatic representation of patient properly positioned for seated posterior fossa operation with knees at heart level and neck not hyperflexed. Monitoring devices are discussed in text. ECG = electrocardiogram; SAP = systemic arterial pressure; PAP = pulmonary artery pressure; CVP = central venous pressure.

a simple method for preventing neck hyperflexion and its attendant complications.

b. Ulnar nerve compression may occur at the elbow if the ulnar groove is in contact with either the edge of the operating table or the arm boards. The ulnar grooves can remain free of pressure if the forearms are crossed over the abdomen and affixed with 4-inch-wide tape running from one elbow to the other. Padding the elbows also minimizes compression.

c. Sciatic nerve damage may be induced by severe flexion of the hips while the knees are held straight. Although optimal venous return to the heart occurs with the knees at heart level, it is best to flex the knees in order to reduce tension on the sciatic nerve.

d. Lateral peroneal nerve compression may occur from pressure from the headrest brackets near the lateral aspect of the knees. Liberal padding should be applied at this point to avoid contact with metal supports.

D. Air embolism

1. **Pathophysiology.** Whenever the operative site is higher than the level of the heart, venous blood falls freely past the incision. In this situation, room air may be entrained into the circulation through surgical openings in the veins. During posterior fossa operations, there is a high incidence (30%–50%) of air embolism because of the large hydrostatic pressure gradient between the occiput and the heart and because dural tacking to bony structures tends to hold the veins open. Air then enters the circulation as a fine stream of bubbles, passes through the right side of the heart, and subsequently lodges in the pulmonary arterioles. Intensive vasoconstriction occurs, resulting in ventilation-perfusion mismatch, interstitial pulmonary edema, and reduced cardiac output as pulmonary vascular resistance increases. Small amounts of air can be excreted through the lungs, but as the capacity of the pulmonary vasculature is exceeded, air bubbles back up into the right side of the heart and prevent cardiac ejection by causing an "air lock" effect.

   During posterior fossa procedures, air embolism develops frequently when the posterior neck muscles are dissected free from the subocciput, when bone is excised, and when a vascular tumor bed is entered. Particular vigilance is necessary at these times so that the surgeon can be alerted to the presence of air embolism and can take appropriate measures to stop entrainment of air.

2. **Diagnosis**

   a. The most sensitive method for detecting air embolism is by monitoring the signal of a 2-Hz precordial **Doppler ultrasound probe** placed over the right atrium. Air bubbles as small as 0.1 ml elicit a distinctive change in Doppler frequency since they reflect the ultrasound beam more effectively than erythrocytes when they pass through the right side of the heart. The Doppler device is not foolproof, however, since it cannot accurately quantitate the volume of air passing through the heart. Conversely, the Doppler may fail to detect a very fine stream of air bubbles or its position may shift during a long operation. It is most effective when used in conjunction with at least one other modality for detection of air embolism.

   b. **Infrared end-tidal CO_2 analysis** is less sensitive than is Doppler monitoring, but does permit quantification of the severity of an air embolus. When enough air has entered the circulation to produce pulmonary vasoconstriction, wasted

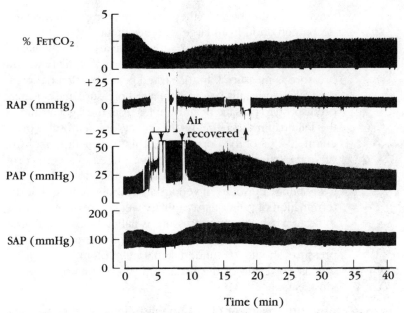

Fig. 11-2. Record of air embolism occurring during posterior fossa exploration. Concomitant with a modest reduction in systemic arterial pressure (SAP) is a marked increase in pulmonary artery pressure (PAP), a fall in end-tidal CO_2 fraction ($FETCO_2$), and a slight increase in right atrial pressure (RAP). Breaks in RAP and PAP traces indicate where a small volume of air (5–10 ml total) was recovered from both the right atrium and pulmonary artery.

ventilation increases and end-tidal CO_2 concentration promptly decreases in proportion. False-positive diagnoses are possible, however, since an abrupt decrease in cardiac output (as caused by an arrhythmia or brainstem compression) will also decrease end-tidal CO_2 and may be misinterpreted as an air embolus (Fig. 11-2).

c. **Pulmonary artery pressure monitoring** affords positive diagnosis of air embolism and also quantifies its severity, since pulmonary artery pressure increases proportionally with the volume of air embolized. Pulmonary artery pressure is not readily affected by sudden changes in cardiac output unless associated with acute left ventricular failure. Pulmonary artery catheters also allow recovery of air from both the pulmonary artery and right atrium, although recovery is rarely necessary if the diagnosis of air embolism is made early and prompt surgical correction is undertaken. Late signs of air embolism, such as premature ventricular beats, a mill-wheel murmur, or systemic hypotension, are of little diagnostic value because they reflect ongoing cardiovascular decompensation from large volumes of air.

Pulmonary artery pressure monitoring also affords an estimate of left atrial pressure when pulmonary capillary wedge pressure is measured. In the seated position, left atrial pressure frequently falls below right atrial pressure and this may predispose to passage of air bubbles from the right atrium to the left atrium through a probe-patent foramen ovale (present in 20-25% of the population). This arterial air embolism, or "paradoxical air embolism," has resulted in severe coronary and cerebral ischemic complications following relatively minor episodes of venous air embolism. Frequent determination of pulmonary capillary wedge pressure can thus indicate when left atrial pressure is falling below right atrial pressure and when measures that will elevate left atrial pressure should be undertaken (e.g., volume loading or gradual lowering of the head of the operating table) (Perkins-Pearson, 1982).

3. **Treatment.** Treatment of air embolism must be directed first at stopping further entrainment of air. The incision should be packed with soaked sponges and the bone edges should be waxed. Compression of the neck veins may be performed to increase venous pressure, temporarily slow air entry, and demonstrate the bleeding site. N_2O must be discontinued promptly so that embolized air bubbles do not expand. Recovery of air from the right side of the heart or pulmonary artery is accomplished by aspirating the mixture of blood and air from the right atrial or pulmonary artery catheter. Systemic hypotension responds readily to ephedrine, 10 to 15 mg IV, but is rarely needed if a prompt diagnosis is made and appropriate surgical intervention is conducted. If arterial hypotension persists, the head of the operating table should be lowered. With increased venous pressure, not only does entrainment of air stop, but active bleeding can indicate where air is entering the circulation and these sites can be cauterized and sealed. The use of 10 cm of positive endexpiratory pressure (PEEP) is not effective in the acute treatment of air embolism.

E. **Cardiovascular changes.** Surgical manipulation near the brainstem and cranial nerves often causes abrupt fluctuations in blood pressure and heart rate. Stimulation of the fifth cranial nerve, the periventricular gray area, the medullary reticular formation, or the nucleus of the tractus solitarius may produce arterial hypertension, whereas stimulation of the vagus nerve causes bradycardia. Compression of the medulla and pons results in sudden arterial hypotension. Differentiating arterial hypotension from an air embolus not heard with a Doppler may be difficult in the absence of pulmonary artery pressure monitoring.

F. **Fluid management.** Since formation of edema at the operative site is potentially fatal, patients should receive balanced salt solution replacement only in volumes compatible with hemodynamic stability. Blood loss is replaced with 5% albumin solution, blood, or both, depending on the hematocrit. Since blood loss may be massive and temporarily uncontrollable, routine use of 2 large-bore peripheral intravenous routes is recommended.

IV. Anesthetic management

A. Induction sequence

1. General anesthesia is induced with thiopental (2 to 4 mg/kg IV), and airway patency is assured by positive pressure ventilation with oxygen by a bag and mask. Pancuronium, 0.1 mg/kg IV, is given and N_2O (50–70% in oxygen) is added if no recent air-contrast study has been done. If N_2O cannot be used, then low concentrations of volatile anesthetic and oxygen are employed. Controlled hyperventilation is maintained until total neuromuscular blockade is observed.

2. Before endotracheal intubation, lidocaine, 1.5 mg/kg IV, and additional thiopental, 2 to 3 mg/kg IV, are given. Laryngoscopy is begun just as arterial pressure begins to decrease in response to these drugs. This, in turn, minimizes the increase that often occurs in both arterial and intracranial pressures after endotracheal intubation.

3. After endotracheal intubation, an esophageal stethoscope and thermister are introduced, the eyes are taped closed, and the endotracheal tube is secured with liberal amounts of adhesive tape.

B. The seated position

1. **Before positioning,** the legs are wrapped from toes to groin with ace bandages, and a urinary catheter is inserted. The operating table is slowly maneuvered into a semiseated position with the patient's hips and knees flexed, legs elevated, and knees at heart level. Both arterial and ICP transducers are secured at head level to verify adequate CPP. The forearms are crossed over the abdomen and secured with tape.

2. If a **pin headholder** is to be used, additional thiopental and lidocaine should first be given to prevent intracranial hyperten-

sion as the pins are secured in the skull. As the head is positioned, care must be taken to avoid hyperflexion of the neck, and the eyes must be checked to ensure that there is no external pressure being applied from the headrest. Once the headrest is in place, the endotracheal tube and circle absorber hoses can be suspended from the headrest bracket to avoid traction on the airway.

3. **After the patient has been placed in the seated position,** the precordial Doppler can be placed over the right atrium and the capnograph line inserted into the endotracheal tube. Care must be taken to avoid skin burns from patient contact with the capnography head, which becomes quite hot with prolonged use.

4. **Once cardiovascular stability has been achieved** in the seated position, the level of anesthesia may be deepened with judicious doses of narcotics or volatile agents (ideally with an ICP monitor in use) before the skin incision. Many prefer to discontinue N_2O immediately before the skin incision is made in an effort to prevent an increase in size of any air emboli that may occur. Intravenous drugs, such as barbiturates, diazepam, and droperidol, should be used with caution, however, since prolonged somnolence may make postoperative neurologic assessment more difficult.

C. Ventilation

1. **Ventilation is controlled** throughout posterior fossa procedures to maintain modest hypocapnia. Changes in blood pressure, heart rate, or both are used as an indication of brainstem ischemia or harmful manipulation. A minority of clinicians believe that changes in depth, pattern, or frequency of respiration during spontaneous ventilation are a more sensitive indicator of brainstem involvement than are cardiovascular changes. The risks of hypercapnia or coughing during operation, however, contraindicate this technique.

2. The patient's requirement for **postoperative mechanical ventilation** should be assessed before the end of the procedure. In general, with patients who have had minimally traumatic procedures, such as microvascular nerve-root decompression, the trachea can be extubated at the conclusion of the operation. Conversely, patients who have had extensive posterior fossa exploration and possible damage to respiratory centers or protective reflex pathways should be observed until they are fully awake. Extubation is then performed only when they are able to breathe and cough adequately.

D. Fluid and medication management

1. Maintenance **IV fluid requirements** during operation are met with balanced salt solutions with dextrose. If cardiovascular instability is associated with either low cardiac filling pressures or poor urinary output, then 5% albumin, whole blood, or both are used for intravascular volume expansion.

2. Patients who are receiving **corticosteroids** preoperatively receive a constant infusion of dexamethasone, 4 mg/kg, throughout the procedure. Mannitol, 0.25 to 0.5 gm/kg, or furosemide, 20 to 40 mg, are given if needed to reduce brain bulk once the craniectomy has been performed.

3. **Serum electrolytes and glucose** are determined every few hours during operation, since hyperventilation and diuretics can profoundly alter sodium and potassium levels and steroid therapy may cause severe hyperglycemia. Arterial blood gases and pH are checked frequently to document the adequacy of ventilation and oxygenation.

V. Postoperative care

A. Ventilation

1. **A patent airway and adequate alveolar ventilation** are prerequisites for accurate assessment of neurologic status. Since respiratory centers or airway protective reflexes may be compromised during extensive posterior fossa dissection, some patients may require intubation postoperatively. Ventilation is assisted or controlled to maintain arterial carbon dioxide tension ($PaCO_2$) at approximately 35 mmHg.

2. Intraoperative **air embolism** may result in interstitial pulmonary edema. Patients who have sustained air embolism should have serial blood gas analyses and chest x-rays postoperatively. The use of oxygen therapy, ventilatory support, or PEEP is dictated by the results of these studies.

3. Choosing the proper time for **extubation** is difficult. Coughing and straining on an endotracheal tube are hazardous because they may precipitate intracranial bleeding. Conversely, aspiration and pneumonitis may result from premature extubation if patients are not alert and able to cough and swallow effectively. Occasionally, patients may require intubation for several days before airway protective reflexes return. Usually these patients can be identified early because they do not react vigorously to prolonged intubation and they require minimal sedation during the postoperative period.

B. Neurologic care

1. Patients are nursed in the 30-degree head-up position to reduce formation of edema around the brainstem and cranial nerves. **Level of consciousness** is the most reliable sign of early brainstem compromise, and for this reason long-acting, nonreversible sedatives, such as diazepam and droperidol, should be avoided. Sudden postoperative deterioration of consciousness may indicate obstructive hydrocephalus or brainstem encroachment by hematoma.

2. **Tension pneumocephalus** has been recognized recently as a potential cause of serious postoperative neurologic dysfunction. As CSF leaks out of the subarachnoid space during posterior fossa operations in the seated position, the cerebral hemispheres can collapse and allow air to enter through the craniectomy and accumulate over the cortex. This effect is probably enhanced further in patients who have functioning lateral ventricular shunts where the hydrostatic pressure gradient between the head and the chest tends to promote loss of CSF. After the incision has been closed, CSF accumulates faster than the air can be absorbed, producing a tension pneumocephalus. If suspected, the diagnosis can be made easily with skull x-ray, and the intracranial air can be released through a small twist drill burr hole placed after local anesthetic infiltration of the area.

3. **ICP monitoring and computerized tomography** (CT) capability are mutually complementary in the postoperative assessment of patients who are slow to awaken. Increased ICP may result from brain edema, obstructive hydrocephalus, or tension pneumocephalus. CT scanning can rapidly identify causes of elevated ICP and indicate which patients require prompt surgical intervention. Patients who remain somnolent despite the absence of a surgically correctable lesion and the reversal of sedatives usually have developed brain edema or vasospasm and require prolonged supportive care until consciousness returns.

C. Cardiovascular control

1. Continuous direct arterial and venous pressure and ECG **monitoring** are necessary for the first 24 to 48 hours postoperatively.

2. **Arterial hypertension** frequently occurs after posterior fossa exploration and should be treated aggressively with vasodilators or sympathetic blocking drugs before brain edema or hematoma formation occurs. Since arterial hypotension may lead to cerebral vasospasm, meticulous maintenance of normal cardiac filling pressures and arterial blood pressure is mandatory.

D. **Fluid and electrolyte management.** Corticosteroid therapy is continued into the postoperative period at doses equivalent to those used preoperatively. Immediately after operation, serum electrolyte concentrations are determined and appropriate fluid replacement with sodium- and potassium-containing solutions is begun. Insulin is given to treat high blood glucose levels. In general, fluid restriction is continued to prevent both brain edema and dilutional hyponatremia secondary to high postoperative ADH levels.

References

1. Albin, M. S., Babinski, M., Maroon, J. C., et al.   Anesthetic management of posterior fossa surgery in the sitting position. *Acta Anaesth. Scand.* 20:117, 1976.
2. Artru, A. A., Cucchiara, R. F., and Messick, J. M.   Cardiorespiratory and cranial nerve sequellae of surgical procedures involving the posterior fossa. *Anesthesiology* 52:83, 1980.
3. Ellis, S. C., Bryan-Brown, C. W., and Hyderally, H.   Massive swelling of the head and neck. *Anesthesiology* 42:102, 1975.
4. Hitselberger, W. E., and House, W. S. A.   Warning regarding the sitting position for acoustic tumor surgery. *Arch. Otolaryngol.* 106:69, 1980.
5. Kitahata, L. M., and Katz, J. D.   Tension pneumocephalus after posterior fossa craniotomy, a complication of the sitting position. *Anesthesiology* 44:448, 1976.
6. Marshall, W. K, and Bedford, R. F.   Evaluation of a pulmonary artery catheter for diagnosis and treatment of air embolism. *Anesthesiology* 52:131, 1980.
7. Paul, W. L., Munson, E. S., and Maniscalo, J. E.   Cerebrospinal fluid pressure during O_2 encephalopathy and N_2O inhalation. *Anesth. Analg.* (Cleve.) 55:849, 1976.
8. Perkins-Pearson, N. A. K., Marshall, W. K., and Bedford, R. F.   Atrial pressures in the seated position: Implications for paradoxical air embolism. *Anesthesiology* 57:493, 1982.

12. Transsphenoidal Procedures

Kalmon D. Post
Philippa Newfield

I. General principles. Although the transsphenoidal operation dates back to 1907, and Cushing (Henderson, 1939) performed over 200 such operations for resection of pituitary tumors, it was not until 1959 that Guiot and Thipaut (1969) popularized the operation using image-intensified fluoroscopy. Hardy and co-workers (1969) further modernized the procedure by introducing the operating microscope, which had the advantages of both magnifying and significantly improving focal illumination. With these advances, the transsphenoidal approach to sellar lesions has become increasingly popular and successful.

A. Advantages of the transsphenoidal approach

1. Morbidity and mortality are extremely low.

2. Trauma to the brain is minimized.

3. Operation is tolerated extremely well by acutely ill and aged patients.

4. Approach allows visual differentiation of small tumors within the gland.

5. Anesthetic and convalescent times are short.

6. Incidence of diabetes insipidus is low.

7. Blood loss is minimal.

B. Disadvantages of the transsphenoidal approach

1. Neural structures adjacent to a large tumor cannot be visualized.

2. Approach is through a nonsterile field (although meningitis is extremely rare).

3. Capabilities are limited if the diagnosis is questionable.

4. Suprasellar extension of the tumor into frontal fossa, middle fossa, or retroclival area that is asymmetric cannot be removed.

II. Indications for transsphenoidal approach to the sellar region. The indications for the transsphenoidal approach are most often limited to sellar and suprasellar lesions such as pituitary tumors, intrasellar and cystic craniopharyngiomas, cerebrospinal fluid (CSF) leaks, and intrasellar masses of uncertain type. The transsphenoidal approach is also used for hypophysectomy performed for breast or prostatic cancer as well as for intrasinus lesions such as tumors or mucoceles. Experience is increasing in the utilization of this approach for clival lesions such as chordomas.

A. Pituitary tumors. Pituitary tumors can be divided into two broad categories, nonfunctional and hypersecreting. In the past, radiation

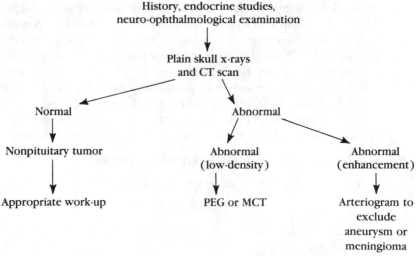

Fig. 12-1. Suggested tests for nonsecretory tumors. CT = computed tomography; MCT = metrizamide computed tomography; PEG = pneumoencephalography.

was the treatment of choice for small tumors when diagnosis was reasonably certain on visual, endocrinologic, and radiologic bases. Craniotomy and primary decompression were reserved for (1) large tumors that compromised vision to 20/200 or worse, (2) cystic adenomas, (3) pituitary apoplexy, or (4) uncertain diagnosis.

1. Nonfunctional tumors (Fig. 12-1)

    a. Diagnosis. Unless they either appear as incidental findings on skull film or cause headaches or mild endocrinopathies, nonfunctional tumors are usually diagnosed when they become large enough to produce a mass effect with visual changes and hypopituitarism secondary to compression of the optic chiasm and pituitary gland, respectively.

    b. Indications for surgery. The size of the nonfunctional tumor may mandate surgical intervention. Any cranial nerve deficit (e.g., intraocular muscle abnormalities from dysfunction of cranial nerves III, IV, VI) other than that of the optic nerve also demands surgical treatment. Progressive visual loss in acuity or fields and other mass effects, such as CSF obstruction with hydrocephalus, a generalized increase in intracranial pressure (ICP) from a large tumor in either the frontal or middle fossa, and specific neuroendocrine deficits because of hypothalamic dysfunction, also mandate surgical removal and decompression. Additional indications include pituitary apoplexy, uncertain diagnosis, tumor recurrence after radiation treatment, and CSF leak.

In autopsies performed on patients who did not have evidence of pituitary dysfunction, as many as 23% had pituitary adenomas (Costello, 1936), presumably nonfunctional and requiring no treatment. (Although they had no signs of Cushing's disease or acromegaly, prolactin secretion could have been present.) Undoubtedly, then, a large proportion of small nonfunctional or prolactin-secreting tumors may have a benign natural history. Therefore, the incidental nonfunctional tumor that produces neither neurologic nor endocrinologic deficit can either be followed conservatively with the use of computed tomography (CT) until evidence of growth is present or it may be treated with radiation therapy to arrest growth; surgery is not usually performed. Occasionally, for psychological reasons, a patient will desire the removal of even a small tumor, and this is done.

2. **Hypersecreting tumors** (Fig. 12-2)

a. **Presentation.** Hypersecreting tumors may produce adrenocorticotropic hormone (ACTH), growth hormone (GH), thyroid-stimulating hormone (TSH), and prolactin, singly or in combination. Because of the effects of the excessive hormone secretion, patients usually seek treatment while the tumors are small, and therefore mass effect with compression of the neural structures is less common as an early manifestation.

b. **Indications for surgery** include all the indications for nonfunctional tumors and the following:

(1) **Cushing's disease.** Cushing's disease is almost always secondary to a pituitary microadenoma, but x-ray studies of the sella are more often normal than abnormal. In a series of 86 patients who had Cushing's disease, only 20 were noted to have abnormalities on sella tomograms or plain skull films. Tyrrell et al. (1978) explored the sella in 20 consecutive cases of Cushing's disease, 8 of whom had normal sellae by x-ray study. In 2, there were technical difficulties that precluded intrasellar exploration, but in 17 of the other 18, a microadenoma was found and

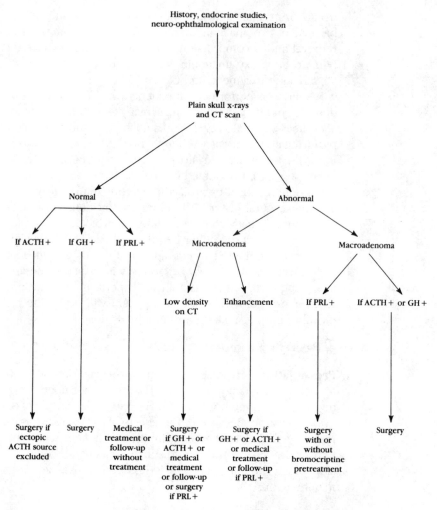

Fig. 12-2. Suggested tests for secretory tumors. ACTH = adrenocorticotropic hormone; CT = computed tomography; GH = growth hormone; PRL = prolactin.

removed. In the other patient, a hypophysectomy was performed and a 1.5-mm adenoma was seen in the specimen. Hypercortisolism was corrected in all but one of these patients.

We recommend sellar exploration of all patients who have Cushing's disease since the systemic effects of excessive ACTH and cortisol, such as hypertension, diabetes mellitus, osteoporosis, obesity, and myopathy, contribute to the five-year mortality of 50%. The low morbidity of pituitary surgery is an advantage compared with adrenalectomy. Additionally, the risk of Nelson's syndrome, reportedly 9% to 10% after adrenalectomy, is negated. The cure rate and rapidity of response after operation have made this modality superior to radiation therapy for children as well as adults.

(2) Nelson's syndrome. Whether developing after adrenalectomy or representing the further growth of an occult tumor initially responsible for Cushing syndrome, Nelson's syndrome has also been treated surgically. This tumor tends to have aggressive growth patterns, and early removal is suggested.

(3) Acromegaly. Excessive GH has many serious adverse systemic effects such as hypertension, diabetes mellitus, cardiomyopathy, cerebrovascular disease, and chronic pulmonary disease. The death rate is almost twice that expected from the general population, making surgical removal of a GH-secreting adenoma imperative. GH-secreting adenomas are not usually as large as nonfunctional tumors when first discovered. Treatment with conventional and heavy-particle irradiation is beneficial, yet there is a significant delay before plasma GH falls and, more importantly, it may never return to normal. Similarly, medical treatment offers some benefits but does not ablate the tumor. Therefore, we consider surgery to be the therapy of choice.

(4) Prolactinomas. Prolactinomas are the most common pituitary tumor, constituting 30% to 70% of most series. If the tumor is large and causes neurologic deficit, surgery is suggested. However, recent studies with bromocriptine show significant shrinkage with relief of neural compression. Male patients who have prolactinomas generally require surgery because of visual-field defects. Women who have amenorrhea-galactorrhea syndromes often are infertile and have hyperprolactinemia and asymmetric sellae on CT scan. The efficacy of bromocriptine in normalizing prolactin and promoting pregnancy is excellent. The cure rate for microadenomas by selective adenomectomy is also high, the morbidity is extremely low, and the mortality is zero. If predictable shrinkage of tumors during treatment with bromocriptine is confirmed, then surgery may be indicated only for those patients who are medical-treatment failures or to remove the residual adenoma after shrink-age. There is no evidence to date that radiation therapy is effective enough against prolactin-secreting tumors to consider irradiation as the primary form of therapy.

3. **Pituitary apoplexy.** The sudden enlargement of a pituitary adenoma secondary to either hemorrhage or hemorrhagic in-farction associated with acute neurologic deficits has been an absolute indication for surgical decompression in our clinic. Although some patients may recover spontaneously, even with the addition of high-dose glucocorticoid therapy the risks of waiting are great in relation to the risks of decompression, even in an acutely ill, elderly patient.

4. **Uncertain diagnosis.** If there is doubt as to the clinical diag-nosis of a sellar lesion, specific tissue diagnosis is mandatory, especially if radiation therapy is considered. Arachnoid cysts, Rathke's cleft cysts, craniopharyngiomas, dermoid and epider-moid tumors, and chordomas may be present, which are refrac-tory to radiation treatment.

5. **Treatment failures.** Patients who have been treated unsuccess-fully with other modalities and show evidence of pituitary tumor growth or persistence of hypersecretion are operative candi-dates.

B. **Sellar or parasellar lesions.** Arachnoid cysts, Rathke's cleft cysts, small or cystic craniopharyngiomas, dermoid and epidermoid tumors, meningiomas, and chordomas may all be approached through the transsphenoidal route.

C. **Cerebrospinal fluid leaks.** Rhinorrhea from leakage through the sphenoid sinus may be secondary to trauma, malignant tumor, be-nign tumor, previous transsphenoidal operations, or increased ICP. Surgery is mandatory in such patients to seal the leak and prevent meningitis. Radiotherapy may also be required.

D. **Sphenoid sinus disorders.** Lesions of the sphenoid sinus such as tumor or mucocele may be approached transsphenoidally.

E. **Metastatic cancer.** Metastatic cancer of either the breast or the prostate may respond to hormonal ablative therapy through total hypophysectomy. Therefore, transsphenoidal surgery is often per-formed in these patients who are frequently debilitated and suffer-ing from other medical problems.

III. **Preoperative evaluation**

A. **Medical assessment.** Preoperative assessment includes attention to specific problems associated with pituitary tumors including diabetes mellitus, hypertension, diabetes insipidus, hypothyroidism (rarely hyperthyroidism), and adrenal insufficiency.

B. Anatomic evaluation of sellar region. The patient's visual fields are evaluated to assess function of the optic nerves and chiasm. Neurologic evaluation is necessary to detect signs of mass effect or local invasion or compression. Otolaryngologic examination of the nasal passages and nasopharynx is important.

Radiologic studies include plain skull films and CT scans. Pneumoencephalograms are rarely performed. Carotid arteriograms are performed to exclude the presence of an aneurysm in all patients except those who have hypersecreting tumors. The CT scan is particularly helpful in assessing the size of the mass lesion and the degree of suprasellar extension and for estimating the ICP.

C. Physiologic endocrine testing. Many tests are available for the evaluation of pituitary function. Certain investigations are indicated in the evaluation of hypopituitarism (Table 12-1), whereas others are of more relevance in presumptive states of pituitary hypersecretion (Table 12-2). The most useful procedures are summarized in Table 12-3. Test procedures detailed in Tables 12-1 and 12-2 can be added or interchanged, especially for pretreatment and posttreatment comparison, whereas Table 12-3 represents the basic profile. In the preanesthetic evaluation, the most informative studies are those for ACTH reserve, thyroid function, and electrolyte balance.

D. Preoperative medications. Because the surgical procedure will involve either manipulation or removal of the anterior lobe of the pituitary gland, patients receive steroid replacement to provide adequate glucocorticoid concentrations during the perioperative period. We give cortisone acetate, 50 mg intramuscularly, on the night before surgery and on call to the operating room. If diabetes mellitus is present, then appropriate insulin coverage will be necessary. For the hypothyroid patient, thyroid replacement is initiated 4 to 6 weeks before elective surgery when possible to achieve an euthyroid state. Diabetes insipidus can be controlled with aqueous pitressin or with desmopressin (1-desamino-8-D-arginine vasopressin; DDAVP).

Premedication consists of diazepam, 10 to 15 mg IM, 1 to 2 hours before surgery. The use of narcotics is rarely necessary and may retard awakening from anesthesia.

E. Nasal passages. A nasal culture is obtained preoperatively to identify the flora in the event of a postoperative infection. Instruction is also given for mouth breathing, because the nasal passages will be occluded with packing for several days after surgery.

Table 12-1. Diagnostic tests especially recommended for the investigation of hypopituitarism

Hormone	Test material (adult dosage)	Time of peak serum response	Comments
GH	L-Dopa (500 mg orally)	60 min	Very safe; nausea occasionally occurs; GH *falls* in acromegaly; PRL is normally suppressed (see also Table 12-2)
	Insulin (0.05-0.3 units/kg body weight IV)	60 min	To obtain a maximum response, adequate hypoglycemia must be achieved. ACTH and PRL reserve can be determined simultaneously
PRL	TRH (500 μg IV)	30 min	Very safe. TSH reserve can be determined simultaneously. A GH rise may occur in acromegaly
	Chlorpromazine (25 mg IM)	60–90 min	May produce hypotension and somnolence in hypopituitary or hypothyroid subjects. Tests for hypothalamic reserve for PRL release

			See above
ACTH	Insulin (see above)	30 min for ACTH: 60 min for cortisol	
	Metyrapone (30 mg/kg body weight orally at 12 midnight). The longer procedure may also be used—750 mg orally every 4 hr for 6 doses	9 A.M. for 11-deoxycortisol and cortisol and/or ACTH	Safe but may cause nausea and vomiting. Unlike the insulin challenge, metyrapone testing is vitiated by concurrent glucocorticoid administration
TSH	TSH (500 μg IV)	30–60 min	See also above under PRL. The test does not reliably separate hypothalamic from pituitary hypothyroidism
Gonadotropins	LH-RH (25–150 μg)	30–60 min	Very safe. A GH rise may occur in acromegaly
	Clomiphene (50 mg b.i.d. for 5–7 days	LH at 5–7 days; also in females at 12–15 days for ovulatory surge	In females can cause ovarian cyst formation and "superovulation." Tests the hypothalamic reserve for gonadotropin release

Source: K. D. Post and I. M. D. Jackson, Endocrinologic Evaluation of Pituitary Tumors. In D. Long and G. Tindall (Eds.), *Contemporary Neurosurgery*, Vol. 2, No. 5. Baltimore: Williams & Wilkins, 1980.

Table 12-2. Diagnostic tests especially recommended for the investigation of states of pituitary hyperfunction

Hormone	Test material (adult dosage)	Time of maximum serum response	Comments
GH	Glucose (50–100 gm PO)	60–120 min	Failure of GH suppression is diagnostic of acromegaly in the appropriate clinical setting
	L-Dopa (500 mg PO)	60–120 min	GH suppression commonly occurs in acromegaly and is suggestive of this diagnosis
	TRH (200–500 μg IV)	30 min	Positive response in acromegaly correlates with therapeutic response to bromocriptine
Prolactin	TRH (500 μg IV) (see also Table 1)	30 min	Failure of PRL rise may occur more frequently in prolactinomas than in other hyperprolactinemia states
	L-Dopa[a] (500 mg PO)	60–120 min	Failure of PRL to fall adequately suggests the presence of a pituitary adenoma
ACTH	Dexamethasone at a dose of 1 mg PO at 12 midnight	Cortisol[b] and/or ACTH at 9 A.M.	Failure of suppression is a useful screening test for Cushing's syndrome

Dexamethasone at a dose of 0.5 mg every 6 hr for 2 days	Cortisol[b] and/or ACTH at 48 hr. Urine for 17-OHCS and/or "free" cortisol can also be determined	Failure of suppression suggests Cushing's syndrome[c]
Dexamethasone at a dose of 2 mg every 6 hr for 2 days	Cortisol[b] and/or ACTH at 48 hr. Urine for 17-OHCS and/or "free" cortisol can also be determined	Suppression occurs in Cushing's disease[d] but not in other causes of Cushing's syndrome
Metyrapone (750 mg PO every 4 hr for 6 doses). The overnight test may also be used (see Table 12-1)	ACTH and/or 11-deoxycortisol at 24 hr or urine 17-OHCS on the next day	Marked rise occurs in Cushing's disease but not in other causes of Cushing's syndrome

[a] Preceded by carbidopa, L-dopa may be helpful in the diagnosis of prolactinomas.
[b] In Cushing's syndrome due to adrenal tumor, the ACTH level is already suppressed.
[c] In some patients with Cushing's disease, "normal" suppression occurs.
[d] In some patients with Cushing's disease, higher doses of dexamethasone are required for suppression.

Source: K. D. Post and I. M. D. Jackson, Endocrinologic Evaluation of Pituitary Tumors. In D. Long and G. Tindall (Eds.), *Contemporary Neurosurgery*, Vol. 2, No. 5. Baltimore: Williams & Wilkins, 1980.

Table 12-3. Suggested tests

Tumor	Tests
Nonfunctional tumor	PRL every 15 min for 3 samples (pooled specimen). Thyroid function: T_4, T_3 resin, TSH, LH, FSH, estradiol, or testosterone. Cortisol (may be combined with Cortrosyn test). Metyrapone or ITT (if <50 years old and no cardiovascular disease)
Prolactinoma	All of the above for nonfunctional tumors, TRH stimulation test (suggestive of tumor if PRL rise is blunted)
Acromegaly	All of the above for nonfunctional tumors, GH, glucose tolerance test, L-dopa test
Cushing's disease	All of the above for nonfunctional tumors, ACTH, dexamethasone suppression test, metyrapone test

Source: K. D. Post and I. M. D. Jackson, Endocrinologic Evaluation of Pituitary Tumors. In D. Long and G. Tindall (Eds.), *Contemporary Neurosurgery,* Vol. 2, No. 5. Baltimore: Williams & Wilkins, 1980.

IV. Anesthesia

A. **Preoperative considerations.** In evaluating a patient who requires anesthesia for transsphenoidal surgery, the most important considerations are the nature of the patient's diagnosis and the reason for the procedure. Patients undergo transsphenoidal operations for treatment of hypersecreting pituitary tumors causing amenorrhea, galactorrhea, Cushing's disease, or acromegaly, nonfunctional pituitary adenomas, craniopharyngioma, hormone-responsive metastatic carcinoma, intractable cancer pain, sphenoid sinus lesions, and CSF rhinorrhea.

Each preoperative condition has its own constellation of systemic disorders and accompanying effects on intracranial dynamics that must be considered when selecting an anesthetic technique. Patients who have Cushing's disease may also suffer from hypertension, diabetes, osteoporosis, obesity, and friability of skin and connective tissue. Patients who have acromegaly may have hypertension, cardiomyopathy, diabetes, and osteoporosis as well as prognathism, cartilaginous and soft-tissue hypertrophy of the larynx, and an enlarged tongue, which may complicate intubation of the trachea. Patients who have panhypopituitarism require preoperative supplementation with appropriate hormones and modulation of doses of anesthetic drugs since they may be hypothyroid. Patients suffering from metastatic malignancies are frequently cachectic and debilitated and may have clotting abnormalities and pleural effusions.

B. **Selection of anesthetic drugs.** The size and location of pituitary and associated tumors determine their effect on intracranial dynamics. The pituitary microadenomas do not act as space-occupying lesions. Craniopharyngiomas and other suprasellar tumors and pituitary tumors with suprasellar extension, however, may be large enough to exert a mass effect. Induction and maintenance of anesthesia are planned so as not to impair cerebral compliance unduly because of any untoward increase in cerebral blood flow (CBF) as a result of intubation during inadequate anesthesia, introduction of inhalation anesthetics before hyperventilation, use of drugs that increase CBF, head-down positioning, or systemic hypertension.

Because residual blood and secretions frequently remain in the posterior pharynx at the conclusion of the operation, it is important that the patient be sufficiently awake to ensure protection of the airway before extubation is accomplished. If the patient is not responsive, the trachea should remain intubated until the patient is awake. Selection of appropriate doses of anesthetic drugs and timing of their administration are particularly important in this regard because transsphenoidal explorations are relatively short procedures (2 to 3 hours) that conclude very abruptly: once the mucosal and abdominal incisions have been closed, the nose is packed and the operation is over.

C. **Monitoring.** The anesthesiologist monitors the patient's blood pressure, heart rate and rhythm, temperature, arterial oxygen and carbon dioxide tensions, and fluid balance. Blood pressure is measured directly when indicated by preexisting medical problems. The use of a urinary catheter is not routine, but may be necessary to aid the management of patients who have diabetes mellitus or diabetes insipidus.

D. **Anesthetic management**

1. **Technique.** In selecting an anesthetic technique, the major concerns are the effect of anesthetic drugs on intracranial dynamics in the presence of a space-occupying lesion, the potential difficulties with tracheal intubation in patients who have acromegaly, the brevity of the procedure, and the patient's medical problems. If the patient has had a pneumoencephalogram with air as the gaseous contrast medium any time up to a week before surgery, nitrous oxide (N_2O) is avoided. When oxygen is used for pneumoencephalography, N_2O may be included in the anesthetic technique.

   The combination of N_2O and oxygen with thiopental, a narcotic (fentanyl), and a muscle relaxant (succinylcholine for intubation and then pancuronium) is a satisfactory technique. Isoflurane or enflurane may be added in low concentrations for blood pressure control or, alternatively, used as the primary anesthetic drug (after establishment of hyperventilation). Halothane is contraindicated because of its potential for inducing ventricular arrhythmias during infiltration of the oral and nasal mucosa with 0.5% lidocaine and epinephrine 1:200,000 or the application of 5% cocaine-soaked pledgets to the mucosa.

The patient is reassured on arrival in the operating room, and is again reminded about the need for mouth breathing postoperatively because of the nasal packs.

2. **Induction.** The induction sequence includes preoxygenation, d-tubocurarine, 3 mg, thiopental, 4–5 mg/kg, succinylcholine, 1.5 mg/kg, and fentanyl, 2–3 μg/kg. The trachea is intubated after administration of lidocaine, 1.5 mg/kg IV. If difficulty with intubation is anticipated, an inhalation induction precedes intubation during spontaneous ventilation. An assortment of tubes and blades and the use of a fiberoptic bronchoscope may be helpful.

After intubation and auscultation of the breath sounds bilaterally, the endotracheal tube is moved to the left corner of the patient's mouth and taped securely across the chin. The esophageal stethoscope and temperature probe are inserted and secured on the lower left as well, leaving the upper lip totally free. An orogastric tube is placed, aspirated, and then put to gravity drainage during the procedure. The oropharynx is then packed with moist cotton gauze. The eyes are first taped closed and then covered with cotton-padded adhesive patches to prevent corneal abrasion and seepage of cleansing solution and blood into the eyes.

3. **Subarachnoid catheter.** Access to the superior margin of a suprasellar tumor is facilitated by placement of a lumbar subarachnoid catheter (epidural catheter or #5 Stamey ureteral catheter through a 14-gauge Tuohy needle) after intubation and intraoperative instillation of preservative-free saline to bring the tumor down into the sella. Alternatively, delineation of the suprasellar component is accomplished by intraoperative injection of 15 to 25 cc of either air or a nitrous oxide-oxygen mixture into the subarachnoid space in 5-cc increments. It is important to avoid an increase in the intracranial volume caused by the different blood-gas solubilities of N_2O and air. Therefore, either filtered nitrous oxide-oxygen from the inspired gas line is injected into the subarachnoid space or air is injected and N_2O is discontinued. The subarachnoid catheter should have a stopcock to prevent the excessive loss of CSF and should be within the anesthesiologist's reach.

4. **Positioning.** The patient's head, supported by a three-point pin headholder, is turned toward his right side, and elevated 20

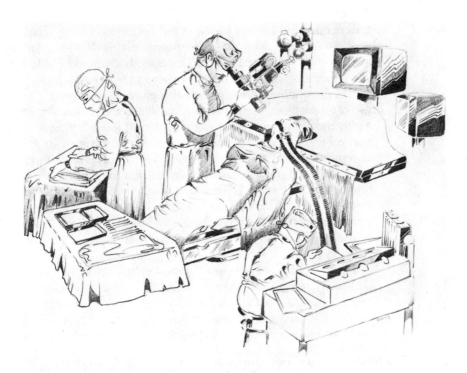

Fig. 12-3. Diagrammatic representation of operative setup for transsphenoidal approach to the sella. Note the position of the patient's head, surgeon, anesthesiologist, fluoroscope with televised image, and operating microscope. (From K. D. Post, I. M. D. Jackson, and S. Reichlin [Eds.], *Pituitary Adenoma*. New York: Plenum, 1980. By permission.)

degrees and centered within a C-arm fluoroscopy unit for x-ray control during surgery. Lead aprons must be used. The hoses from the anesthesia circuit are firmly secured to prevent disconnection and extubation during the operation (Fig. 12-3). The patient's arms are placed at his sides and padded to avoid injury to the ulnar nerves. Prophylactic antibiotics (vancomycin, 1 g IV, and tobramycin, 80 mg IM) and corticosteroids (Solu-Cortef 100 mg/1000 ml crystalloid solution) may be given at this point.

5. **Maintenance.** Anesthesia is maintained with N_2O and oxygen, fentanyl (2–4 µg/kg), pancuronium (0.05 mg/kg), and enflurane or isoflurane. Ventilation is controlled to keep the arterial carbon dioxide tension ($PaCO_2$) between 32 and 37 mmHg to prevent a decrease in brain volume, which may withdraw the suprasellar part of the tumor out of the surgeon's reach by the transsphenoidal approach. In the presence of a large space-occupying mass or obstructive hydrocephalus, the $PaCO_2$ should be reduced to 26 to 32 mmHg. The use of mannitol is rarely necessary.

6. **Emergence.** At the conclusion of the operation, muscle relaxation is reversed with either neostigmine (0.04–0.05 mg/kg) and atropine (0.02–0.025 mg/kg), or edrophonium (0.5 mg/kg) and either atropine (0.01 mg/kg) or glycopyrrolate (3.5 µg/kg). N_2O is discontinued and the patient is given 100% oxygen. The use of an analgesic such as fentanyl facilitates the patient's quiet emergence from anesthesia and his ability to tolerate the endotracheal tube without coughing or straining. The orogastric tube is removed while suction is applied, the oropharynx is thoroughly cleared of blood and secretions, and the throat pack is taken out. The trachea is extubated when the patient is able to respond to commands. Neurologic examination including grasp, movement of the extremities, pupil size and reaction, and visual acuity is performed in the operating room and again in the recovery room.

If the patient is not responsive, the tube remains in place until the patient regains consciousness. Cardiovascular status permitting, the patient's head is elevated 30 degrees. Close monitoring including neurologic evaluation is continued in the recovery room and subsequently on the ward.

E. **Fluid management.** Administration of fluids during transsphenoidal procedures is calculated to include maintenance requirements and replacement of blood loss and fluid deficit. Some patients may have taken nothing by mouth for as long as 12 to 15 hours before surgery. It is therefore important that they receive additional fluid during induction of anesthesia as replacement of their deficit and in anticipation of blood loss. Operative blood loss is usually 200 to 300 ml, but can be extensive and acute. Blood should be available. If diabetes insipidus is present, the urinary losses must be replaced as well.

Ringer's lactate solution with or without 5% dextrose is a suitable crystalloid solution. Blood is given as necessary in the form of either whole blood or packed red cells reconstituted with equal volumes of normal saline. There is little indication for administration of colloid (plasmanate, albumisol, albumin).

F. **Intraoperative problems**

1. **Use of cocaine and epinephrine.** The topical use of cocaine and the oral and nasal submucosal injection of local anesthetic solutions containing epinephrine help constrict gingival and mucosal vessels and dissect the nasal mucosa away from the cartilaginous septum. Epinephrine may produce hypertension, arrhythmias, or both; cocaine interferes with the intraneuronal uptake of catecholamines and can thus augment both the hyper-

tensive and arrhythmogenic properties of epinephrine. The use of epinephrine is relatively safe, however, if the following conditions are met: halothane is avoided, ventilation is adequate, epinephrine is given in combination with lidocaine instead of saline, epinephrine concentrations of 1:100,000 to 1:200,000 are used, and total dose does not exceed 10 ml of 1:100,000 solution in 10 minutes for a 70-kg adult. A total dose of 250 mg of cocaine should not be exceeded. Persistent arrhythmias may require treatment with lidocaine. Hypertension may be controlled with an inhalation anesthetic or small intravenous doses of hydralazine.

2. **Bleeding.** Although an infrequent occurrence, the potential for rapid, copious blood loss from entry into either the cavernous sinus or the carotid artery is present, especially in acromegalic patients. In patients who have Cushing's disease, a steady ooze may be encountered. It is therefore important to administer adequate amounts of crystalloid solution during the early part of the procedure to prevent a significant decrease in intravascular volume should hemorrhage occur. Careful serial calculation of blood loss and immediate recognition of brisk bleeding are imperative. Replacement with crystalloid solution is usually adequate unless the patient's preoperative hematocrit is low, blood pressure is difficult to maintain, or blood loss becomes excessive.

   Some anesthesiologists induce hypotension to control bleeding. In our experience, however, excessive blood loss is not sufficiently common to warrant the use of controlled hypotension. Raising the patient's head 20 degrees helps to reduce bleeding as well.

3. **Arterial injury.** If the carotid arteries are compressed or injured within the sella or cavernous sinus, thrombotic occlusion may occur and cause cerebral ischemia.

4. **Air embolism.** Since the site of operation is above the heart during transsphenoidal procedures, the possibility of air embolism exists. The point of entry into the venous system is the vascular ring formed by the cavernous sinuses, which lie lateral to the pituitary gland, and the communicating intercavernous connections between the sinuses, which are anterior, posterior, and inferior to the gland. The opening of the veins along the path of surgical entry through the mouth and nose may also introduce intravenous air. Monitoring for air embolism with either the use of the Doppler ultrasonic precordial transducer or the measurement of end-tidal carbon dioxide tension will alert

the anesthesiologist and the surgeon to entrainment of intravenous air so that the site may be identified and occluded and appropriate treatment may be instituted.

Because air embolism may occur during transsphenoidal procedures, the possibility of intravenous air should be included in the differential diagnosis of intraoperative hypotension, tachycardia, arrhythmias, hypoxia, hypercapnia, and bronchospasm.

5. **Dural manipulation.** Manipulation of the dura either anteriorly or, even more frequently, laterally along the medial aspects of the cavernous sinus often causes bradycardia. This may be due to either a trigeminal or vagal reflex. With cessation of manipulation, the bradycardia resolves.

6. **CSF leakage.** An arachnoid pouch may extend into the sella and partially obscure the operative field. This may cause herniation of the pituitary gland or increase the risk of a dural tear and resultant leakage of CSF. The surgeon may ask the anesthesiologist to remove various amounts of CSF through the subarachnoid catheter to alleviate these problems.

7. **Visual evoked responses.** Some centers use visual evoked responses (VER) to monitor optic nerve function during surgical manipulation. Decompression of the optic nerve enhances VER, and trauma to the optic nerve distorts or abolishes them.

8. **Diabetes insipidus.** Diabetes insipidus is not an uncommon sequela of transsphenoidal procedures, particularly hypophysectomy. Although the onset is usually on the first or second postoperative day, diabetes insipidus will occasionally occur during anesthesia or in the recovery room. Measurement of urine output is important but insertion of a urinary catheter is usually unnecessary. Initial treatment includes fluid replacement with a balanced salt solution containing 5% dextrose. Five percent dextrose in water is not given because cerebral edema may be induced by the creation of an osmotic gradient between the brain and the intravascular compartment. If diabetes insipidus persists or it becomes difficult to match urinary losses, the patient may receive aqueous pitressin, pitressin tannate oil, or desmopressin. Diabetes insipidus that occurs after most transsphenoidal procedures is usually self-limited and resolves within one week to ten days.

V. Postoperative considerations

A. Immediate postoperative care

1. **Airway.** Because the nasal passages are packed, maintenance of a clear airway is of paramount importance.

2. **Nausea and vomiting.** During transsphenoidal dissection, blood and secretions run down the posterior pharynx and accumulate in the stomach. Since the presence of blood in the gastrointestinal tract is irritating, patients frequently experience nausea and vomiting in the recovery period. This can be alleviated to a certain extent once the airway has been secured by packing the pharynx with moist cotton gauze to prevent migration of blood to either the stomach or the tracheobronchial tree during surgery. The throat pack must be removed before extubation of the trachea. Aspiration of the stomach with an orogastric tube before extubation will also remove some of the accumulated air, gastric secretions, and blood, thus reducing the incidence of postoperative nausea and vomiting.

3. **Hypertension.** Patients who have a history of hypertension (as well as some who do not) may be hypertensive in the recovery period, despite normal preoperative blood pressures. If analgesics are ineffective, blood pressure may be controlled by administering incremental doses of hydralazine, 5 mg IV, at 5-minute intervals, until the desired pressure is reached. If the heart rate is greater than 70 and there is no history of either asthma or congestive heart failure, each dose of hydralazine may be given in combination with propranolol, 0.5–1 mg IV, both for therapeutics and prevention of reflex tachycardia.

4. **Bleeding.** Bleeding from either the nose or the sublabial incision and either expectoration or vomiting of copious amounts of blood require that the neurosurgeon assess the situation and replace the nasal packing, if necessary. The application of pressure and replacement of nasal packing is usually sufficient to stop the bleeding. The nasal packing may also require adjustment if it has worked its way into the posterior pharynx, causing the patient to gag and cough.

5. **Fluids.** Urinary output and specific gravity are measured frequently to diagnose and treat diabetes insipidus. Serum and urine osmolarities are also measured. The treatment of diabetes insipidus is discussed in Chapter 7.

6. **Medications**

   a. Corticosteroid coverage is mandatory until postoperative testing shows an intact pituitary-adrenal axis. Dexamethasone is often given in the immediate postoperative period and then changed to prednisone.

   b. Thyroid replacement is given if the patient had been hypothyroid before surgery. If euthyroid preoperatively, patients need not receive replacement medication in the immediate postoperative period.

c. Antibiotics are given in our clinic for 48 hours after surgery.

B. Long-term postoperative care

1. Anterior and posterior pituitary function must be evaluated completely.

2. Sinus complaints may occur and are treated symptomatically.

3. Other modes of therapy may be necessary such as radiation therapy or medication, depending on the nature of the process.

References

1. Bergland, R. M., Ray, B. S., and Torack, M.   Anatomical variations in the pituitary gland and adjacent structures in 225 human autopsy cases. *J. Neurosurg.* 23:93, 1968.
2. Costello, R. T.   Subclinical adenoma of the pituitary gland. *Am. J. Pathol.* 12:205, 1936.
3. Guiot, G., and Thibaut, B.   L'extirpation des adenomes hypophysaires par voir transsphenoidale. *Neurochirurgia (Stuttgart)* 1:133, 1969.
4. Hardy, J.   Transsphenoidal microsurgery of the normal and pathological pituitary. *Clin. Neurosurg.* 16:185, 1969.
5. Henderson, W. R.   The pituitary adenomata: Follow-up study of surgical results in 338 cases (Dr Harvey Cushing's series). *Br. J. Surg.* 26:811, 1939.
6. Kernohan, J. W., and Sayre, G. P.   Tumors of the pituitary gland and infandibulum. In *Atlas of Tumor Pathology*, 1st series, Fascicle 36. Washington, D.C.: U.S. Armed Forces Institute of Pathology, 1956.
7. Kjellberg, R. N., Shintani, A., Frantz, A. G., et al.   Proton-beam therapy in acromegaly. *N. Engl. J. Med.* 278:690, 1968.
8. Laws, E. R., Jr., Kern, E. B.   Complications of transsphenoidal surgery. *Clin. Neurosurg.* 23:401, 1975.
9. Messick, J. M., Jr., Laws, E. R., Jr., and Abboud, C. F.   Anesthesia for transsphenoidal surgery of the hypophyseal region. *J. Anesth. Analg.* 57:206, 1978.
10. Newfield, P., Albin, M. S., Chestnut, J. S., et al.   Air embolism during transsphenoidal pituitary operations. *Neurosurgery* 2:39, 1978.
11. Post, K. D., Jackson, I. M. D., and Reichlin, S. (Eds.).   *Pituitary Adenoma.* New York: Plenum, 1980.
12. Post, K. D., and Jackson, I. M. D.   Endocrinologic Evaluation of Pituitary Tumors. In D. Long and G. Tindall (Eds.), *Contemporary Neurosurgery,* Vol. 2, No. 5. Baltimore: Williams & Wilkins, 1980.
13. Post, K. D., and Stein, B. M.   Technique for spinal drainage: A technical note. *Neurosurgery* 43:255, 1979.
14. Post, K. D., and Wolpert, S. M.   Radiologic Evaluation of Pituitary Adenomas. In D. Long and G. Tindall (Eds.), *Contemporary Neurosurgery,* Vol. 2, No. 6. Baltimore: Williams & Wilkins, 1980.
15. Renn, W. H., and Rhoton, A. L., Jr.   Microsurgical anatomy of the sellar region. *J. Neurosurg.* 43:288, 1975.
16. Roth, J., Gorden, P., and Brace, K.   Efficacy of conventional pituitary irradiation in acromegaly. *N. Engl. J. Med.* 282:1385, 1970.

17. Tyrell, M. B., Brooks, R. M., Fitzgerald, P. A., et al.   Cushing's disease: Selective transsphenoidal resection of pituitary microadenomas. *N. Engl. J. Med.* 298:753, 1978.
18. Wilson, C. B., and Dempsey, L. C.   Transsphenoidal microsurgical removal of 250 pituitary adenomas. *J. Neurosurg.* 48:13, 1978.
19. Wright, A. D., Hill, D. M., Lowy, C., et al.   Mortality in acromegaly. *Q. J. Med.* 39:1, 1970.

13. Head Trauma

Management

Derek A. Bruce

Accidents and homicides remain the major cause of death in children and adolescents: trauma takes more lives in all people less than 45 years of age than any other single cause. Severe head injuries occur in approximately 600,000 people each year; 50,000 or more die, and some significant residual disability remains in more than 20% of survivors. Head trauma, either with or without co-existing injury to other organs, is the most commonly reported injury among motor vehicle accident victims. Other causes of trauma include falls, firearm accidents, criminal assault, birth trauma, and sporting accidents. Clearly, the ideal way to treat this problem is to eliminate the injuries. This has proved impossible in our automobile-oriented society, and thus the burden is on the medical profession to improve the outcome of the patient who has sustained head trauma.

I. **Pathophysiology.** Improvement in the understanding of the pathophysiology of head injuries has resulted in significant changes in the treatment of patients who sustain severe craniocerebral trauma. In the past, transient concussion has been separated conceptually from prolonged unconsciousness. We now believe that there is a continuum of injury ranging from amnesia to transient concussion to prolonged traumatic unconsciousness to sudden death from disruption of the brainstem. Even transient concussion is associated with some damage to the neurons and white matter. Severe acceleration-deceleration injury will produce damage in a radial fashion from the cortex to the brainstem, usually involving both areas pathologically.

A. **Brainstem contusion.** Primary brainstem injury that causes disruption of the pontomedullary junction, severe hemorrhage into the brainstem, or acute vascular damage to the basilar and vertebral arteries usually proves rapidly fatal before the patient even reaches the hospital. Prolonged unconsciousness (associated with bilateral, fixed, dilated pupils and/or decerebrate posturing) is rarely the result of the primary brainstem injury but rather is caused by diffuse damage to the white matter of the hemispheres and brainstem. These unconscious patients have often received inadequate care in the past because the diagnosis of a brainstem contusion implied that no therapy was available. However, such patients can develop brain swelling and brain edema leading to increased intracranial pressure (ICP) and secondary brain injury, all of which are amenable to treatment. There is no clinical value in considering an injury to be a primary brainstem contusion, since many of the secondary injuries can be successfully treated.

B. Intracranial hemorrhage

1. **Epidural.** Epidural hematomas are most frequently due to laceration of branches of the middle meningeal artery. They are usually caused by an impact injury, most frequently to the temporal region. Venous epidural hematomas from laceration of the dural sinuses present with signs and symptoms of increased ICP and can occur from several days to two weeks after injury. In adults, skull fractures are seen in association with epidural hematomas in approximately 80% of cases, whereas in children, the incidence is approximately 50%.

2. **Subdural.** It is useful to separate subdural hematomas into acute, subacute, and chronic.

   a. **Acute subdural hematomas** are usually the result of acceleration-deceleration injury to the mobile head and are associated with injury and swelling of the underlying cerebral hemispheres. Although bleeding may be venous from torn bridging or cortical veins, it is more frequently arterial from an area of lacerated cerebral cortex. The presence of acute subdural hematoma is associated with increased mortality and poor outcome. Survival may be improved, however, by rapid intervention to decompress the brain (Seelig, 1981). Acute subdural hematomas are similar to other expanding mass lesions in presentation. They often occur after a lucid interval after injury and can be small and spread over much of the hemisphere, or large and focal.

   b. **Subacute subdural hematomas** are similar to acute hematomas but are usually the result of venous bleeding. The hematoma is suspected clinically more than 24 hours after injury. In these patients, the degree of hemispheric injury is frequently less and the outcome is better than in acute hematomas since the most significant factor producing clinical deterioration is the expanding mass effect of the clot rather than any severe diffuse brain injury.

   c. **Chronic subdural hematomas** are liquified hematomas that frequently present with little or no definite history of specific trauma. They are generally associated with some brain atrophy and therefore tend to occur in either the elderly or the chronically alcoholic patient. The mechanism is believed to be slow accumulation of blood in the subdural space as a result of tearing of bridging cortical veins. Once the subdural blood has begun to accumulate, episodes of minor head trauma, coughing, sneezing, or straining (all of

Table 13-1. Glasgow coma scale

Observation	Points
Eye opening	
Spontaneous	4
To speech	3
To pain	2
None	1
Best verbal response	
Oriented	5
Confused	4
Inappropriate	3
Incomprehensible	2
None	1
Best motor response	
Obeys commands	6
Localizes pain	5
Withdraws from pain	4
Flexes to pain	3
Extends to pain	2
None	1

which produce venous engorgement and raise the intracranial venous pressure) can exacerbate the bleeding from either the initially damaged vein or the thin-walled vessels within the external membrane of the subdural hematoma. These lesions become important in acute trauma because fresh bleeding into the chronic hematoma results in new trauma. It is common to see acute hemorrhage in a chronic subdural hematoma on computed tomographic (CT) scan. These chronic lesions present in a multiplicity of ways from transient ischemic attacks to progressive dementia.

3. **Subarachnoid.** Subarachnoid hemorrhage is extremely common after head trauma, especially in children. Eighty percent of children who have Glasgow coma scores (Table 13-1) of less than 5 during the first 48 hours after injury have evidence of subarachnoid hemorrhage on CT scan. Subarachnoid hemorrhage is an indication of the severity of the injury and, when extensive, increases the risk of delayed hydrocephalus.

4. **Intracerebral.** Intracerebral hematoma is an uncommon finding after head trauma (5% in children) and usually occurs only with severe injuries. With the use of the CT scan, however, small or even large hematomas may be seen in the absence of neurologic deficit. The typical cause of intracranial hemorrhage is a shearing injury that tears the cerebral substance and causes

hemorrhage into the white matter. Frequently, more than one small hematoma is present. These lesions are generally not amenable to surgical intervention, but in patients who have high levels of alcohol, delayed hemorrhage is probably much more common than had been previously suspected. If there is further deterioration or a delayed increase in ICP, intracerebral hemorrhage must be considered. Delayed hemorrhage will also occur occasionally with the onset of signs of increased ICP from 5 to 14 days after trauma. Local hematomas occur below the area of skull fracture, after impact to the skull, particularly with depressed fractures. While they frequently do not require operation, large localized lesions producing pressure symptoms may require surgical removal.

C. **Acute brain swelling.** Acute brain swelling occurs more frequently, but not exclusively, in children from birth to 16 years of age. Noted even after relatively trivial injury, acute brain swelling may or may not be associated with a lucid period after trauma. While formerly thought to be due to severe acute brain edema and often referred to as malignant edema, the entity has been well defined pathologically. The brain is severely swollen and there is vascular engorgement of the white matter but rarely are any signs of primary impact injury present. Recent studies with CT scan and measurement of cerebral blood flow (CBF) suggest that acute brain swelling is due to sudden intracerebral vascular congestion and hyperemia, which can be controlled if treated early (Bruce, 1981). The recognition of the presence of acute brain swelling has important implications for the initial treatment of the brain-injured child and young adolescent.

D. **Cerebral edema.** Cerebral edema is an increase in the water content of the brain, usually in the extracellular spaces of the white matter. On the initial CT scan after trauma, cerebral edema is rarely seen. Edema occurs most frequently more than 24 hours after trauma either in the areas around cerebral contusions or intracerebral hematomas or in multiple sites after diffuse impact injury. Cerebral edema is usually progressive over several days, and it is common to see a small contusion on day 1 become a large area of edema by day 3 or 4 (Fig. 13-1).

E. **Cerebral ischemia.** Cerebral ischemia can occur after head injury as a result of occlusion of a major vessel, vascular spasm, hypotension, shock, or severe intracranial hypertension with compression of vessels. The most common area of ischemia in the distribution of the large vessels is in the area fed by the posterior cerebral arteries.

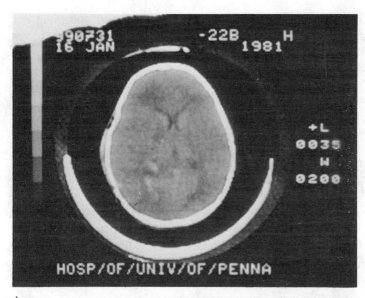

A

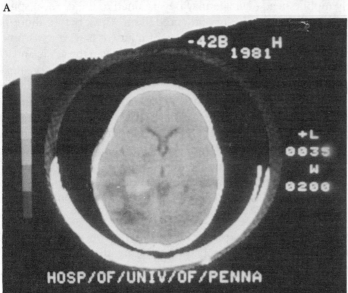

B

Fig. 13-1. *A.* CT scan in 2-year-old 24 hours posttrauma shows small deep hemorrhage in the left parieto-occipital region. The hemorrhage was seen after evacuation of an epidural hematoma. *B.* Marked increase in edema in deep parietal white matter 4 days later.

Ischemia occurs here as a result of herniation of the brain and compression of the posterior cerebral arteries. The second most common area is the anterior inferior frontal area, which is compromised by compression of the anterior cerebral arteries. It is common, particularly in children, to see areas of apparent infarction scattered thoughout the thalami.

In children less than 1 year of age, focal areas of decreased density are frequently seen on the first CT scan after trauma. These usually represent areas of ischemia rather than of edema. It is important to realize that the decreased density seen soon after head trauma is of ischemic origin. A careful search should be made for vascular compression, intracranial hypertension, or systemic hypotension. The therapy and prognosis of these ischemic areas are clearly different from those for edema since edema can be expected to resolve with little problem whereas ischemia and infarction are likely to leave significant cerebral injury.

F. **Craniospinal injury.** When an acceleration force is applied to the freely mobile head, damage may be sustained to the cervical spine as well as to the cerebrum and cerebellum. Thus, before there is any available history as to the nature of injury, it is wise to assume that craniospinal trauma has occurred, especially in the adult, and to take all reasonable precautions to prevent excessive extension, flexion, or lateral rotation of the patient's neck during retrieval from the site of accident, transport, and resuscitation. A good history, and, if necessary, cervical spine films to include the C-7 vertebra should be obtained as soon as possible and before further movement (e.g., to the operating room or CT scanner). Evidence of spinal trauma may be identified on neurologic examination but may be difficult to diagnose in the comatose patient. Spinal trauma may only become clinically apparent as the patient begins to recover from the cerebral injury.

G. **Multiple trauma.** Multiple trauma will not be specifically addressed in this chapter except to emphasize that isolated cranial trauma does not produce hypotension and tachycardia. When hypotension occurs, a careful search for another source of blood loss is necessary, which will most frequently be in the abdomen or fractured long bones. In children less than 1 year old, a large epidural hematoma can cause hypovolemia and anemia in the presence of an associated skull fracture, which permits decompression of the hematoma into the subperiosteal or subgaleal space (Fig. 13-2). Abdominal lavage may also be necessary to identify a source of bleeding. Fluid not recovered from the abdomen during the lavage has to be taken into account when calculating the desired fluid balance for that 24-hour period.

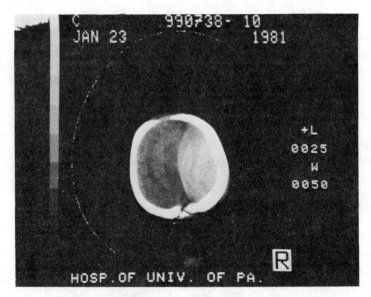

Fig. 13-2. CT scan in 9-month-old child with evidence of massive right parietal epidural hematoma and active bleeding. This child was awake and alert and had only a mild left hemiparesis.

H. Primary versus secondary injury

1. **Primary injury.** Head trauma causes primary and secondary injury to the brain. The primary injury occurs within a few milliseconds after the traumatic force is applied to the head. This injury involves the relative movement of structures inside the head, which causes immediate damage to the white matter, tearing of the arteries and veins, and contusion of the brain. What happens to neurons, dendrites, and synapses is not known. The pathology of this impact injury as it relates to the white matter includes shearing injury, tearing of axons and myelin, transient conduction abnormalites, and petechial hemorrhages. Exactly what happens to the gray matter neurons and dendrites is, at present, not understood at all. There is no treatment for this primary injury, although an artery that is torn at the moment of impact (and is therefore part of the primary injury) may cause an expanding hematoma minutes to hours later. There is overlap between the primary injury and secondary injury.

2. **Secondary injury.** The secondary injuries are a series of progressive pathophysiologic changes that can produce more damage to the brain. They are due to events set in motion by the primary insult, and do not produce their deleterious effects until

minutes to hours after impact. The factors contributing to the secondary injury are hypoxia, hypercapnia, systemic hypotension, and intracranial hypertension. The apparent common denominator of the secondary injury is cerebral ischemia, both focal and global. Included within this secondary injury are the various syndromes of transcallosal, transtentorial, and cerebellar tonsillar herniation.

II. **Emergency management.** Current emergency management of head-injured patients is based on maximal effort from the earliest possible time to prevent the secondary injury. All of the events that lead to secondary injury of the brain can, theoretically, be prevented, setting the stage for maximal recovery.

   A. **Airway.** From the first moments of resuscitation, a patent airway must be assured. In severely head-injured patients, opening the airway will usually result in moderate hyperventilation, although hypoxia may persist. First, the mouth must be cleaned out manually to remove debris, vomitus, or teeth, and the tongue must be kept forward. In adults, preservation of an open airway without an artificial airway is frequently difficult, whereas in children an airway can usually be easily maintained. Hyperextension of the neck should be avoided in both groups, if possible, until the integrity of the cervical spine has been ascertained. There is no need to hyperextend the child's neck to ventilate, whereas it may be difficult to establish an adequate airway in an adult (especially someone who has a short, fat neck) without moderate hyperextension or an artificial airway.

   Although endotracheal intubation may be the ideal method of airway control in the severely head-injured patient, the trachea must be intubated only when suction and oxygen are available, and when the dangers of a cervical fracture, a full stomach, and intracranial hypertension are taken into account. Until preparations can be made for endotracheal intubation, ventilation with bag and mask and supplemental oxygen (40%–60%) is usually adequate, the object being to maintain the arterial carbon dioxide tension ($PaCO_2$) between 30 and 35 mmHg and the arterial oxygen tension (PaO_2) above 80 mmHg. In the presence of severe facial injuries, an emergency tracheotomy may be necessary. Beside this situation, there are few other indications for tracheotomy, and attempts at nasal or oral endotracheal intubation should be made.

   Much of the secondary injury results from poor ventilation. Decrease in the PaO_2 below 50 mmHg increases cerebral blood flow (CBF), cerebral blood volume (CBV), and intracranial pressure (ICP). Increased $PaCO_2$ also increases CBF, CBV, and ICP. Brain swelling, brain edema, and mass lesions all raise ICP, which is further aggravated by hypercapnia and hypoxia. Most adults and children who have Glasgow coma scores of less than 8 (see Table 13-1) will require endotracheal intubation at least in the early post-injury period. Endotracheal intubation not only permits control of arterial gas tensions but also enables the patient to be transported safely from the emergency room to the CT scanner, intensive care unit (ICU), or operating room and allows the use of muscle paralysis to obtain good CT scans. Whether to continue intubation beyond this time is based on each patient's needs. Both the level of consciousness and the results of the CT scan will help in making this decision.

In unconscious patients (Glasgow coma scores of 8 or less), endotracheal intubation is performed after administration of 100% oxygen, succinylcholine, thiopental, and the use of cricoid pressure to prevent gastric regurgitation and aspiration. Uncuffed endotracheal tubes that permit a small leak are used for children. Once the endotracheal tube is secured, the stomach is emptied with a large-bore nasogastric tube. The nasogastric tube is then left in place and connected to straight drainage.

It is our practice to obtain a lateral x-ray film of the cervical spine if time permits before endotracheal intubation, particularly in patients who have sustained acceleration-deceleration injuries. The seventh cervical vertebra must be seen, and although the x-ray film does not definitively rule out spinal injury, it will identify dislocations or fractures and may suggest that nasotracheal intubation may be preferable, particularly in adults, to avoid hyperextension of the neck. The adult who has a short neck and cervical spine injury may require tracheotomy to establish an airway safely.

Once the endotracheal tube is in place, we continue moderate hyperventilation to a $PaCO_2$ of 30 mmHg in adults and 25 mmHg in children. Since it is likely that areas of disruption of the blood-brain barrier are present, the higher the end-capillary pressure and the blood flow, the greater the amount of edema that will form. Decreasing the $PaCO_2$ will reduce CBF by producing arteriolar constriction and decreasing end-capillary pressure and will prevent edema formation. Hyperventilation will also decrease cerebral blood volume and lower ICP. Children who have had acceleration-deceleration injuries develop a true hyperemia in about 50% of cases. This acute brain swelling is due in large part to vasodilatation; because of this, we prefer to keep $PaCO_2$ between 25 and 30 mmHg.

B. **Cardiovascular status.** The head injury itself is rarely the cause of hypotension and the source of bleeding must be sought. Resuscitation from shock should be accomplished with isotonic fluid, normal saline or Ringer's lactate solution, or colloid if blood is not readily available. Glucose and water should not be used as this decreases serum osmolality and can aggravate the cerebral swelling. The ideal replacement, of course, is blood. Since the cerebral vessels are already dilated because of the hypotension, rapid restitution of the normal arterial pressure will precipitate brain swelling. It is extremely valuable to insert an ICP monitor during resuscitation in the emergency room so that both systemic arterial pressure and ICP can be measured and controlled, thus avoiding severe elevations of ICP, which can be fatal.

It is frequently necessary to take children directly to the operating room because of intra-abdominal hemorrhage. Here again, the ability to measure and control ICP during the resuscitation, transport, and surgery is only possible when ICP is monitored directly. In patients who have circulatory collapse, the insertion of an intra-arterial cannula and an ICP monitor is vital early in the course of resuscitation: only then can the correct balance between arterial pressure and ICP be maintained.

C. **History and examination.** Frequently, there is little or no history available when the patient arrives in the emergency room and when the resuscitation must be begun. It is always valuable to assign one person to talk to whatever witnesses are available or to the ambulance personnel. The history should be brief but should include, if possible, the type of injury (e.g., fall, pedestrian or automobile injury); the course of events since the time the patient was first observed (i.e., improving, worsening, or the same); and the presence of any period of apnea or evidence of seizure activity. Usually any past history is unobtainable at this point.

1. **The neurologic examination** of the comatose patient is, of necessity, limited and can be performed in a few minutes and need not interfere with the resuscitative efforts. The Glasgow coma score (see Table 13-1) is a good initial measurement of the degree of insult sustained. Once the patient is stabilized, the scale is helpful in making some predictions of likely outcome. The simplicity of the scale makes interobserver agreement on examination possible. The results of the assessment of pupillary responses, cold caloric responses, spontaneous ventilation, and gag reflexes will define the state of the brainstem, pons, and medulla, as well as the hemispheres. The symmetry of the motor examination, both side-to-side and proximal-to-distal, also gives information on the localization of the lesion within the brain, spinal cord, and peripheral nervous system. After head trauma, a single examination is less helpful than repeated examinations over a period of time. Changes in the patient's score can be used to define neurologic deterioration or improvement.

2. **Pupillary responses** are tested by using a bright light, and both **direct** and **consensual** responses must be assessed in each eye. The presence of equal and reactive pupils indicates that the upper brainstem, mesencephalon, and second and third cranial nerves are all intact. Unilateral loss of direct response with preservation of consensual response suggests optic nerve injury. Loss of unilateral response is usually caused by injury either to the area of the superior colliculus or to the optic nerve bilaterally. When the third nerve is involved, the pupils are usually large. With lesions in the tegmentum, the pupils are frequently in the midposition and unreactive. Small unresponsive pupils signify pontine lesions, whereas small reactive pupils are most commonly seen with hemorrhage into and around the third ventricle.

3. **Oculovestibular responses.** Because of the risk of cervical spine injury, we prefer to use the cold caloric test to assess the oculovestibular response instead of the doll's eyes or oculocephalic maneuver, in which the head is rotated from side to side and the movements of the eyes are noted. Cold caloric testing is performed with cold water irrigation of the ears. Before the test, the ear canals must be examined. If there is no leakage of cerebrospinal fluid (CSF), if the eardrum is intact, and if the canal is not filled with blood or wax, the test can be performed safely. Ideally, the head should be elevated 30 degrees from the horizontal, but this may be contraindicated if there is any question of cervical spine injury. Ice water, 100 to 200 ml, is used to irrigate each ear over several minutes to obtain maximal stimulation. A response is expected within 2 to 3 minutes. If no response is obtained, several minutes must elapse before the other side is tested.

   The normal conscious response is mild deviation of the eyes to the cooled side with rapid nystagmus back to the midline. In comatose patients, the nystagmus component is lost and an intact response involves bilateral tonic deviation to the cooled side. Lesions of the medial longitudinal fasciculus will prevent the adducting eye from crossing the midline; this may be observed either unilaterally or bilaterally. More destructive lesions will result in bilateral loss of eye movement in response to either unilateral or bilateral cooling. These findings signify severe involvement of the pons and midbrain but may be associated with recovery from head injury, especially in children.

4. **Ventilatory and gag responses.** The lowest pathways in the medulla involve the gag response and spontaneous ventilation. These responses should always be evaluated. Care must be taken

when checking the gag response not to induce vomiting before endotracheal intubation. Gag response is tested by gently stimulating either side of the posterior soft palate or by placing a cotton-tipped applicator against the posterior pharyngeal wall. Spontaneous ventilation is tested by ensuring an open airway and observing the patient's spontaneous ventilatory efforts. If resuscitation has been performed and hyperventilation has been part of that resuscitation, CO_2 will have to rise to the normal range before the absence of spontaneous ventilation can be satisfactorily diagnosed. Patients who do not have spontaneous ventilatory effort will rarely, if ever, make a significant recovery, and the absence of spontaneous ventilation coupled with the absence of the other brainstem responses signifies brain death.

III. **Special studies.** Once the patient's condition is stabilized, the next step is to determine the need for further diagnostic studies. The patient's level of consciousness, the clinical examination, and the history of the trauma are all considered in selecting necessary studies.

A. **Plain x-ray films of skull and spine.** In those patients who have Glasgow coma scores of 8 or more, skull x-ray films can diagnose linear or depressed fractures, the presence of which will heighten concern about possible epidural hemorrhage. X-ray studies may demonstrate pneumocephalus, which indicates a basal fracture, and in children (particularly those less than 1 year), plain skull x-ray films after trauma may show evidence of splitting of the sutures. The combination of split sutures and a linear skull fracture is frequently associated with an intracranial mass lesion, most commonly an epidural hematoma, and should be an indication for obtaining a CT scan. Skull x-ray films are rarely helpful in patients who have coma scores of less than 8. These patients require CT scan (or arteriogram if CT scan is unavailable). All patients who are unconscious after head trauma who do not show signs of rapid recovery require neuroradiologic investigation to rule out the presence of a mass lesion.

To establish normal alignment of the cervical spine, lateral x-ray films of the spine, including C-7, are obtained as soon as possible in any patient who has had acceleration-deceleration trauma. While a single lateral x-ray film will not rule out all cases of cervical fracture or dislocation, it is a good screening test before the head is moved to facilitate intubation of the trachea.

B. **CT scan.** The CT scan is the single most useful study for the examination of patients who have severe head injury or a deteriorating level of consciousness. In demonstrating the state of the soft tissues, sinuses, bones, brain, and CSF spaces, the CT scan clearly defines hematomas and contusions. In restless patients, a good scan cannot be obtained because of movement artifact. The danger of missing a significant mass lesion on the CT scan is small, but the presence of motion artifact can obscure small subdural or epidural hematomas, cortical contusions, or both. If the scan is necessary, then either sedation or endotracheal intubation and general anesthesia will be required. It is dangerous to accept a poor scan: a false sense of security may be imparted to those caring for the patient.

With the new rapid scanners, the problem of movement artifact has been minimized. The CT scan is now capable of demonstrating all of the pathologic lesions associated with head injury from diffuse impact injury to intracerebral hematomas. We do not generally use contrast during the first CT study.

C. **Arteriography.** When the CT scan is available, arteriography is rarely used in the study of acute head trauma patients. If a CT scan is unavailable, however, then cerebral arteriography remains the investigation of choice in the unconscious, severely head-injured patient. The arteriogram does not define the traumatic pathology as well as the CT scan, but it demonstrates the vascular pathology much more effectively. Thus, in patients in whom either cerebral arterial spasm or arterial occlusion is suspected, arteriography may still be the procedure of choice. When arteriography is considered necessary, the integrity of the cervical spine must be established. The patient must be stable enough to undergo the procedure. The safest way to accomplish the study is with the use of an endotracheal tube, muscle paralysis, controlled ventilation and sedation with narcotics. Under these conditions, good arteriograms without movement artifact are obtained, and the patient's airway, blood pressure, and ventilation are carefully controlled during the procedure.

IV. **Further management.** After emergency resuscitation with the establishment of an airway and the correction of any cardiovascular instability, the further management of the patient is determined by the results of the neurological examination and the CT scan, as well as any associated injuries.

A. **Scalp lacerations.** All scalp lacerations should be liberally irrigated and gently examined, using a gloved finger to seek evidence of a depressed skull fracture. If a depression is present, the wound is covered with sterile saline-soaked sponges and x-ray films are obtained. If indeed there is a compound depressed skull fracture, surgical correction is required. If either no fracture or a linear fracture is present, surgery is rarely necessary, and the wound is then closed primarily.

B. **Skull fractures.** The majority of skull fractures need no therapy. Fractures involving the base of the skull with CSF otorrhea or rhinorrhea rarely necessitate any kind of emergency surgery. Usually these CSF leaks will stop over several days, and rarely do they require surgical repair. The major disagreement in management of these basal fractures involves the administration of antibiotics. It is not our practice to administer prophylactic antibiotics to patients who have CSF leaks.

Depressed skull fractures and compound depressed fractures are likely to require surgical correction. Usually these fractures occur in patients whose neurologic state is quite good since the fractures result from localized injuries to the head. Closed depressed skull fractures rarely require emergency operation. It is often better to allow 24 to 48 hours to pass to enable the patient's level of consciousness to recover before subjecting the patient to a surgical procedure.

There are two reasons for operating on closed depressed skull fractures: if cosmetic repair is necessary in the frontal areas (if the fractures are depressed beyond the thickness of the table of the skull, there is also a high likelihood of dural laceration) or if the patient has evidence of a focal neurologic deficit owing to injury of the brain underlying the fracture site. In these circumstances, the CT scan can be valuable in demonstrating the degree of depression of the inner table of the skull and the condition of the underlying brain.

Compound depressed skull fractures frequently require emergency surgical correction. The decision to undertake surgery depends upon the patient's neurologic state, the degree of skin laceration, and the position and location of the fractures. The CT scan is helpful before surgery for compound depressed skull fractures to determine the degree of internal displacement of the bone fragment, the condition of the underlying brain, and, equally important, evidence of any other associated cerebral injury. Our technique of repairing compound depressed skull fractures is as follows: (1) try to save all fragments of bone; (2) perform a circular craniotomy that includes the area of fracture; (3) remove the bone pieces: (4) debride the brain; (5) repair the dura (an important step); and (6) replace the various pieces of bone after they have been steeped in antibiotic solution. If the dura is left open, significant cerebral herniation can occur through the defect with secondary ischemia, infarction, and increase in cerebral damage.

C. **Physiologic monitoring.** In adults who have Glasgow coma scores of 8 or less and in children who have Glasgow coma scores of 5 or less (see Table 13-1), it is advisable to insert an intra-arterial cannula and ICP monitor when the patient is in the emergency room. The blood pressure and ICP can then be monitored on portable equipment during transfer to CT scan, operating room, or ICU. For children in whom we recommend a low $PaCO_2$ as part of the early management, it is useful to have a portable capnograph to monitor end-tidal CO_2. This group of patients will also require a urinary catheter provided there is no evidence of perineal trauma. If perineal trauma is present a urethrogram may be necessary before catheterization to rule out urethral fracture. All unconscious patients require at least one large-bore intravenous catheter. A nasogastric tube is usually inserted after the endotracheal tube is in place; the only real contraindication is the presence of severe facial, frontal, or basal skull fractures.

Once the patient's condition is stabilized in the ICU, further monitoring may include the use of a Swan-Ganz catheter if there is any cardiovascular instability or evidence of pulmonary edema. The insertion of a jugular bulb catheter permits measurement of cerebral blood flow (CBF) and cerebral metabolic rate ($CMRO_2$), which may be helpful if extreme hyperventilation ($PaCO_2$ of 20–25 mmHg) is necessary to control brain swelling.

Continuous monitoring of the EEG is not useful in patients who have head injury. The monitoring of visual, somatosensory, and brainstem evoked responses is relatively new, but there are suggestions that useful information may be obtained (Greenberg, 1977). At the same time, blood should be drawn for type and crossmatch and base-line serum electrolytes, amylase, and osmolality. In comatose children, inappropriate antidiuretic hormone secretion is a common problem, and a sudden drop in serum sodium can occur within the first 24 to 48 hours despite fluid restriction. Thus, frequent measurement of serum electrolytes and osmolality and careful control of fluid balance are necessary in this particular group of patients.

D. **Management of increased ICP.** In unconscious patients it is extremely difficult to judge whether ICP is elevated. Therefore, all early therapy during resuscitation is designed to lower raised ICP or, at least, to prevent further increases in ICP. Simple maneuvers such as a 15- to 20-degree **head-up tilt,** keeping the head in the midline position and not rotated to either side to maintain open jugular veins, relative restriction of fluid intake, and maintenance of normal, rather than increased, arterial pressure will all help control ICP. **Endotracheal intubation** is performed using adequate supplemental oxygen and medication to ensure good oxygenation and low $PaCO_2$ and to prevent coughing and straining during laryngoscopy and intubation.

In the noncomatose patient, there is rarely need for any specific medication or therapy to reduce ICP. If the patient requires a CT scan, the findings will determine whether therapy is required (e.g., corticosteroids because of an intracerebral hematoma). In patients who have a deteriorating level of consciousness after admission, it is imperative to ascertain the cause of the altered neurologic state. Is the patient having seizures? Is the deterioration from intracranial hypertension, systemic hypotension, or hypoxia? Is there evidence that an increasing mass lesion is producing herniation with either pupillary dilatation or contralateral hemiparesis or hemiplegia? Therapy should be directed toward the cause of the problem (e.g., adequate ventilation and anticonvulsant drugs for a patient who is having seizures) rather than specifically concerned with lowering ICP (e.g., mannitol).

In patients in whom intracranial hypertension is suspected, either from an epidural or subdural hematoma or diffuse brain swelling, emergency treatment to reduce ICP is vital. A definitive study to identify the cause of the clinical deterioration is conducted afterwards. The first and most rapidly effective therapy is **hyperventilation.** In a patient who has multiple trauma and reduced blood volume, care must be taken during controlled ventilation to avoid increasing the intrathoracic pressure, thus decreasing cardiac return and producing secondary hypotension. Corticosteroids (dexamethasone or methylprednisolone) are of little benefit in trauma, and, certainly, these drugs should not be relied on to lower the ICP rapidly.

Although **mannitol** will effectively lower the ICP within minutes after administration, its use remains controversial. The drug is indicated, however, when either elevated ICP or a mass and herniation are responsible for the patient's deteriorating state. The risk of increasing the size of hematoma is negligible compared to the disastrous effects of untreated progressive uncal herniation. If decompression of transtentorial herniation is delayed, secondary hemorrhage into the brainstem can occur and cause irreversible neurologic deficit. Once mannitol is given and the ICP is reduced, the specific intracranial disorder must be identified as soon as possible to prevent a recurrence of the patient's deterioration.

Occasionally, the diagnosis of an epidural hematoma will be obvious and immediate operation will be required because of rapid deterioration of the patient's level of consciousness. More frequently, the use of hyperventilation and mannitol gives the surgeon time to obtain a CT scan to define the intracranial disorder. The use of exploratory burr holes is not advocated, because if no definitive lesion is found, the patient still requires further neurodiagnostic studies. If a surgical lesion is found after additional diagnostic procedures, the patient must again be returned to the operating room.

The extra time may also be detrimental since good recovery depends on the rapidity with which a hematoma is evacuated. The CT scan is clearly invaluable in the efficient diagnosis and treatment of severely head-injured patients.

In children, acute deterioration is much less frequently due to surgically correctable lesions. Such deterioration is most often caused either by generalized brain swelling and increased ICP or by seizure activity. Thus, the use of radiologic study before any surgical intervention in children is even more important than in adults. Since acute deterioration seems to be associated with a swollen congested brain rather than with cerebral edema, we do not recommend mannitol for children unless the presence of an epidural hematoma is strongly suspected. The initial therapy for deterioration in children, then, is hyperventilation and head-up tilt of 15 to 30 degrees. If an epidural hematoma is suspected, mannitol may be given after the CO_2 has been lowered.

In both adults and children, the initial dose of mannitol is 0.5 to 1 gm/kg given over 3 to 5 minutes by intravenous infusion rather than by direct intravenous bolus injection. When mannitol is given rapidly to unanesthetized patients, a rise in blood pressure usually occurs and is frequently accompanied by a rise in ICP. This elevation of blood pressure and ICP can be prevented if the drug is given slowly. The reason for avoiding mannitol or other osmotic diuretics in children during the early resuscitative period is that mannitol increases cerebral blood flow (CBF) independent of its effect on ICP. If the diffuse swelling in children is due to hyperemia, it is possible that mannitol could exacerbate this condition and produce a further increase in ICP and clinical deterioration. The best way to treat the initial deterioration is to monitor the ICP of comatose patients from the earliest phase of resuscitation. In this way, the ICP, its response to therapy, and the need for further intervention can be measured accurately, and appropriate treatment can be initiated.

E. **Corticosteroids.** Corticosteroids have not been demonstrated to be of value in improving the outcome after head injury. Although the complications of corticosteroid therapy are minor over the first few days (hyperglycemia is the most frequent problem in adults), a number of centers have abandoned the administration of large doses of dexamethasone or methylprednisolone to comatose patients as part of the early treatment.

F. **Barbiturates.** The use of barbiturates in large doses to reduce ICP in head-injured patients is not part of the initial resuscitation. Their administration is usually reserved for situations in which other measures to control the ICP have failed. Large doses of barbiturates are dangerous because they interfere with peripheral resistance and

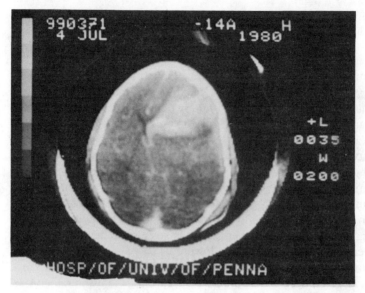

Fig. 13-3. CT scan in 8-year-old who was ejected 100 feet in the air from the cockpit of an airplane. CT scan reveals large right frontal intracerebral hemorrhage, subarachnoid hemorrhage, and brain swelling. Despite surgical evacuation, hyperventilation, barbiturates, and hypothermia, intracranial pressure rose to equal systemic arterial pressure and the child died of intracranial hypertension.

cardiovascular function, which commonly results in hypotension. This reaction occurs most often in hypovolemic patients. Therefore, we do not suggest the routine use of these drugs.

If the patient shows signs of rapid deterioration in the emergency room because of intracranial hypertension, the insertion of an ICP monitor and intra-arterial cannula allows sensible management. Under these circumstances, if hyperventilation and osmotic agents fail to lower the ICP, barbiturates, initially thiopental and then pentobarbital, may be administered. In children who have severe diffuse injury, marked swelling, and high ICP, the use of barbiturates will frequently reduce the ICP when other methods have proven ineffective. If the damage to the brain is too extensive, the ICP will rise again rapidly (Fig. 13-3). In patients whose injuries are less severe the ICP will be controlled. Barbiturates in large doses should not be used to treat intracranial hypertension unless systemic arterial pressure, central venous pressure, and ICP are monitored continuously.

G. Hypothermia. Hypothermia to 32°C is associated with a 40% to 50% decrease in the cerebral metabolic rate and a concomitant reduction in CBF, cerebral blood volume, and ICP. When barbiturates are given in large doses, the patient's temperature frequently falls to the 32° to 34°C range; we make no effort to restore the temperature to normal. The benefits of hypothermia thus include a reduction in ICP and potentially some protective effect as a result of the decreased metabolic rate, which allows the brain to tolerate episodes of ischemia (e.g., pressure waves) better. The dangers of hypothermia, however, are multiple: peripheral vasoconstriction, impaired white cell phagocytosis, increased incidence of pneumonia, decreased ciliary function of the bronchi, and, if the temperature goes below 30°C, an increased risk of cardiac arrhythmia. Nonetheless, we believe that hypothermia, whether induced or as a concomitant of barbiturate therapy, is a useful adjunct in patients whose ICP is difficult to control by other means.

V. **The anesthesiologist's role in severe head injury.** The anesthesiologist's involvement in the care of the head-injured patient begins immediately on arrival of the patient in the trauma unit, or, if there is an outgoing ambulance retrieval system, at the site of the collection of the patient. The need to stabilize the patient before transfer from hospital to hospital is axiomatic; yet frequently, patients are transferred without provision of an adequate airway, in shock with no large-bore intravenous catheter, or with clear evidence of abdominal bleeding. Under these circumstances, the transfer is frequently detrimental to the patient's welfare. In children, not only is there a problem with inexperienced examiners' overlooking significant blood loss but frequently smaller hospitals do not have the equipment required for endotracheal intubation of small tracheas.

Our policy at the Children's Hospital of Philadelphia is to send our own transport team directed by an anesthesiologist who works with a pediatric resident and a nurse to collect the child at the outlying hospital. Equipment for ventilation and suction is carried in the ambulance. The child is not transported before an adequate airway, intravenous infusion, and intra-arterial pressure monitoring are established. It is likely that such transport support will become increasingly prominent in the critical care of brain-injured patients. In some areas of the country, well-trained paramedics can perform a similar sort of stabilization before transfer from the site of the accident. Good on-the-spot care has been shown to decrease the incidence of hypoxia on arrival in the emergency room significantly and should be the goal in all communities.

Systemic Effects
Jane Matjasko

The systemic effects of head injury are diverse and affect nearly all organs. In addition, they may be responsible for morbidity and even mortality in the

Table 13-2. Peripheral sequelae of acute head injury

Cardiopulmonary
  Abnormal breathing patterns
  Airway obstruction
  Hypoxia
  Shock
  Adult respiratory distress syndrome (ARDS)
  Neurogenic pulmonary edema (NPE)
  Fat embolism
  Venous thromboembolism
  Electrocardiographic changes
Hematologic
  Inhibition of neutrophil phagocytosis
  Trauma and coagulation
  Disseminated intravascular coagulation (DIC)
Endocrinologic
  Anterior pituitary insufficiency
  Posterior pituitary dysfunction
    Diabetes insipidus
    Syndrome of inappropriate ADH (SIADH)
Metabolic
  Cerebrospinal fluid metabolic changes
  Nonketotic hyperosmolar hyperglycemic coma (NHHC)
Gastrointestinal
Skeletal
  Cervical spine injuries
  Maxillofacial injuries

severely head-injured patient. They thus require active prevention and prompt, thorough treatment. Table 13-2 lists the organs and disease processes that are related to head injury.

I. Cardiopulmonary effects of head injury

    A. Initial management and resuscitation. Severe head injury may cause apnea and hypoxia at the time of concussion or after the development of massive brain swelling which can lead to intracranial hypertension and tentorial herniation. Airway obstruction may occur from neck flexion, loss of muscle tone, or the presence of debris in the mouth. Aspiration of gastric contents predisposes the patient to chemical pneumonitis, atelectasis, and bronchopneumonia. There seems to be no relation between abnormal breathing patterns and the site or extent of neurologic injury; persistent spontaneous hyperventilation from either cerebrospinal fluid (CSF) lactic acidosis or brainstem dysfunction carries a poor prognosis.

    When admitted to the hospital, 30% to 50% of head-injured patients will have a PaO_2 of less than 60 mmHg in the absence of airway obstruction or prior pulmonary disease. Minute ventilation may be twice normal, particularly if CO_2 production is above normal, as it is in the decerebrate patient. Severe refractory hypoxia is associated with a poor prognosis. A large intrapulmonary shunt ($\dot{Q}s/\dot{Q}t$) indicates an ill-defined effect of acute intracranial hypertension on ventilation-perfusion relationships.

The primary concern is to establish ventilatory support and a patent, protected airway using a cuffed endotracheal tube and controlled ventilation. Neurologic and cardiopulmonary resuscitation includes:

1. **Intubation:** cuffed endotracheal tube (low-pressure cuff)

2. **Mechanical ventilation**

   a. PaO_2, 100 mmHg; $PaCO_2$, 25 to 30 mmHg; optimal positive end-expiratory pressure (PEEP) if neurologic condition permits

   b. Consider sedation or muscle relaxation in restless or decerebrate patients

3. **Cardiovascular support**

   a. Maintain cerebral perfusion pressure (CPP) at normal levels with crystalloid or colloid

   b. Blood transfusion to maximize O_2 carrying capacity

   c. Inotropic and vasopressor drugs as indicated

4. **Monitoring.** Mean arterial pressure (MAP), intracranial pressure (ICP), CPP, PaO_2, $PaCO_2$, hemoglobin, neurologic status, fluid and electrolyte balance, and chest x-ray

5. **Drugs**

   a. Intubation. Rapid sequence induction with thiopental, 1 to 3 mg/kg IV, and/or lidocaine, 1 mg/kg, to prevent an acute rise in ICP during laryngoscopy, and succinylcholine, 1.5 mg/kg

   b. Mannitol. 0.25 to 1 gm/kg rapidly

   c. Pancuronium. 0.1 mg/kg initially; then 0.02 to 0.03 mg/kg each hour if muscle paralysis is to be maintained

   d. Sedation. Diazepam, 5 to 10 mg every 2 to 3 hours, and fentanyl, 0.7 to 1.4 μg/kg each hour

B. **Shock and adult respiratory distress syndrome (ARDS).** As many as 50% of head-injured patients will have multisystem trauma and hemorrhagic shock; as many as 10% may have concomitant cervical spinal cord injury and spinal shock. Cardiogenic shock may be caused by either direct or secondary myocardial injury or by a protracted low flow state from hemorrhagic shock. Neurogenic shock related to collapse of the vasomotor center rarely occurs and is almost always fatal. ICP and pupil size should be monitored in head-injured patients who are anesthetized for emergency operations of the abdomen, face, chest, or extremities since progressive neurologic deterioration may otherwise be undetectable.

1. Approximately 20% of head-injured patients may develop **ARDS** characterized by

   a. Progressive hypoxia

   b. Reduced functional residual capacity (FRC)

   c. Reduced compliance

   d. Pulmonary hypertension

   e. Diffuse patchy consolidation on chest x-ray film

   f. Hyaline membrane formation

   g. Pulmonary fibrosis

2. The **combination of hypoxia and shock** may exacerbate the initial neurologic injury because the resultant reduction in CPP causes cerebral ischemia. Treatment includes

   a. Optimal inspired oxygen tension (FIO_2).

   b. Careful fluid balance based on measurement of pulmonary capillary wedge pressure (PCWP), central venous pressure (CVP), cardiac output, and urine output.

   c. Chest physiotherapy and prompt treatment of pulmonary infection.

   d. Optimal PEEP, the lowest positive end-expiratory pressure that will produce maximum oxygen availability (arterial oxygen content × cardiac output). The increased airway pressure produced by PEEP may increase intrathoracic pressure, increase CVP, and hence increase ICP while simultaneously reducing CPP because of reduced cardiac output and MAP. When PEEP is discontinued, the sudden increase in central blood volume and MAP may increase cerebral blood volume and cerebral edema, particularly when cerebral autoregulation is impaired. The effect of PEEP is most critical in patients who have reduced intracranial compliance. Optimal PEEP implies achieving the greatest increase in PaO_2 without either reducing cardiac output or raising ICP.

3. Criteria for **weaning from mechanical ventilation**

   a. Vital capacity of greater than 10 ml/kg

   b. Maximum inspiratory force of greater than -20 cm H_2O

   c. VD/VT of less than 0.6

   d. $P(A-a)O_2$ of less than 300 mmHg

   e. Cardiovascular stability

   f. Normal metabolic state

C. **Neurogenic pulmonary edema.** Various forms of noncardiogenic pulmonary edema have been explained by the presence of hypoxic pulmonary vasoconstriction that causes pulmonary arterial hypertension, pulmonary arteriolar wall rupture, and leakage of protein-rich edema fluid into the interstitium and alveoli. There are similarities between the pathologic and clinical pictures of ARDS and neurogenic pulmonary edema (NPE). Perfusion of the brain with hypoxic blood leads to a lung lesion that is pathologically similar to shock lung and is associated with increased pulmonary venular resistance, vascular congestion, and interstitial and intraalveolar edema and hemorrhage. NPE is associated with a high mortality, and it is not clear whether reversal of the pulmonary hypertension in its early stages by the use of vasodilators such as sodium nitroprusside or nitroglycerin could be beneficial.

1. **Characteristics**

   a. Association with a variety of insults to the central nervous system (CNS) including head injury

   b. Presence of intracranial hypertension

   c. Marked pulmonary vascular congestion of rapid onset

   d. Massive neural discharge from injured brain or hypothalamus leading to pulmonary hypertension

   e. Increased pulmonary blood volume and pulmonary edema and hemorrhage

2. **Therapy**

   a. Immediate reduction in ICP through pharmacologic or surgical intervention, or both

   b. Hyperventilation: $PaCO_2$ of 25 to 30 mmHg with continuous positive pressure ventilation and high inspired oxygen tension

D. **Fat embolism.** Fat embolism may occur in the hours or days after the fracture of any bone containing marrow. Failure to recover consciousness after general anesthesia may suggest this diagnosis; secondary deterioration in a head-injured patient may be a consequence of fat embolism. No laboratory test is pathognomonic.

1. **Characteristics**

   a. Hypoxia

   b. Fluffy infiltrates on chest x-ray film

   c. Anemia, thrombocytopenia, hypocalcemia

2. **Symptoms and signs** appear 24 to 48 hours after trauma.

   a. Changes in mental status ranging from restlessness to coma

   b. Seizures, paralysis

   c. Evanescent petechial rash (anterior axillary folds, neck, abdominal wall, conjunctiva)

3. **Treatment.** Therapy is directed primarily to correct hypoxia with PEEP and increased FiO_2. Massive fat embolism is associated with high mortality.

E. **Venous thromboembolism.** The incidence of fatal pulmonary embolism in head-injured patients is unknown. There is a higher incidence of thromboembolic complications among patients who have suprasellar masses than among those who do not have suprasellar masses; a relationship between suprasellar masses and hypothalamic-associated hypercoagulability has been implied. Dehydration, obesity, and/or immobilization, all of which may be associated with hypothalamic malfunction, also predispose the patient to thromboembolism.

Minidose heparin therapy (5000 units SC every 12 hours as long as the patient is bedridden) can be used safely after a variety of surgical procedures. Whether this approach can prevent deep-vein thrombosis and pulmonary embolism in the neurosurgical population, including head-injured patients, without increasing the incidence of hematoma, is unknown.

F. **Electrocardiographic changes.** Arrhythmias and cardiac arrest may occur after head injury. Bradycardia, shortened Q–T interval, elevated S–T segment, nodal rhythm, increased T wave amplitude, and atrial fibrillation have occurred after head injury, in the presence and absence of intracranial hypertension. The pathogenesis is obscure. Atropine (for bradycardia), digoxin (for atrial fibrillation), and correction of metabolic and electrolyte abnormalities may be required.

II. Hematologic abnormalities

A. **Inhibition of phagocytosis.** Many disease states, including anoxic brain damage and head injury, are associated with the inhibition of the phagocytic function of neutrophilic granulocytes. Severe disturbances in phagocyte function have been observed in some head-injured patients who have clear consciousness and post-traumatic diabetes insipidus, implying a hypothalamic mechanism. There is a correlation between elevated serotonin levels in the CSF of head-injured patients and the inhibition of phagocytosis. Corticosteroids also stimulate serotoninergic metabolism in the brain.

B. **Trauma and coagulation.** The patient may be in a hypercoagulable and fibrinolytic state during the first few hours after trauma, probably from the release of tissue thromboplastin for hemostatic purposes. An abrupt rebound antifibrinolysis may also occur to facilitate hemostasis. Multiple transfusions, shock, sepsis, and unknown factors can also influence coagulation. Aspirin, phenylbutazone, chlorpromazine, penicillin, general anesthetics, furosemide, and many other drugs, as well as head trauma, impair platelet aggregation.

C. **Disseminated intravascular coagulation (DIC).** DIC is a physiologic response to a variety of stimuli that provoke a generalized activation of the hemostatic mechanism, leading to the intravascular consumption of clotting factors with subsequent thrombosis, bleeding diathesis, or both. DIC can be the result of three processes: endothelial cell injury, tissue injury, or red cell or platelet injury. The pathogenesis of DIC in cases of head injury is uncertain. The severity of the coagulopathy correlates with the severity of the head injury and systemic trauma. Shock, sepsis, extensive surgery, and fat embolism have all been associated with DIC. In addition, the brain is rich in tissue thromboplastin, and high levels of fibrinolytic activity are present in the highly vascular connective tissue of the choroid plexus and meninges. The mortality from DIC associated with head injury is high; death may be a consequence of intractable cerebral edema, intracerebral or intraventricular hemorrhage, multiple organ failure from microthrombosis, uncontrollable systemic hemorrhage, or a combination of these factors.

1. **Diagnostic criteria for DIC** include abnormal results of at least three screening tests: prothrombin time, fibrinogen, and platelets. If only two of these three factors are abnormal, one of

the following should be abnormal to establish the diagnosis: thrombin time, euglobulin clot lysis, or fibrin split products.

2. Management

a. Coagulation profile routinely on admission of head-injured patients

b. Treatment of the underlying disease process

c. Administration of cryoprecipitate (fibrinogin, factor VIII), fresh frozen plasma (factor V), platelet concentrates, and fresh red blood cells to correct the hemostatic defects

d. Heparin therapy

(1) May produce dramatic effects within a few hours, raising fibrinogen and plasminogen levels to normal, shortening thrombin time, and allowing resynthesis of consumed clotting factors

(2) May predispose the head-injured patient to intracranial hemorrhage

III. Endocrinologic abnormalities

A. Anterior pituitary insufficiency. Signs of anterior pituitary insufficiency after head trauma are rare; recognizable pituitary or hypothalamic damage is commonly found postmortem, however. Anterior pituitary insufficiency may be caused by traumatic rupture of the pituitary stalk, interruption of the vascular supply to the stalk at the time of head injury, traumatic hemorrhage into the pituitary gland, or systemic vascular collapse from hemorrhagic shock. More likely to occur in a patient who has a fracture of the middle cranial fossa, anterior pituitary insufficiency is frequently accompanied by transient or permanent diabetes insipidus. The diagnosis of anterior pituitary insufficiency should also be considered when there is a basal skull fracture, secondary amenorrhea, galactorrhea, or regression of secondary sexual characteristics or the persistence of poor recovery, posttraumatic psychosis, or general malaise. Appropriate replacement therapy is indicated when specific deficiencies are proved through endocrinologic testing: prednisone, 5 mg orally each morning and 2 to 5 mg each afternoon; levothyroxin (Synthroid) 0.1 to 0.15 mg orally each day.

B. Posterior pituitary dysfunction

1. Diabetes insipidus. Diabetes insipidus commonly occurs after craniofacial trauma and skull fracture. It can be permanent or transient and may be related to hypoxic brain damage, drug overdose, hemorrhagic shock, or fat embolism. **Signs** of antidiuretic hormone (ADH) deficiency are as follows:

a. Polyuria (2–15 L/day)

b. Polydipsia (unless hypothalamus is destroyed)

c. Hypernatremia

d. Serum hyperosmolality (320–330 mOsm/L)

e. Dilute urine (sp gr 1.001–1.005, 50–150 mOsm/L)

f. Urine/serum osmolality of less than 1

The **diagnosis** is usually obvious but it can be confirmed by determining the plasma level of ADH or neurophysin (ADH carrier protein) in relation to changes in plasma and urine osmolality induced by water restriction or administration of synthetic ADH.

Essentials of **management** include determination of daily weight, careful fluid balance, and serial measurement of serum BUN, electrolytes, and osmolality, and urine specific gravity and osmolality. The hourly urine output and the usual estimate for insensible fluid loss are replaced with solutions containing water and little or no electrolytes. Administering sodium-containing solutions may lead to severe hypernatremia. Water intoxication (lethargy, confusion, seizures, and coma) can occur if excess vasopressin is administered. When the patient is awake and able to take fluids orally, fluid balance can often be maintained satisfactorily. If urinary output exceeds either 250 ml/hr for two consecutive hours or 6 to 7 L/day, or if the patient is unable to maintain fluid balance, then aqueous vasopressin (5 to 10 IU IM or IV every 4 to 6 hours) or vasopressin tannate in oil (5 IU IM every 24 to 72 hours) may be used. A long-acting synthetic vasopressin nasal spray (desmopressin; DDAVP) is convenient for patients who develop permanent diabetes insipidus. It is supplied in 2.5 ml bottles of 100 μg/ml; the usual dose is 10 to 20 μg intranasally every 12 to 24 hours.

2. Syndrome of inappropriate ADH (SIADH). Many disorders of the CNS have been associated with SIADH. Anesthesia and surgery can cause elevation of plasma ADH secondary to pain, stress, and various drugs. In neurosurgical patients, all the features of SIADH may be produced by the administration of aqueous vasopressin during overvigorous therapy of diabetes insipidus. SIADH after head trauma probably results from either the overproduction or excessive release of ADH in response to irritation of the hypothalamic-pituitary axis. Secretion of ADH may also be increased by stimulation of the intrathoracic volume receptors when patients are nursed in the head-up position; this position may exacerbate SIADH as well. Fluid restriction may prevent the syndrome from becoming full-blown.

The typical **signs** of SIADH include:

a. Hyponatremia

b. Serum hypoosmolality

c. Urine/serum osmolality of greater than 1

d. Normal renal and adrenal function

e. Absence of signs of volume depletion (normal skin turgor and blood pressure)

f. Signs of water intoxication (anorexia, nausea, vomiting, irritability, neurologic abnormalities, i.e., muscle weakness or convulsions)

Treatment involves water restriction, with or without the administration of hypertonic saline. In patients whose serum sodium is less than 110 mEq/L, hypertonic saline may be necessary (3% saline, 513 mEq/L). Hyponatremia can also occur after prolonged diuresis from mannitol if sodium losses are not replaced, but total osmolality is increased and circulatory volume is reduced.

IV. Metabolic abnormalities

A. Water and electrolyte balance. Sodium retention is a normal response to bodily injury; it generally lasts from 2 to 4 days and appears to be related to hypothalamic stimulation, aldosterone secretion, and subsequent release of ACTH. There is no relationship between the severity of the sodium retention and the location of the brain damage. Major trauma may also cause a mild degree of ADH-mediated water retention, which lasts for 2 or 3 days. Despite the sodium retention, head-injured patients may be mildly hyponatremic because of the concomitant water retention.

B. Glucose metabolism. Glucose intolerance commonly develops after trauma. High catecholamine levels inhibit the release of insulin. ACTH, serum cortisol, and growth hormone levels may be elevated posttrauma, as well. Exogenously administered corticosteroids are diabetogenic since they promote gluconeogenesis and increase hepatic production of glucose. Severe diabetes mellitus develops in only a few patients receiving corticosteroids; and only in those patients who have a reduced insulin reserve (e.g., the adult-onset diabetic) is the diabetogenic action of corticosteroids extreme. Latent diabetes mellitus may be unmasked by trauma, and may be detrimental to the patient's recovery if it goes unrecognized.

C. **Cerebrospinal fluid metabolic changes.** Brain injury results in CSF lactic acidosis. The severity of CSF acidosis relates directly to the severity of the head injury, and seems to be dependent on the amount of lactic acid produced by the injured and hypoxic brain tissue. Marked intracranial hypertension causes a reduction in cerebral blood flow (CBF) and is accompanied by long-lasting but reversible lactic acidosis of cerebral tissue. Low CSF pH promotes spontaneous hyperventilation. Serotonin levels in the CSF rise after head trauma in proportion to the severity of the trauma. CSF cAMP levels are lowest in patients in the deepest grades of coma after either head injury or spontaneous intracranial hemorrhage.

D. **Nonketotic hyperosmolar hyperglycemic coma.** Nonketotic hyperosmolar hyperglycemic coma (NHHC) complicates many primary illnesses, including neurologic disorders, in diabetic and nondiabetic patients. The average age of patients who have NHHC is 57 years; two-thirds have no previous history of diabetes mellitus. Many predisposing factors to NHHC are present in neurosurgical patients: they are receiving corticosteroids, prolonged mannitol therapy, hyperosmolar tube feedings, and limited water replacement. The mortality is 40% to 70%. Causes of death include renal failure, arrhythmias, cerebrovascular accidents, and systemic thromboembolic complications.

1. **Diagnostic criteria for NHHC**

   a. Hyperglycemia (400 to 2700 mg/100 ml)

   b. Glucosuria

   c. Absence of ketosis

   d. Hyperosmolality (greater than 330 mOsm/L)

   e. Dehydration

   f. CNS dysfunction

2. **Characteristics.** Severe potassium depletion may result from the osmotic diuresis. Patients may also exhibit leukocytosis, hemoconcentration, and azotemia with a BUN-to-creatinine ratio of greater than 30:1. Many patients are febrile, in shock, and in coma; they may or may not have focal neurologic signs. Coma and subsequent death are attributed to either total-body sodium depletion or cellular dehydration, particularly in the brain.

3. **Pathogenesis.** The pathogenesis of NHHC is not clear. The

absence of ketosis may reflect either the antiketogenic effects of severe hyperglycemia or the effect of insulin on fat and carbohydrate metabolism. At low concentrations of insulin in the plasma, insulin has no effect on the uptake of glucose by cells, but can still inhibit the release of free fatty acids from adipose tissue. Before initiating therapy, appropriate laboratory data must be obtained (serum Na^+, osmolality, pH, BUN, glucose, K^+, lactate). Plasma osmolality can be estimated and followed during therapy (Posm = $2 Na^+$ + glucose 18).

4. **Treatment.** Hypovolemia and hypertonicity are the immediate threats to life. Hypotonic saline administration may not improve sodium and water deficits rapidly enough; therefore, normal saline may be used until blood pressure and urine output are stabilized. If a patient is in hypovolemic shock, administration of isotonic sodium chloride or plasma may be necessary, regardless of the osmolality. The volume of hypotonic fluid necessary varies, depending on the individual patient, but it is usually greater than 5 liters during the first 12 hours of treatment and averages 500 to 1300 ml/hr until the plasma osmolality reaches 325 mOsm/L.

Hyperglycemia usually responds dramatically to the administration of relatively small doses of insulin. Large doses of insulin reduce the serum glucose rapidly and may increase mortality by decreasing the plasma volume before there has been adequate fluid and salt repletion. The recommended dose is 25 units of regular insulin each hour until sodium deficits have been replaced.

V. **Gastrointestinal abnormalities.** Seventeen percent of head-injured patients may have esophageal, gastric, or duodenal ulceration and hemorrhage. The frequency of gastrointestinal bleeding is positively correlated with the severity of injury: severely injured patients receiving glucocorticoids have a higher incidence of bleeding than have less severely injured patients receiving corticosteroids. Hypothalamic stimulation, gastric mucosal disruption, ingestion of aspirin or ethanol, hyperacidity, and hemorrhagic shock are among the etiologic factors. Signs and symptoms include epigastric pain, abdominal distention, ileus, hypotension, hematemesis, and melena. In the unconscious patient, perforation of a viscus may be asymptomatic.

Treatment includes nasogastric suction, cold saline lavage, fluid and blood replacement, and cimetidine (to block histamine H_2 receptor and reduce parietal cell hydrogen ion secretion). Cimetidine may offer preventive therapy in patients who have preexisting ulcer disease or predisposing conditions, since it reduces acid secretion and elevates gastric pH. In one study, however, prophylactic antacid therapy was found to be more efficacious in the general category of stress ulceration, although cimetidine seemed to offer advantages to neurosurgical patients (MacDougall, 1977).

VI. Skeletal abnormalities

A. Cervical spine injuries. Ten percent of head-injured patients have associated cervical spine injury. Fifty percent of patients who have cervical spine fracture also have concurrent evidence of head trauma. Head-injured patients should therefore be considered to have cervical spine injury until it is proven otherwise. Hyperextension of the neck during laryngoscopy and endotracheal intubation may displace an unstable fracture and cause or exacerbate spinal cord compression. All diagnostic and therapeutic maneuvers must therefore be performed with extreme caution until the stability of the cervical spine is established.

High transection of the spinal cord (above the C-3 level) is most often fatal owing to the cessation of diaphragmatic and intercostal muscle function and to subsequent hypoventilation and secondary infection. The absence of sympathetic tone leads to hypotension, bradycardia (cardiac output may be high, low, or normal), and an increase in alveolar dead space from a reduction in pulmonary perfusion.

Mechanical ventilation may be indicated for the management of ventilation-perfusion abnormalities (atelectasis secondary to hypoventilation, infection, "shock lung") and hypercapnia (increased alveolar dead space without compensation). Continuous application of positive pressure breathing may decrease cardiac output by reducing venous return in a patient who cannot compensate by increasing venous tone. Treatment includes replacement of intravascular volume and maintenance of adequate hemoglobin levels. Minute volume, PEEP, and chest physiotherapy are adjusted to achieve maximum acceptable oxygen availability with minimal interference with venous return. Weaning of such patients must be accomplished on an individual basis, although the usual criteria apply (see section **I.B.3**).

B. Maxillofacial injuries. Blunt trauma in the cervical region can cause carotid artery injury. Compression or stretching of the vessel may lead to thrombosis, transient ischemic attacks, Horner's syndrome, or hematoma of the lateral neck and airway obstruction. Horner's syndrome may develop after neck trauma as a result of pressure or direct injury to the sympathetic neural supply to the face. The unilateral pupillary constriction that results or the pupillary dilatation that accompanies direct trauma to the eye may lead to confusion and overtreatment of a suspected intracranial mass. Subcutaneous emphysema resulting from frontal or ethmoid sinus fractures must be distinguished from emphysema resulting from thoracic injury. Fractures of the cribriform plate may allow a nasogastric tube to enter the intracranial space; these tubes must be placed through the mouth under direct vision; gastrostomy may be indicated.

Anesthesia
Robert D. McKay

The anesthesiologist has an important role in the care of head-injured patients in the emergency room, operating room, and neurosurgical intensive care unit (ICU). The anesthesiologist's skills in airway management, fluid resuscitation, monitoring, and support of the cardiac and respiratory systems are invaluable. Many patients who have head injury will require anesthesia; the procedures may be neurosurgical or nonneurosurgical, such as repair of long bone fractures, facial fractures, or laparotomy for hemorrhage. A successful outcome in these situations depends on both the anesthesiologist's knowledge and application of relevant physiologic, pathophysiologic, and neuropharmacologic principles and his or her meticulous attention to detail.

I. Pathophysiology

A. **Primary head injury** is damage sustained as a direct, immediate result of the trauma (Bruce, 1980). Acceleration-deceleration head injuries without impact tend to produce subdural hematomas from tearing of bridging veins, as well as diffuse cortical injury with contusions or lacerations from impact of the brain with bony prominences or sharp edges of the falx cerebri or tentorium. Injury from skull impact is more likely to consist of skull fracture with associated contusion of the brain. Hematoma formation is not uncommon, particularly if the fracture line crosses either an artery or a venous sinus. Categories of primary head injury are listed in Table 13-3.

B. **Secondary head injury** is any injury to the brain that occurs after the initial traumatic event. It is potentially preventable so that theoretically the patient should survive, the quality of survival being determined by the severity of the primary injury. The factors involved in secondary head injury may be initiated either by intracranial or systemic events. Factors that produce secondary head injury include the following:

Table 13-3. Categories of primary head injury

Scalp
  Contusion
  Abrasion
  Laceration
  Subgaleal hematoma
Skull fractures (open or closed)
  Linear
  Comminuted
  Depressed
  Stellate
Meninges
  Epidural hematoma
  Subdural hematoma (acute, subacute, chronic)
  Basal dural tear
  Rhinorrhea
  Otorrhea
  Pneumocephalus
Brain
  Concussion
  Contusion
  Laceration
  Hematoma

---

1. **Disturbances in the regulation of cerebral blood flow.**
   Cerebral blood flow (CBF), normally coupled closely with cerebral metabolism, is regulated by several mechanisms including neurogenic (the autonomic nervous system), myogenic (autoregulation), metabolic (changes in the concentrations of acid metabolites such as lactic acid), and chemical (arterial oxygen and carbon dioxide tensions). Head trauma may disrupt some or all of these regulatory mechanisms, leading to imbalances in the delivery of O_2 to brain tissues relative to the O_2 demanded by those tissues.

   CBF in excess of metabolic demands (hyperemia or luxury perfusion) may lead to increases in cerebral blood volume, intracranial pressure (ICP), and edema formation. If autoregulation is impaired, CBF becomes a passive function of cerebral perfusion pressure (CPP), the difference between mean arterial pressure and ICP (MAP-ICP). Inadequate CBF, produced by hypotension, compression of the arterial supply, or vasospasm, causes a shift from aerobic to anaerobic metabolism, increased lactate production, and vasomotor paralysis. Failure of chemical regulation of CBF after head trauma is associated with loss of CO_2 reactivity by the cerebral vessels. In addition, sympathetic stimulation as a homeostatic response to hemorrhage may constrict cerebral vessels and reduce CBF.

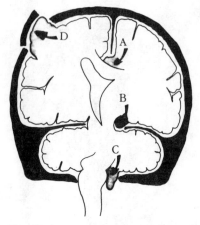

Fig. 13-4. Four sites of brain herniation. *A.* Cingulate. *B.* Uncal. *C.* Cerebellar or tonsillar. *D.* Transcalvarial.

2. **Hypoventilation.** Hypoventilation from brainstem injury, airway obstruction, aspiration, thoracoabdominal injury, or shock may contribute to secondary brain injury. Resultant hypoxia and hypercapnia both increase CBF and cerebral blood volume.

3. **Cardiovascular dysfunction.** Cardiovascular dysfunction may produce secondary brain injury, particularly when autoregulation is impaired. Hypertension will increase CBF and cerebral blood volume, causing brain swelling, whereas hypotension will lower CPP and exacerbate cerebral ischemia and acidosis.

4. **Cerebral swelling.** Cerebral swelling is an increase in CBF. Cerebral edema, an increase in brain tissue water, and intracranial mass lesions such as epidural, subdural, and intracerebral hematomas all reduce intracranial compliance and increase ICP. The relationship among the intracranial fluid volumes—brain tissue, brain tissue water, cerebrospinal fluid (CSF), and cerebral blood volume—and ICP is defined by the Munro-Kellie doctrine: an increase in the volume of one of the fluid compartments must be matched by a decrease in one or all of the remaining volumes or the ICP will rise.

5. **Increased ICP.** An increase in ICP causes further compression of tissue, decreases CPP, and increases ischemia. If this reduction of CPP is not reversed, a vicious cycle may develop, culminating in either inadequate cerebral perfusion (ICP greater than MAP) or herniation and compression of vital structures (Fig. 13-4).

II. **CNS effects of anesthesia.** Anesthetic drugs have substantial effects on CBF and cerebral metabolism. Other interventions such as intuba-

Table 13-4. Effects of anesthetic drugs on CBF, ICP, MAP, and CPP

Drug	CBF	ICP	MAP	CPP
Thiopental	↓ ↓	↓ ↓	↓	↑
Fentanyl	↓	↓	SL ↓	↑
Diazepam	↓	↓ ?	SL ↓	↑ ?
Droperidol	↓	↓	↓	SL ↓
Ketamine	↑ ↑ ↑	↑ ↑ ↑	↑	↓
Halothane	↑ ↑	↑	↓	↓
Enflurane	↑	↑	↓	↓
Isoflurane	↑	↑	↓	↓
N_2O	↑	↑	NC	↓

tion, positioning, and airway pressure may also affect the central nervous system (CNS).

A. **Intravenous anesthetics.** With the exception of ketamine, the intravenous anesthetics tend to decrease ICP, as long as CO_2 retention is prevented. CBF remains coupled with cerebral metabolism. The systemic and CNS effects of these drugs are summarized in Table 13-4 and Fig. 13-5.

1. The **barbiturates** produce the greatest reduction in CBF and $CMRO_2$. Autoregulation remains intact and the formation of cerebral edema after experimental head injury is limited. The metabolic depression with barbiturates affects the cells' energy requirements for neuronal function, rather than the requirements to maintain cellular integrity. The primary cardiovascular effects of thiopental are hypotension from venodilatation, decreased CNS sympathetic outflow, and decreased cardiac output. Reflex attempts to correct hypotension include increases in heart rate and total peripheral resistance. The hypotension may be attenuated by slow administration. The decrease in ICP from the fall in CBF is usually greater than the decrease in MAP, resulting in an increased CPP. This may not be true in the hypovolemic patient; in this situation the decrease in MAP may exceed the decrease in ICP and cause a reduction in CPP.

2. **Narcotics** in anesthetic doses cause a modest decrease in CBF and $CMRO_2$ when CO_2 retention is prevented; this decrease tends to reduce ICP. As with the barbiturates, autoregulation remains intact, and formation of edema in response to injury is reduced. Cardiovascular changes associated with narcotics include mild hypotension, primarily from venodilatation and bradycardia. Morphine produces more hypotension than does fentanyl. ICP is decreased to a greater extent than MAP, how-

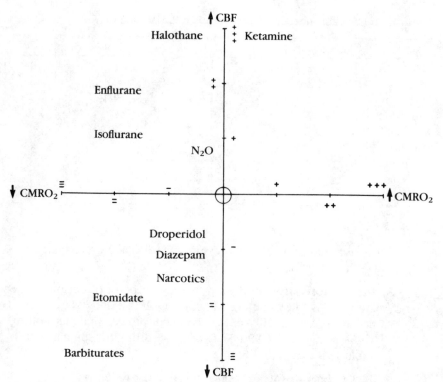

Fig. 13-5. Effect of anesthetic agents on the relationship between cerebral blood flow (CBF) and metabolism (CMRO$_2$). Increases and decreases in CBF are indicated along the vertical axis while increases and decreases in CMRO$_2$ are indicated along the horizontal axis. A drug that has no effect on CBF or CMRO$_2$, such as sodium chloride, would occupy the intersection point.

ever, so the end result is an increase in CPP. Hypertension is not an uncommon development during anesthesia with a narcotic. The administration of naloxone to reverse the narcotic may result in hypertension and tachycardia as well as an increase in CBF, CMRO$_2$, and ICP.

3. **Diazepam, midazolam, and lorazepam** cause a modest decrease in CBF and CMRO$_2$, theoretically decreasing the ICP. The reduction of CBF and CMRO$_2$ with diazepam may be potentiated by N$_2$O. The cardiovascular effects of these drugs are mild; the slight decrease in MAP is more than offset by the reduction in ICP, resulting in an increase in CPP. However, a recent report found no change in ICP when diazepam was used as the induction drug; CBF was not measured (Tateishi, 1981).

4. **Droperidol** causes a moderate reduction in CBF and ICP. The metabolic effects of this drug are not as well documented.

$CMRO_2$ is either unchanged or slightly decreased. Droperidol produces hypotension primarily through alpha-adrenergic blockade and also by decreasing CNS sympathetic outflow. The degree of hypotension is variable. In some cases, particularly in hypovolemic patients, the reduction in MAP may exceed the reduction in ICP and cause a decrease in CPP.

5. **Etomidate,** in induction doses of 0.2 to 0.3 mg/kg, decreases CBF and ICP. The minimal cardiovascular effects of this drug result in an unchanged or increased CPP (Moss, 1979).

6. **Ketamine** is the only intravenous anesthetic that increases CBF; this increase is of a most impressive magnitude. The effect of ketamine on cerebral metabolism is not as dramatic; there is either a slight increase or no change in $CMRO_2$. The increase in MAP by ketamine does not compensate for the increased ICP so that the CPP is reduced. The effects on CBF may be either reversed or blocked by diazepam and thiopental.

B. **Inhalation anesthetics.** The inhalation anesthetics increase CBF while reducing $CMRO_2$. This uncoupling of flow and metabolism does not occur with the intravenous anesthetics. The CNS and cardiovascular effects of the inhalation anesthetics are shown in Table 13-3 and Fig. 13-5.

1. **Halothane** causes a significant dose-related increase in CBF and a significant decrease in $CMRO_2$. The increased CBF increases cerebral blood volume and ICP. This rise in ICP is dose-related and may be attenuated by introducing the drug only after hyperventilation to a $PaCO_2$ of 25 to 30 mmHg for 10 minutes. The increase in ICP with halothane can be reduced by thiopental. Halothane also impairs autoregulation in a dose-dependent fashion. Formation of edema in response to experimental cerebral cold injury is increased. The effects of halothane on the cardiovascular system include myocardial depression and vasodilatation, leading to hypotension. This, combined with the increase in ICP, causes a fall in CPP. Halothane also sensitizes the heart to catecholamines, which is important if infiltration of the scalp with a solution containing epinephrine is planned.

2. **Enflurane** is a weaker cerebrovasodilator than halothane but a more potent depressant of cerebral metabolism. ICP may be increased and, because its effect on MAP is similar to halothane, CPP is reduced. Enflurane may also produce seizures, particularly in the presence of hypocapnia. These seizures can cause increases in both CBF and $CMRO_2$.

3. **Isoflurane** increases CBF and ICP while decreasing $CMRO_2$.

The increase in ICP is not as great as with halothane. Hyperventilation instituted simultaneously with isoflurane may be adequate to block the increase in ICP. Isoflurane also causes hypotension and decreases CPP. The effect on MAP appears to be primarily from vasodilatation rather than from reduced cardiac output. Isoflurane may exert a protective effect in the presence of cerebral hypoxia.

4. **Nitrous oxide** (N_2O) is similar to the volatile anesthetics in that it is a cerebrovasodilator and thus can increase ICP. The increased ICP with N_2O can be prevented by prior administration of diazepam and thiopental. Aside from its effects on CBF, N_2O can increase ICP in the presence of pneumocephalus by diffusing into the trapped air faster than nitrogen can diffuse out.

C. **Muscle relaxants** differ in their CNS effects. With controlled $PaCO_2$ and MAP, succinylcholine does not increase ICP. The use of curare may be associated with a rise in electrical impedance and ICP, most likely because of histamine release. The release of histamine also plays a role in producing systemic hypotension. Pancuronium does not seem to affect ICP; it may produce hypertension and tachycardia. Dimethyl curare also does not increase ICP, at least in doses where histamine release is not seen.

Succinylcholine causes potassium release. Elevations of serum potassium sufficient to cause lethal arrhythmias have been reported when succinylcholine was administered to head-injured patients. The time between injury and onset of susceptibility to hyperkalemia has not been established. Patients who have flaccid paralysis, spasticity, or clonus after head injury may be susceptible, as may be those who move extremities in response to pain but not to command. In the absence of massive muscle trauma, the use of succinylcholine in the head-injured patient within three days of injury should not cause significant hyperkalemia.

D. **Nonpharmacologic interventions**

1. **Laryngoscopy and intubation,** in addition to significantly raising the blood pressure, may cause a substantial increase in ICP. This response can be demonstrated in the absence of coughing and straining, which will aggravate the increase in ICP.

2. Placing the patient in **Trendelenburg position** with the head down will decrease cerebral venous return, increase ICP, and promote the formation of cerebral edema. Cervical rotation or flexion may compress a jugular vein, which will have the same effect. Care must be taken when inserting internal jugular intravenous catheters. Puncture of the carotid or vertebral artery and

laceration of the jugular vein may create a hematoma that com-presses the jugular vein, again decreasing venous return and increasing ICP.

3. **Positive airway pressure** may be transmitted to the pleura and vena cava, which may decrease jugular venous return. The effect of positive end-expiratory pressure (PEEP) on ICP is unpredict-able so that the need for PEEP in a head-injured patient is an indication for ICP monitoring. While PEEP *may* increase ICP, it should be remembered that hypoxia *will* increase ICP. The posi-tive airway pressure may also reduce venous return enough to decrease stroke volume, cardiac output, MAP and CPP; these reductions will be of greater magnitude in the hypovolemic patient.

III. **The anesthesiologist's evaluation.** The anesthesiologist should evaluate the patient on arrival in the emergency room, without waiting to see whether the patient will come to the operating room. The anes-thesiologist can make a significant contribution to the patient's care through airway management, fluid resuscitation, cardiorespiratory sup-port, and monitoring, even if surgery is not necessary.

A. **Evaluate the airway.** This is of paramount importance and is dis-cussed in section **IV.**

B. **Evaluate the CNS status.** The Glasgow coma scale (see Table 13-1) has been an important advance in the neurologic evaluation and monitoring of the head-injured patient. The value of this system is its reproducibility from observer to observer, the ease with which changes can be documented, and the demonstration of trends in recovery or exacerbation. Other pertinent neurologic findings in-clude focal deficits, signs of herniation, or signs of brainstem dys-function. Spinal cord injury not uncommonly accompanies head injury.

C. **Obtain patient history.** If the patient is awake, a history should be obtained. Many patients will unfortunately be unable to provide any information because of the severity of their injury, the influence of alcohol, prescription drugs, or street drugs, or a combination of these factors.

1. Ascertain time and nature of **last oral intake.**

2. Obtain **description of the injury** if the patient can recall. The description may provide clues as to potential associated injuries. Approximately 1 out of 3 patients who have head injury will also have at least one other associated injury.

Arterial line

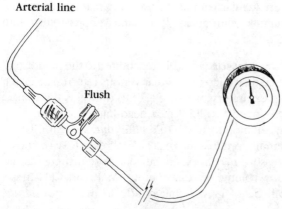

Flush

Fig. 13-6. A gas sterilized aneroid manometer connected to an arterial line. This system may be useful for monitoring blood pressure during transport. The needle fluctuations correspond to mean arterial pressure.

 3. Obtain **drug and alcohol** history from family members, friends, or witnesses. Ethanol intoxication worsens the prognosis of severe head injury.

 D. Perform physical examination. A thorough physical examination is essential because positive nonneurologic findings will suggest sites of associated injury. For example, fractured ribs may indicate lung contusion, or ecchymosis over the right upper quadrant may suggest liver laceration. An estimate of the patient's intravascular volume should be made, using the "Tilt test" (determination of pulse and blood pressure while the patient is supine and then with the head elevated).

 E. Monitor the patient. After initial evaluation and stabilization, many patients undergo computerized tomography (CT) or cerebral angiography during which time the anesthesiologist should establish monitoring, ensure adequate intravenous access, and check on laboratory results and blood bank support. These patients will be closely monitored in the operating room and neurologic ICU; they should receive the same close attention while in transport or in the radiology suite. Precordial or esophageal stethoscope and blood pressure cuff should be routine. If an arterial cannula is in place, a portable transducer and oscilloscope or an aneroid manometer (Fig. 13-6) can be used to monitor MAP.

IV. Airway management

 A. Basic principles. Securing the airway of the head-injured patient may present many potential problems. Since 5% to 10% of patients will also have cervical spine injuries, hyperextension of the neck should be avoided when opening the airway. The possibility of an unsuspected fracture of the basal skull or the cribriform plate makes the insertion of nasopharyngeal airways, nasogastric tubes, or nasotracheal tubes hazardous, since the object may pass intracranially rather than into the pharynx. Fractures into nasal sinuses that are accompanied by dural tears and CSF rhinorrhea present another problem: positive pressure ventilation transmitted to the nasal sinuses may push contaminated material into the CNS, creating a serious infection.

Mask fit may be difficult in the patient who has serious craniofacial trauma; the mouth may not open well and laryngoscopic exposure may be poor because of bleeding into the airway. A hematoma in the neck can compress and shift the larynx and trachea, making visualization and intubation difficult. Preexisting conditions such as receding mandible, protruding teeth, or a short, thick neck may also make intubation difficult.

Awake intubation has hazards also. Attempts at awake intubation may cause coughing and straining, leading to increases in ICP or spinal cord injury from unstable fractures or dislocations of the cervical spine. A rapid sequence induction may be associated with wide swings in blood pressure or inability to insert the endotracheal tube or ventilate the patient once anesthesia and muscle relaxation have been induced.

B. Criteria for airway support. In the absence of pulmonary complications, airway injury, thoracoabdominal injury, or shock, patients who are awake and following commands will not need endotracheal intubation. Unresponsive patients who have an impaired gag reflex will require intubation. Patients who fall in between these points on the spectrum need close evaluation. The Glasgow coma scale (see Table 13-1) may be helpful in making the decision: endotracheal intubation of all patients who have a Glasgow coma score of 7 or less is a safe approach.

C. Establishing the airway. Airway management must begin at the scene of the accident, since hypoxia and hypercapnia are important factors in secondary head injury. Clearing the airway of mucus, blood, vomitus, and broken teeth, pulling the jaw forward, and administering supplemental oxygen will usually correct hypercapnia and hypoxia.

   1. Assisted ventilation. If air exchange is inadequate, then respirations must be assisted. An oropharyngeal airway or esophageal obturator and oxygen delivery with positive pressure may be used. The esophageal obturator should not be removed until the trachea is intubated because of the likelihood of regurgitation after its removal. If an oral airway is used, then cricoid pressure will minimize gastric distension and regurgitation. All patients who have head injury have a full stomach. Once the airway is secure, radiologic evaluation of the cervical spine including C-7 can then be performed. Care is indicated to avoid spinal cord injury if the radiographs showing no evidence of a fracture or dislocation are incomplete.

2. **Monitoring.** Basic monitoring should be established, using precordial stethoscope, blood pressure cuff, and electrocardiogram (ECG).

3. **Intubation**

   a. **Stable vital signs.** If vital signs are stable, if hypovolemia is not present, and if intubation does not appear difficult, anesthesia can be induced with thiopental, 3 to 6 mg/kg. Muscle relaxation can be achieved using either succinylcholine (after pretreatment with a nondepolarizing muscle relaxant to prevent fasciculations) or pancuronium. A nerve stimulator should be used to ensure the presence of good muscle relaxation before laryngoscopy. Lidocaine, 1.5 mg/kg IV, 90 seconds before intubation may prevent an increase in ICP with laryngoscopy and intubation.

   b. **Unstable vital signs.** If the vital signs are unstable or if significant hypovolemia is suspected, a smaller dose of thiopental (1–2 mg/kg) should be used. Diazepam, 0.1 to 0.2 mg/kg, or etomidate, 0.2 to 0.3 mg/kg, are suitable alternatives. These drugs can be given with lidocaine and a muscle relaxant. A flow chart for the airway management of a head-injured patient is illustrated in Fig. 13-7. Adequate preparation for intubation includes suction, monitoring, oxygen, and a selection of laryngoscopes, blades, and endotracheal tubes.

   c. **Difficult intubation.** If a difficult intubation is suspected, muscle relaxants should not be used until either the larynx has been visualized or the endotracheal tube has been placed. Sedation with droperidol, fentanyl, and/or diazepam may be used. Superior laryngeal nerve blocks or transtracheal instillation of lidocaine should not be used with a full stomach. Lidocaine, 1.5 mg/kg IV, may be used to minimize coughing and rise in ICP. Nasotracheal intubation while the patient is awake may be used in the absence of a direct communication between the nasal passages and the brain. A "blind" approach may be used or the tube may be

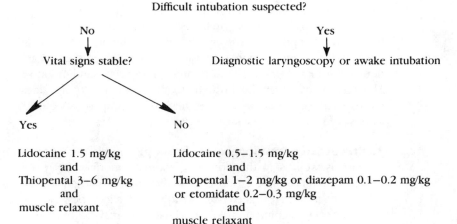

Difficult intubation suspected?

No — Vital signs stable?

Yes — Diagnostic laryngoscopy or awake intubation

Yes

Lidocaine 1.5 mg/kg
and
Thiopental 3–6 mg/kg
and
muscle relaxant

No

Lidocaine 0.5–1.5 mg/kg
and
Thiopental 1–2 mg/kg or diazepam 0.1–0.2 mg/kg
or etomidate 0.2–0.3 mg/kg
and
muscle relaxant

Fig. 13-7. Airway management of the head-injured patient.

placed under direct vision. Alternatively, a suction catheter, ureteral catheter, or other guide can be inserted through the larynx and the tube passed over it. Flexible fiberoptic instruments, optical stylets, prisms, and the retrograde technique have all been used successfully. Tracheotomy or cricothyroidotomy is necessary when there is no access to the larynx perorally or pernasally or when the trachea communicates with the outside. Once the endotracheal tube is in place, intravenous sedatives, narcotics, and muscle relaxants should be administered to prevent coughing and straining, and to facilitate controlled ventilation.

V. Anesthetic management for neurosurgical procedures. Operative procedures include craniotomy for epidural, subdural, or intracerebral hematoma, placement of ICP monitors, elevation of depressed skull fractures, and decompression operations such as craniectomies or excision of portions of the frontal or temporal lobe.

A. Monitoring. Monitors can be divided into two classes, noninvasive and invasive. Invasive monitors are indicated when the benefit of the information to be gained outweighs the risk to the patient that the monitor entails, or more simply, when the risk of not having the information outweighs the risk of getting the information. Noninvasive monitors pose minimal risk to the patient; the decision to use them is based in part on the cost-effectiveness of the monitor. Ideally, the considerations for monitoring the patient during emergency neurosurgical procedures should be the same as those for the patients undergoing more elective procedures. However, the patient who has an epidural hematoma and impending herniation has compromise of viable brain tissue. Delay in evacuating the hematoma may produce irreversible damage. The best way to avoid delay in the operating room is to use the time in the emergency and neuroradiology areas to establish intravenous access and monitors. The patient can then be brought to the operating room, anesthetized (if not already under anesthesia), and prepared as quickly as possible for the surgical procedure.

1. **Precordial or esophageal stethoscope** is useful during transport as well as in the operating room to monitor heart and breath sounds. The esophageal stethoscope is particularly important in neurosurgery because the connections between the anesthesia machine and endotracheal tube may be hidden by drapes.

2. **The ECG** is essential since patients who have head injury may manifest electrocardiographic changes. The ECG may also show abnormalities from basic medical problems and cardiovascular complications of trauma.

3. **Blood pressure** may be measured by an indwelling arterial catheter or a blood pressure cuff; placement of a Doppler device may facilitate the cuff measurements. Direct arterial measurement offers several advantages, including beat-to-beat pressure monitoring capability, monitoring in transit, and accessibility of blood for arterial blood gases, hematocrit, blood chemistries, and coagulation profiles.

4. **A urinary catheter** provides measurement of urine output and urine samples for determination of specific gravity, osmolality, and chemistries.

5. **CVP and pulmonary artery catheters.** An indication of preload can be helpful. In the absence of left ventricular dysfunction, measurement of central venous or right atrial pressure is adequate. A Swan-Ganz pulmonary artery (PA) catheter should be used when there is left ventricular dysfunction or high cervical spinal cord injury. This catheter can also provide cardiac output measurements and information necessary to calculate peripheral and pulmonary vascular resistance, which can be useful information, particularly in patients receiving high doses of barbiturates. A central venous catheter can be easily exchanged for a pulmonary artery catheter using the Seldinger technique. Acceptable veins for placing the catheters include antecubital, subclavian, internal and external jugular, and femoral.

6. **Esophageal thermistor.**

7. **Ventilator monitors** include FIO_2 analysis, a disconnect alarm, and end-tidal CO_2.

8. Monitors for the **detection of venous air-embolism** (Doppler, end-tidal CO_2, Swan-Ganz catheter) are indicated for procedures in which veins in the operative site are above the level of the heart. Surgical positioning (particularly the seated position), hypovolemia with low venous pressure, potential venous sinus injury, or other factors may cause venous air embolism.

B. **Induction of anesthesia** in neurosurgical emergencies is inseparable from securing the airway (see section **IV**). If succinylcholine is used for intubation, pancuronium should be administered before the patient has recovered enough neuromuscular function to cough or strain.

C. **Maintenance of anesthesia.** Close attention to the airway is required during positioning and preparation to avoid dislodging, kinking, or advancing the tube into a main stem bronchus.

1. **Ventilation** should be controlled. A $PaCO_2$ of 25 to 30 mmHg will promote brain relaxation for surgical exposure without producing ischemia from hypocapnic vasoconstriction. A higher $PaCO_2$ (30–35 mmHg) is recommended for patients who require burr holes for evacuation of chronic subdural hematomas, particularly after decompression, since a slack brain may encourage recurrence. The $t_{1/2}$ for CSF adaptation to hypocapnia is 6 hours.

2. **Anesthetic drugs** of choice for head-injured patients are the intravenous agents (excluding ketamine) in combination with N_2O-O_2 and muscle relaxants. Narcotics, benzodiazepines, and barbiturates all reduce CBF, CMRO$_2$ and ICP. Cautious administration of these drugs to avoid decreasing MAP will result in a rise in CPP. Although N_2O can increase ICP, this effect can be abolished by prior administration of diazepam and thiopental.

The volatile anesthetics increase ICP, particularly during normocapnia. Although hyperventilation will attenuate the increase in ICP, in the head-injured patient, cerebrovasoconstriction in response to hypocapnia is not a dependable response. The introduction of volatile agents in these patients may increase ICP and exacerbate formation of edema. The volatile anesthetics may have a role in the treatment of intraoperative hypertension, however.

Muscle relaxation should be maintained with pancuronium and monitored by a peripheral nerve stimulator. Administration of 100% oxygen only to unresponsive patients with unstable cardiovascular systems should be avoided. Surgical decompression may improve these patients' level of consciousness enough for them to cough, with disastrous consequences.

Patients who have chronic subdural hematoma and are alert and responsive may have burr holes for evacuation with local anesthesia and moderate sedation. Some depressed skull fractures may also be elevated under local anesthesia with sedation. This technique must be used cautiously in the patient placed in the pin headholder who has a full stomach.

3. **Administration of fluid** should be limited to the amount required to maintain satisfactory organ perfusion, as indicated by heart rate, blood pressure, urine output, and cardiac filling pressures. The fluid of choice is an isotonic salt solution such as Ringer's lactate solution, either with or without 5% dextrose, which will not provide the free water to promote formation of edema. Significant blood loss should be replaced with blood products to avoid hemodilution.

VI. **Anesthetic management for nonneurosurgical procedures.** The same considerations for anesthesia for neurosurgical procedures apply to nonneurosurgical procedures. These patients may be at even greater risk than patients undergoing neurosurgical procedures. The brain of a patient undergoing a neurosurgical procedure may be decompressed by the operation whereas the patient who has severe head injury and is undergoing a nonneurosurgical procedure gains no improvement in intracranial dynamics. This is not the situation in which to administer an inhalation anesthetic with spontaneous ventilation.

The use of **regional anesthesia** in these patients is controversial. Peripheral nerve blocks (such as digital or ankle blocks) or blocks of a major plexus (such as brachial, sciatic, or femoral) may be acceptable as long as sedation is not so heavy that respiratory depression occurs, unless of course the patient has an endotracheal tube and the ventilation is controlled. Care must also be taken to avoid a local-anesthetic-induced seizure. In the absence of patient cooperation, a nerve stimulator can be used to identify nerves. Spinal anesthesia would appear to be unsuitable, since there is potential for sudden changes in CSF volume and pressure. Epidural anesthesia shares this potential problem because of possible entry into the subarachnoid space. In addition, epidural injection may reduce intracranial compliance by compressing the spinal subarachnoid space, diminishing the ability of this space to accept CSF translocated from above.

The need to administer anesthesia for a nonneurosurgical procedure to a patient after craniocerebral trauma is a strong indication to monitor ICP. Only then can elevations of ICP be diagnosed and treated appropriately. Monitoring of EEG and evoked potentials may prove useful in these situations.

VII. Pediatric considerations. The brains of children and teenagers have significantly better recuperative powers than adults; the mortality after severe head injury in patients under 19 years of age is only a quarter of that for adults. The reason for this difference is not completely clear, although some differences in pathophysiology are apparent. Within 24 hours after head injury, children manifest cerebral swelling from hyperemia more frequently than adults. Whereas this makes mannitol less useful, hyperventilation to a $PaCO_2$ of 20 to 25 mmHg may be effective in reducing ICP without causing cerebral ischemia. Children who are unresponsive in the emergency room and who have dilated pupils and gasping respiration may respond after intubation and ventilation alone. The time to peak formation and resolution of cerebral edema is also much shorter in children than in adults.

The choice of anesthetic technique for the pediatric patient who has severe head injury is the same as for adults. Close attention to the position of the endotracheal tube, fluid and blood replacement, and temperature control is essential. Moderate hypothermia is acceptable and perhaps even beneficial.

Small children can lose a significant percentage of their blood volume into an intracranial hematoma. Initially, hypotension may not be apparent because of the hypertension induced by an increase in ICP. The surgical evacuation of the hematoma and subsequent decompression of the brain under anesthesia may unmask the hypovolemia and cause severe hypotension.

VIII. Treatment of intraoperative complications

A. Hypotension in the presence of increased ICP will reduce cerebral perfusion. The most likely causes of intraoperative hypotension in patients who have severe head injury are hypovolemia, anesthetic overdose, and neurogenic changes. Cardiogenic, anaphylactic, endocrinologic, and septic causes are rare. Hypovolemia may be compensated by increased sympathetic nervous system activity as a response to increased ICP. Surgical decompression can then reduce the hypertension, producing serious hypotension. Sudden hypovolemic hypotension may also be caused by rupture of a subcapsular splenic hematoma or an aortic dissection.

Treatment of hypovolemia consists of restoring the circulating blood volume with balanced salt solutions and blood products, guided by heart rate, blood pressure, urine output, and cardiac filling pressures. Treatment of hypotension secondary to anesthetic

Table 13-5. Pharmacologic agents useful in the treatment of hypertension during surgery in head-injured patients

↑ ICP	No ↑ ICP
Hydralazine	Alpha-adrenergic blockers
Sodium nitroprusside	Trimethaphan
Nitroglycerin	
Volatile anesthetic agents	

overdose and neurogenic causes combines fluid therapy with pharmacologic intervention such as ephedrine, 0.1 to 0.5 mg/kg, or calcium chloride, 5 to 10 mg/kg.

B. **Arterial hypertension** is caused by hypercapnia, light anesthesia, Cushing response to increased ICP, excessive fluid resuscitation, preexisting hypertension, or surgical stimulation of the cerebellum or the sensory branches of the trigeminal nerve. The heart rate may be helpful in determining the cause because bradycardia is usually associated with the Cushing response and trigeminal stimulation, whereas tachycardia can accompany hypercapnia, light anesthesia, and fluid resuscitation. With preexisting hypertension, the heart rate is variable.

Hypertension secondary to hypercapnia can best be treated by lowering $PaCO_2$. The ideal drug to treat other forms of hypertension during anesthesia for head-injured patients—potent, fast-acting, and of short duration—should not increase ICP or alter the neurologic status. Unfortunately such an agent is not yet available. The drugs in current use have cerebrovascular effects: those that increase CBF may increase ICP in the head-injured patient (Table 13-5). The vasodilating drugs may also induce intracerebral steal and impair autoregulation.

Figure 13-8 illustrates a flow chart for the treatment of hypertension during anesthesia for the head-injured patient. The initial treatment consists of the intravenous anesthetics that are cerebrovasoconstrictors; some of them are alpha-adrenergic blocking drugs as well; next would be propranolol and/or phentolamine. If these are ineffective, trimethaphan is the next suitable agent. Disadvantages of this drug include tachyphylaxis and cycloplegia, which may prevent the use of the pupils as neurologic monitors postoperatively. If trimethaphan is ineffective or undesired, the volatile anesthetics can be used in concentrations of less than 0.5 MAC in the hyperventilated patient ($PaCO_2$ 25 to 30 mmHg). The volatile anesthetics are preferable to the direct-acting vasodilators since the depression in $CMRO_2$ accompanying use of the volatile anesthetics

Thiopental, fentanyl, and/or droperidol

       If ineffective

       ↓

Propranolol or phentolamine

       If ineffective

       ↓

Trimethaphan

       If ineffective

       ↓

Volatile anesthetic agent, 0.5 MAC
(isoflurane, enflurane, or halothane)

       If ineffective

       ↓

Sodium nitroprusside, hydralazine, or nitroglycerin

Fig. 13-8. Treatment of intraoperative hypertension in head-injured patients. Treatment assumes hypocapnia (25–30 mmHg) has already been achieved.

may be advantageous. If the blood pressure remains elevated, the direct-acting vasodilators such as sodium nitroprusside, nitroglycerin, or hydralazine may be used. The increase in ICP caused by nitroprusside and the other vasodilators may be attenuated by hypocapnic and hyperoxic conditions and a slow rate of administration. If at all possible, cerebrovasodilating drugs should be used either in conjunction with monitoring of ICP or after the dura has been opened. Then at least the ICP will not increase although brain swelling may produce poor operating conditions. A more detailed discussion of the pharmacologic treatment of hypertension is presented in Chapter 6.

C. **Intracranial hypertension** is a possible complication in every head-injured patient. The diagnosis is suspected when headache, papilledema, unilateral pupillary dilatation, oculomotor or abducens palsy, respiratory irregularities, hypertension, or bradycardia is present. Many of these signs are masked by general anesthesia. The diagnosis is confirmed either by the measurement of an elevated ICP or the finding of a tense, swollen brain at craniotomy, which can make the neurosurgical procedure extremely difficult. Failure to control intracranial hypertension will result in cerebral hypoperfusion and possible herniation. The anesthetic techniques that have been presented are designed to reduce ICP and preserve CPP after

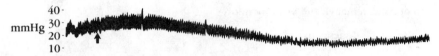

Fig. 13-9. Reduction of elevated intracranial pressure by barbiturates. Pentobarbital, 200 mg, was administered intravenously at the arrow. The reduction occurred approximately 5 min after the pentobarbital was given.

the institution of adequate hyperventilation ($PaCO_2$ of 25–30 mmHg in adults, 20–30 mmHg in children).

If, in spite of these techniques, intracranial hypertension persists, there remain avenues of therapy that can produce a rapid effect. Two or more of these therapies may be used simultaneously.

1. **Augmentation of anesthesia.** Thiopental or pentobarbital, 1.5 to 5 mg/kg, as a bolus injection has been shown to be effective in the reduction of increased ICP (Fig. 13-9). Although the CPP in most patients will increase because the magnitude of the decrease in ICP exceeds the magnitude of the decrease in MAP, close monitoring of both pressures is indicated. In situations in which there is either hypotension or hypovolemia, lidocaine, 1.5 mg/kg, may be useful in reducing ICP while maintaining MAP. Failure of intracranial hypertension to respond to barbiturates usually indicates a poor prognosis.

2. **Diuretics.** Loop diuretics such as furosemide and ethacrynic acid have been used to reduce ICP. Mechanisms of action include general diuresis, decreased rate of CSF production, and resolution of cerebral edema. The osmotic diuretics work primarily by removing water from normal brain tissue. Of the osmotic diuretics, mannitol is the most widely used for acute control of intracranial hypertension (Fig. 13-10). Rapid administration may lead to vasodilatation, increased CBF, and a transient rise in ICP. The reduction of ICP begins shortly after administration and lasts 4 to 6 hours, depending on the dose. The usual dose of mannitol is 0.25 to 1.0 gm/kg. Continued use of mannitol

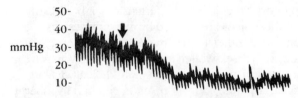

Fig. 13-10. Reduction in elevated intracranial pressure by mannitol, 0.8 gm/kg, administered intravenously at arrow.

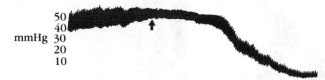

Fig. 13-11. Reduction in elevated intracranial pressure by mannitol, 0.4 gm/kg, and furosemide, 0.6 mg/kg, administered intravenously at arrow.

may lead to hyperosmolality and electrolyte imbalance. This problem may be reduced when the loop diuretics are combined with mannitol (Fig. 13-11).

D. **Hypoxia.** The causes of hypoxia during anesthesia for head-injured patients include aspiration, atelectasis, decreased cardiac output, pneumothorax, neurogenic pulmonary edema, lung contusion, fluid overload, embolism of fat or thrombi, and mechanical problems such as a kinked endotracheal tube or endobronchial intubation. As an initial step in treatment, the FIO_2 should be increased to provide adequate oxygenation. If this cannot be achieved by an FIO_2 of less than 0.55, the use of positive-end expiratory pressure (PEEP) may be indicated. Optimal management includes monitoring the effect of PEEP on ICP, MAP, and CPP since PEEP may increase ICP and decrease MAP and CPP. This effect may be attenuated by elevation of the head and the presence of alveolar pathology.

E. **Diabetes insipidus** is suspected when polyuria with dilute urine occurs. The differential diagnosis includes diabetes mellitus, complications of diuretic therapy, ethanol intoxication, mineralocorticoid deficiency, and mobilization of fluids given during volume resuscitation for multiple trauma. Diagnostic studies include urine and serum chemistries and osmolalities and a monitor of right-sided or left-sided cardiac filling pressures. Failure to treat diabetes insipidus will result in serum hypernatremia and hyperosmolality. Urinary output is replaced with 0.45 normal saline since 5% dextrose in water may lead to superimposed diabetes mellitus or increased cerebral edema. Aqueous vasopressin, 5 IU subcutaneously, will usually relieve the symptoms of diabetes insipidus for 3 to 4 hours. Overzealous treatment with vasopressin may cause water intoxication, which will promote formation of edema.

IX. **Postanesthetic care.** An important question regarding the transition between the operating room and recovery area is whether the patient should go to the recovery room first or directly to the neurologic ICU. This decision depends on the level of care offered, availability of monitoring, and distances involved.

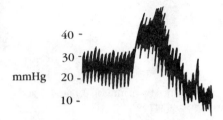

Fig. 13-12. Increased intracranial pressure in response to painful stimulus.

A. **Airway management.** Whether to maintain controlled ventilation, endotracheal intubation, or both in the postoperative period is influenced by many factors including age, preexisting pulmonary disease, thoracoabdominal trauma, severity of the head injury, anticipated level of consciousness, and anticipated edema formation. There is a spectrum ranging from, for example, the young patient undergoing elevation of a depressed skull fracture, who was alert and responsive before anesthetic induction and has minimal underlying brain contusion to the older patient who had evacuation of a large subdural hematoma and who has severe underlying brain injury.

If extubation is planned, the muscle relaxant should be reversed and the trachea extubated when spontaneous ventilation is adequate. Administration of narcotic anesthetics may facilitate tolerance of the endotracheal tube. Lidocaine, 1.5 mg/kg, may attenuate the coughing response to the tube but may also potentiate the action of the nondepolarizing muscle relaxants, possibly interfering with reversal. Controversy exists as to whether recovery from anesthesia and extubation should be in the operating room or special care unit. If it is to be in ICU, precautions should be taken to prevent the patient from coughing and straining during transport. Appropriate monitoring is required during transit. If hypothermia has developed, shivering should be prevented. As the patient recovers from anesthetic effects, painful stimulation should be minimized to prevent elevation of ICP (Fig. 13-12).

B. **Communication** in this transition phase is important. Discussion of the postoperative plans and equipment needs with the special care unit will ensure that a monitor and ventilator will be ready when the patient arrives in the unit. Communication between the anesthesiologist and the neurosurgeon is also essential to delineate and facilitate understanding of the effects of fluid balance, ventilator settings, vasoactive drugs, residual anesthetics, and muscle relaxants. Meticulous attention to detail is necessary for successful outcome in patients who have severe head trauma.

References

Management

1. Adams, H., Mitchell, D. E., Graham, D. I., et al.   Diffuse brain damage of immediate impact type. Its relationship to "primary brain-stem damage" in head injury. *Brain* 100:489, 1977.
2. Bruce, D. A., Alavi, A., Bilaniuk, L. T., et al.   Diffuse cerebral swelling following head injuries in children: The syndrome of "malignant brain edema." *J. Neurosurg.* 54:170, 1981.
3. Bruce, D. A., and Schut, L.   The value of CT scanning following pediatric head injury. *Clin. Pediatr.* 19:719, 1980.
4. Bruce, D. A., Gennarelli, T. A., and Langfitt, T. W.   Resuscitation from comas due to head injury. *Crit. Care Med.* 6:254, 1978.
5. Davis, K. R., Taveras, J. M., Robeson, G. H., et al.   Computed tomography in head trauma. *Semin. Roentgenol.* 12:53, 1977.
6. Dolinskas, C. A., Bilaniuk, L. T., Zimmerman, R. A., et al.   Computed tomography of intracerebral hematomas. 1. Transmission CT observations of hematoma resolution. *Am. J. Roentgenol.* 129:681, 1977.
7. Galbraith, S. C.   Age distribution of extradural hemorrhage without skull fracture. *Lancet* 1:1217, 1973.
8. Greenberg, R. P., Becker, D. P., Miller, J. D., et al   Evaluation of brain function in severe human head trauma with multimodality evoked potentials. Part 2: Localization of brain dysfunction and correlation with posttraumatic neurological conditions. *J. Neurosurg.* 47:163, 1977.
9. Greenberg, R. P., Mayer, D. J., Becker, D. P., et al.   Evaluation of brain function in severe human head trauma with multimodality evoked potentials. Part I: Evoked brain-injury potentials, methods, and analysis. *J. Neurosurg.* 47:150, 1977.
10. Lewis, A. J.   *Mechanisms of Neurological Disease.* Boston: Little, Brown, 1976.
11. Lindenberg, R., Fischer, R. S., Durlacher, S., et al.   The Pathology of the Brain in Blunt Head Injuries of Infants and Children. In *Proceedings of the Second International Congress of Neuropathology.* Amsterdam: Excerpta Medica, 1955. Vol. 1. Pp. 477–479.
12. Ommaya, A. K., and Gennarelli, T. A.   Cerebral concussion and traumatic unconsciousness: Correlation of experimental and clinical observations on blunt head injuries. *Brain* 97:633, 1974.
13. Seelig, J. M., Becker, D. P., Miller, J. D., et al.   Traumatic acute subdural hematoma: Major mortality reduction in comatose patients treated within four hours. *N. Engl. J. Med.* 304:1511, 1981.
14. Windle, W. F., Groat, R. A., and Fox, C. A.   Experimental structural alterations in brain during and after concussion. *Surg. Gynecol. Obstet.* 79:561, 1944.
15. Zimmerman, R. A., Bilaniuk, L. T., and Gennarelli, T. A.   Computed tomography of shearing injuries of the cerebral white matter. *Radiology* 127:393, 1978.

Systemic Effects

1. Aidinis, S. J., Lafferty, J., and Shapiro, H. M.   Intracranial responses to PEEP. *Anesthesiology* 45:275, 1976.
2. Feeley, T. W., and Hedley-Whyte, J.   Weaning from controlled ventilation and supplemental oxygen. *N. Engl. J. Med.* 292:903, 1975.
3. Fox, J. L., Falik, J. L., and Shalhoub, R. J.   Neurosurgical hyponatremia: The role of inappropriate antidiuresis. *J. Neurosurg.* 34:506, 1971.
4. Matjasko, M. J.   Peripheral Sequelae of Acute Head Injury. In J. E. Cottrell and H. Turndorf (Eds.), *Anesthesia and Neurosurgery.* St. Louis: Mosby, 1980. Pp. 211–247.
5. MacDougall, B. R. D., Bailey, R. J., and Williams, R. H_2-receptor antagonists and

antacids in the prevention of acute gastrointestinal hemorrhage in fulminant hepatic failure. *Lancet* 1:617, 1977.
6. McLaurin, R. L., and King, L. R.   Recognition and treatment of metabolic disorders after head injuries. *Clin. Neurosurg.* 19:281, 1972.
7. Shucart, W. A., and Jackson, I.   Management of diabetes insipidus in neurosurgical patients. *J. Neurosurg.* 44:65, 1976.
8. Theodore, J., and Robin, E. D.   Pathogenesis of neurogenic pulmonary edema. *Lancet* 2:749, 1975.

Anesthesia

1. Albin, M. S.   Anesthetic management of the patient with head injury. *Int. Anesthesiol. Clin.* 15:297, 1977.
2. Bedford, R. F., Marshall, W. K., and Persing, J. S.   Rapid reduction of intracranial pressure: Thiopental versus lidocaine. *Anesth. Analg.* (Cleve.) 59:528, 1980.
3. Bormann, B. E., Smith, R. B., Bunegin, L., et al.   Does succinylcholine raise intracranial pressure? *Anesthesiology* (Suppl.) 53:262, 1980.
4. Bruce, D. A.   Management of Severe Head Injury. In J. E. Cottrell and H. Turndorf (Eds.), *Anesthesia and Neurosurgery*. St. Louis: Mosby, 1980. Pp. 183–210.
5. Burney, R. G., and Winn, R.   Increased cerebrospinal fluid pressure during laryngoscopy and intubation for induction of anesthesia. *Anesth. Anal.* (Cleve.) 54:687, 1975.
6. Butler, S. H., and Freund, P. R.   Regional anesthesia as a safe alternative to general anesthesia in the multiple-trauma patient. *Reg. Anesth.* 6:26, 1981.
7. Cotev, S., and Shalit, M. N.   Effects of diazepam on cerebral blood flow and oxygen uptake after head injury. *Anesthesiology* 43:117, 1975.
8. Horton, J. M.   The anaesthetist's contribution to the care of head injuries. *Br. J. Anaesth.* 48:767, 1976.
9. Marsh, M. L., Dunlop, B. J., Shapiro, H. M., et al.   Succinylcholine-intracranial pressure effects in neurosurgical patients. *Anesth. Analg.* (Cleve.) 59:550, 1980.
10. Moss, E., and McDowall, D. G.   ICP increases with 50% nitrous oxide in oxygen in severe head injuries during controlled ventilation. *Br. J. Anaesth.* 51:757, 1979.
10a. Moss, E., Powell, D., Gibson, R. M., and McDowall, E. G.   Effect of etomidate on intracranial pressure and cerebral perfusion pressure. *Br. J. Anaesth.* 51:347, 1979.
11. Phirman, J. R., and Shapiro, H. M.   Modification of nitrous oxide-induced intracranial hypertension by prior induction of anesthesia. *Anesthesiology* 46:150, 1977.
12. Smith, A. L., and Marque, J. J.   Anesthetics and cerebral edema. *Anesthesiology* 45:64, 1976.
13. Stevenson, P. H., and Birch, A. A.   Succinylcholine-induced hyperkalemia in a patient with a closed head injury. *Anesthesiology* 51:89, 1979.
14. Tateishi, A., Maekawa, T., Takeshita, H., et al.   Diazepam and intracranial pressure. *Anesthesiology* 54:335, 1981.
15. Teasdale, G., and Jennett, B.   Assessment of coma and impaired consciousness. *Lancet* 2:81, 1974.

14. Spinal Cord Injury

James E. Cottrell
Philippa Newfield
Joseph P. Giffin
Barbara Shwiry

Each year approximately 1,500,000 people sustain traumatic injuries in the United States, and 100,000 die. Of these, 11,200 victims (more than half under the age of 30) have spinal cord injury; 4200 die before, and another 1150 die during, hospitalization. These who survive require multiple surgical procedures. Spinal cord injuries therefore constitute less than 1% of the total injuries but are responsible for 5% of the mortality from trauma. Among patients who have spinal cord injury, the death rate is 47.7%, as compared to 6.7% for all trauma patients.

These injuries exact tremendous economic, social, and psychological costs as well. By conservative estimates, care for the average victim costs more than $300,000 from the time of injury to the time of death. A two-billion-dollar debt is incurred each year because of new spinal cord injuries in the United States alone.

I. **Pathophysiology.** Our understanding of the pathophysiology of acute spinal cord injury has increased significantly in the past decade. Most spinal cord injuries are accompanied by fracture of the spinal column and/or disruption of the intervertebral discs or the supporting soft tissue around the vertebral column. It is clear, however, that trauma usually does not cause immediate physical transsection of the cord. The traumatizing forces—compression, torsion, stretching, or laceration—injure small vessels (Dohrmann, 1971) and cause both hemorrhage into the gray matter and edema of the white matter of the cord. Tator (1979) and Osterholm (1979) believe that the initial insult leads to delayed ischemia and edema which, several weeks later, result in cavitating necrosis. The necrosis produces a syndrome of anatomic transsection not present at the time of the insult.

Hemorrhagic necrosis of the spinal cord completely disrupts all anatomic structures at the site of the injury. Hematomyelia (blood within the substance of the cord) may extend in either direction from the level of the injury and may be accompanied by edema of both the gray and white matter above and below the level of the lesion. Spinal cord blood flow may be severely reduced for as long as 24 hours after injury, causing further ischemic damage to the injured cord (Sandler, 1976).

Rapid treatment of posttraumatic compression, ischemia, and edema either to prevent or to minimize subsequent cord infarction is of great importance. Tator and Rowe (1979) report that 4 of 20 monkeys recovered after 3 hours of cord compression, whereas 11 of 20 did so when compression was relieved after 1 hour. Similar improvement has been reported when hypothermic irrigation of the injured spinal cord was performed sooner (after 4 hours) rather than compared later (after 8 hours) (Albin, 1978).

Posttraumatic ischemia, decreased cord blood flow, reduced spinal arterial oxygen tension, cord lactic acidosis, and proximal and distal extension of the ischemia in gray and white matter are all involved in the posttraumatic process. Vasospasm from release of norepinephrine and other vasoactive peptides and shunting and thrombosis have been suggested as possible mechanisms. In any event, the attribution of cord necrosis to any of these secondary processes that occur within a specific time frame (rather than to direct mechanical destruction of axons) offers hope that cord injury can be reversed by early intervention.

A. Spinal shock. Pathophysiologic consequences of injury to the spinal cord include spinal shock or total absence of neural activity (Schneider, 1973). Spinal shock occurs immediately after functional disruption of the cord and lasts for a period varying from a few hours to three weeks. The syndrome results from the loss of impulses from higher centers, which reinforce the activity of spinal neurons. Characteristics include flaccid paralysis and loss of reflexes below the level of the lesion, paralytic ileus, and loss of visceral and somatic sensation, vascular tone, and vasopressor reflex. Spinal shock is not usually related to actual anatomic transsection of the cord.

Interruption of the sympathetic outflow with spinal shock can cause vasodilatation, pooling of blood in peripheral vascular beds, and orthostatic hypotension when the patient is tilted head-up. Maintaining the patient in the supine position will reduce the risk of hypotension, but vasopressors may be necessary. The hypotensive phase is usually preceded by a rise in systemic pressure over 3 to 4 minutes as a result of widespread initial sympathetic activation. This phenomenon is of particular significance in the presence of head injury, since cerebral autoregulation may be overcome with a concomitant increase in cerebral blood flow (CBF) and exacerbation of cerebral edema.

Reflex bradycardia from nasopharyngeal or tracheal suctioning or endotracheal intubation can quickly cause cardiac arrest when the cardiac accelerator nerves, which arise from thoracic segments T1–2, have been interrupted. Electrocardiographic (ECG) monitoring and administration of atropine, 0.6 mg every 4 hours, may be necessary.

The spinal cord–injured patient may also have hemorrhagic shock when there has been multiple trauma. However, either hemorrhagic or neurogenic effects will predominate. The key to diagnosis is the presence of bradycardia (usually less than 60) in neurologic shock and a relative tachycardia (pulse more than 100) in hemorrhagic shock.

B. Autonomic hyperreflexia

1. **Pathophysiology.** A stage of reflex automatism occurs after spinal shock during which afferent impulses arising from the peripheral nerves in skin, tendons, muscles, ligaments, joints, and viscera begin to exert their excitatory influence on the neural elements within the isolated cord. No longer restrained by supraspinal inhibitory influences, the cord now reacts to afferent impulses with complex efferent responses.

   Transverse lesions of the cord above the seventh thoracic segment (the splanchnic outflow) functionally separate the sympathetic outflow from the moderating influence of the nuclei in the brainstem and hypothalamus, resulting in loss of sympathetic integration. Activity below the lesion becomes reflex in nature and is characterized by autonomic hyperreflexia, a syndrome of unbridled sympathetic discharge in response to pain, bladder and anal distention, and surgical stimulation. The syndrome occurs in patients who have viable distal cord segments below the level of the lesion.

2. **Signs and symptoms.** Reflex automatism is characterized by hyperreflexia, rigidity and spasticity of muscles, late return of extensor reflexes, and initiation of a mass reflex by cutaneous, proprioceptive, and visceral stimuli resulting in autonomic and motor hypertonus. Signs include pilomotor erection, nausea, agitation, sweating, flushing of the face and neck, severe headache, congestion of mucous membranes, bradycardia, heart block, ventricular arrhythmias, and hypertension (Thompson, 1968). If uncontrolled, the hypertension can lead to loss of consciousness, convulsions, and death from cerebral hemorrhage.

   Reflex sympathetic overactivity in the areas of the body supplied by the isolated spinal cord below the level of the lesion causes vasoconstriction. With lesions above T 7, such a significant portion of the vascular bed is affected that hypertension ensues. Hypertension stimulates the aortic and carotid sinus pressure receptors, which in turn leads to bradycardia, ventricular arrhythmias, or heart block from increased vagal activity.

   Flushing of the face and neck is caused by reflex vasodilatation above the level of the lesion in response to afferent impulses relayed from the aortic arch and carotid sinus receptors to the vasomotor center. Piloerection and sweating occur below the level of the lesion because the centers for segmental control of sweating that exist in the cord are reflexly stimulated (Kendrick, 1953).

3. **Control of autonomic dysfunction.** Autonomic hyper-reflexia usually reaches a peak 4 weeks after spinal cord injury and then subsides. It can, however, recur anytime, even after many years of quiescence, in which case procedures such as subarachnoid instillation of phenol or alcohol, sacral neurotomy, posterior rhizotomy, or cordotomy may be indicated for control. Instillation of alcohol into the lumbar subarachnoid space is simple, fast, and effective since impulses from pelvic structures are the major cause of autonomic hyperreflexia.

II. Treatment of spinal cord injury

A. **Surgical.** Surgical procedures to relieve cord compression, ischemia, and edema must be accompanied by steps to realign, stabilize, and immobilize the injured elements of the vertebral column (Sussman, 1978). Traction and immobilization of the cord are achieved by cervical traction (skull tongs or halo for cervical injury, halo-pelvic or halo-tibial traction for thoracic and lumbar injuries) and by adjustments in posture using bolsters of different shapes and sizes. Surgical reduction may be indicated for dislocations that cannot be reduced by traction, manipulation, or both because of bone fracture and impaction, extensive disruption, or incorporation of soft tissue into the dislocated elements. When instability persists, surgical fixation is also necessary after an adequate period of immobilization by external fixation.

Whereas the role of decompression in the management of cord injury is controversial (Burke, 1976; Heiden, 1975), neurosurgeons agree that decompression and exploration of the spinal canal are indicated when a foreign body is present in the canal and when patients who have incomplete spinal cord injuries deteriorate neurologically. In the latter instance, the evacuation of a subdural or epidural hematoma may reverse the patient's deficit.

In most cases of trauma, the spinal canal is compromised anteriorly. Consequently, the anterior approach is preferable when spinal decompression is necessary, both for accomplishing decompression and for achieving spinal stability. If the laminae or facets have been fractured and driven into the canal, posterior surgical decompression is required. Surgical decompression within 2 hours after injury may increase the chances of recovery, although such attempts are generally unsuccessful when performed after 6 to 12 hours. Some investigators believe, however, that decompressive surgery is of no benefit if the cord is intact, may increase instability of the spine, and may be harmful if the blood supply to the cord is disturbed.

In some series, the incidence of postoperative spinal instability and chronic spinal pain is greater after early decompression than after nonsurgical treatment. Surgical exploration is also not indicated for patients who have a complete loss of cord function after injury. Myelotomy or evacuation of hemorrhagic cavities may be useful, however, in view of evidence that a midline myelotomy or posterior rhizotomy will interrupt the neural reflex loops involved in the release of norepinephrine and other transmitter substances.

If anatomical reduction can be achieved and maintained, the healing of the fractured bone and torn ligaments often produces a stable spine within 3 to 6 months.

B. **Pharmacologic.** Pharmacologic attempts to preserve spinal cord function parallel the approach to preservation of the brain after head injury. A number of animal studies have demonstrated that corticosteroids given before or shortly after injury appear to reduce the degree of spinal cord damage (Kuchner, 1976; Young, 1982). Despite the absence of well-controlled clinical trials, neurosurgeons agree that corticosteroids should be given as soon as possible after spinal injury.

Mannitol, used to treat spinal cord edema, has also produced beneficial effects in animal models of cord injury (Parker, 1973). Vigorous osmotic diuresis requires the prior achievement of hemodynamic stability and adequacy of intravascular volume, however, to ensure perfusion of the cord.

Evidence for the necessity of maintaining spinal cord perfusion pressure—analogous to cerebral perfusion pressure (CPP)—is provided by data from animal models indicating that elevation of blood pressure can reverse the loss of function caused by compression of the cord (Hardy, 1972). In view of the effects of cervical and upper thoracic cord injury on blood pressure and heart rate, however, hemodynamic stabilization can be a problem. Maintenance of pulse and blood pressure are essential because hypoperfusion in the presence of spinal cord edema and ischemia is a major threat to whatever possibility exists for recovery of cord function and must be treated aggressively. Once hemorrhage has been ruled out, the hypotension should be reversed with vasopressor drugs rather than large volumes of intravenous fluid.

C. **Experimental.** Experimental methods of preserving cord function include the use of hypothermia, hyperbaric oxygenation, catecholamine antagonists, dimethyl sulfoxide (DMSO), and endogenous opiate antagonists (naloxone and thyrotropin releasing hormone).

1. **Hypothermia.** Localized cooling of the spinal cord will reduce

cord metabolism at the site of injury (Albin, 1968). Optimal results are obtained when cooling is instituted within 2 hours after injury. The effects of hypothermia are temporary, however, so that spinal cord damage may subsequently progress.

2. **Hyperbaric oxygenation.** In animals that sustained impact injury to the cord, hyperbaric oxygenation (3 atm) resulted in improvement when compared to controls (Hartzog, 1971).

3. **Norepinephrine antagonists.** Pharmacologic agents that inhibit the synthesis, release, or accumulation of norepinephrine may be valuable. Phenoxybenzamine, reserpine, L-dopa, and 1-methyltyrosine are currently being investigated.

4. **Dimethyl sulfoxide.** Dimethyl sulfoxide has been shown to decrease central hemorrhage and edema of the white matter in experimental spinal cord injury (Kajihara, 1973).

5. **Naloxone.** Evidence suggests that endorphins are released after spinal injury (Faden, 1980). The endorphins exacerbate posttraumatic ischemia by causing a reduction in spinal cord blood flow, which is associated with systemic hypotension. Treatment with naloxone improves both spinal cord blood flow and neurologic outcome in animal models by blocking these endorphin-mediated effects (Faden, 1981). Opiate antagonists may also offer some protection by counteracting the systemic hypotension that occurs after trauma. Opiate antagonists may have the adverse effect, however, of increasing posttraumatic pain.

6. **Thyrotropin releasing hormone.** Thyrotropin releasing hormone (TRH) has recently been investigated for use in place of opiate antagonists. In addition to its function in regulating the secretion of thyrotropin from the pituitary gland, TRH has been shown experimentally to act as a partial opiate antagonist. TRH differs from pharmacologic opiate antagonists, however, in two ways: it does not act at the opiate receptor and it reverses many of the behavioral and autonomic effects of opiates while sparing their analgesic properties.

III. **Airway management.** A patient who has a fracture of the vertebral column and either established or potential spinal cord injury requires skilled, meticulous care at the site of the accident, during transport, and in the hospital. Adequacy of airway, oxygenation, and perfusion pressure must be maintained to avoid additional injury to the spinal cord from hypoxia or shock. With complete cervical or upper thoracic lesions, blood pressure may fall because of loss of sympathetic tone;

blood pressure should be restored by vasopressor drugs once hemorrhage has been excluded as a cause of hypotension.

The commonest cause of early death after cervical spinal cord injury is acute respiratory failure. The mortality within the first 3 months after injury has decreased from 10% to 15% in 1965 to 5% today largely because of the skill of emergency medical technicians in dealing with ventilatory failure during the rescue, resuscitation, positioning, and transportation of injured patients.

The comatose, apneic patient requires immediate ventilatory support by means of an oropharyngeal airway, face mask, and self-inflating bag with supplemental oxygen. It must be assumed that comatose patients have unstable spine injuries until x-ray films exclude such lesions. Consequently, if aspiration or marked airway obstruction at the scene of the accident necessitates either intubation or passage of an esophageal obturator, flexion and extension of the neck must be avoided to prevent catastrophic exacerbation of cervical cord injury. When the patient has a normal level of consciousness, intact pharyngeal reflexes, and a patent airway, the rescue team should provide supplemental oxygen and assist ventilation as necessary with bag and mask. These patients require observation, however, to detect progressive loss of ventilatory ability as a result of evolving diaphragmatic or intercostal muscle paralysis.

During transport, the patient is immobilized on a short or long backboard with head and spine properly splinted to minimize movement of the potentially unstable spine. For unstable cervical injuries, axial traction using either a halter device or skeletal fixation with skull tongs should be applied as early as possible.

Obtunded patients who breathe spontaneously may require an oropharyngeal airway only; during insertion, care is necessary to avoid regurgitation, aspiration, and movement of the neck. Patients who resist intubation may suffer further neurologic injury. Gentle neck traction will provide stability for cervical fractures during careful intubation by experienced personnel.

Fracture of the cervical spinal column and resultant cord injury may occur as an isolated entity after diving accidents and gunshot wounds of the neck. Cervical cord trauma also occurs in the patient who has multiple injuries, especially when other structures of the neck, face, and head are affected. Since the patient who has multiple trauma may require surgery under general anesthesia, the presence of a cervical spine fracture (always suspected until radiographically proven otherwise) must be considered during intubation.

An attempt to maintain the stability of the neck may preclude conventional orotracheal intubation. Awake nasotracheal intubation, performed either blindly or guided by a fiberoptic bronchoscope, will permit passage of the tube without motion of the neck. A catheter inserted with a Touhy needle through the cricothyroid membrane and directed up to the nose may serve as a guide for placement of the endotracheal tube.

IV. Monitoring. Since the heart of a spinal cord–injured patient cannot compensate for overtransfusion or increased venous return, careful monitoring is mandatory. A Swan-Ganz pulmonary artery catheter will facilitate assessment of cardiac function and intravascular volume. Observation of the pulmonary capillary wedge pressure (PCWP) will help determine the patient's circulating blood volume. Intravascular volume can be increased by rapid infusion of lactated Ringer's solution, 50 ml/min in 250-ml increments, until an increase in PCWP of greater than 2 mmHg is achieved. Raising the legs is an alternative to infusing fluid and has the advantage of being reversible when the legs are lowered.

There are three possible ways to use the **change in PCWP** to assess cardiac function.

A. One possibility is that the **PCWP increases 3 to 4 mmHg and then decreases** within 5 minutes to a level 2 mmHg above baseline. This indicates that the patient is adequately hydrated considering the prevailing vascular tone. The treatment should then be to maintain the PCWP within this range for optimal cardiac function.

B. The second possibility is that the **PCWP continues to rise** after infusion ceases, which indicates that the heart is unable to increase its contractility to deal with the increased filling pressures. The treatment is to restrict further fluid infusion, eliminate or avoid myocardial depressant drugs, and consider the use of inotropic agents such as dopamine if the trend does not reverse.

C. The third possibility is that **PCWP either does not change or it rises** immediately and then returns to the baseline, which means that the heart is able to deal with a greater circulatory volume than the patient already has. If the patient is oliguric or has a low mixed venous oxygen tension, inotropic agents should not be given. Instead, intravenous fluids should be infused to augment the circulating blood volume.

V. Anesthetic management

A. Preoperative evaluation. The paraplegic patient may require repeated operative intervention for treatment of complications of the original injury, urologic manipulations for stones and infections, or plastic procedures for decubitus ulcer and infection. All operations are complicated by electrolyte imbalance, anemia, sepsis, negative nitrogen balance, hypoproteinemia, amyloidosis, drug dependence, adrenocortical insufficiency, hypovolemia, and emotional instability.

Thus, in addition to correcting fluid and electrolyte balance, the anesthesiologist should evaluate the patient's renal function, myocardial conduction system, respiratory competency (FEV_1/FVC), chest roentgenogram (if atelectasis or pneumonia is suspected), temperature control, skeletal integrity (to rule out pathologic fractures and secondary osteomyelitis), and excretory ability (to prevent postoperative pneumonia or atelectasis from elevation of the diaphragm). Any history of previous episodes of autonomic hyperreflexia should be investigated as well.

Because the patient may be suffering from illness-induced emotional difficulties (including severe depression and psychological instability), it is important to establish good rapport with the patient. It may be difficult to achieve adequate sedation in spinal cord–injured patients, as they may have developed tolerance to sedatives and narcotics.

B. Induction. Since the sympathetic function of patients who have spinal cord injury (especially those with lesions above T 7) is unpredictable, anesthesia is induced slowly. Autonomic excess or deficiency is treated by infusion of direct-acting vasoconstrictors (phenylephrine), vasodilators (nitroprusside or nitroglycerine), or positive (isoproterenol) or negative (propranolol) chronotropic drugs. Sympathetic agonists or antagonists that act indirectly to release catecholamines are avoided.

C. Muscle relaxants. The use of succinylcholine deserves special consideration. The occurrence of succinylcholine-induced ventricular fibrillation was reported in 1970 in spinal cord–injured patients (Smith, 1970), and other cases have since been described. Starting within the first week and continuing over a period of 6 months or more, the muscle cell becomes supersensitive so that the entire cell membrane behaves like the end plate: in response to a depolarizing drug, the cell membrane will depolarize as a unit and release large amounts of potassium into the circulation (Gronert, 1975). The high plasma concentration of potassium causes ventricular fibrillation, which can occur up to 18 months after the original injury. Giving small doses of nondepolarizing muscle relaxants before the succinylcholine will not completely block the hyperkalemic response. Nondepolarizing relaxants are effective and safe alternatives to succinylcholine.

The use of succinylcholine in patients recently injured—even after pretreatment with a nondepolarizing muscle relaxant—is also not advisable, since the time course for the development of extrajunctional receptor sites is not clearly defined during the immediate postinjury period. The trachea should be intubated after topical anesthesia without relaxation while the patient is awake or by the use of a nondepolarizing relaxant such as pancuronium, 0.1 mg/kg, or a moderately deep level of inhalation anesthesia.

D. **Intraoperative autonomic hyperreflexia.** Autonomic hyper-reflexia most frequently occurs when anesthesia is insufficient. Characterized by paroxysmal hypertension, autonomic hyper-reflexia is initiated either by stimuli applied below the level of the lesion or by bladder or bowel distention. Bradycardia and heart block may be reflexly induced as a baroreceptor response to vaso-constriction above the level of the lesion. The pattern usually con-sists of an initial fall in blood pressure during induction and then a precipitous rise with the initiation of surgery. Control is achieved by a cessation of the stimulus, deepening of anesthesia, and administra-tion of direct-acting vasoactive drugs.

Reflex muscle spasm and autonomic hyperreflexia are effectively prevented by spinal and epidural anesthesia, which block affer-ent visceral pathways. The problems with spinal and epidural anes-thesia are manifold, however. In addition to technical difficulties, the level of the block is unpredictable because of anatomic distor-tion. Severe hypotension may occur, especially when intravascular volume is decreased. Muscle spasms may be eliminated by adminis-tering neuromuscular blocking drugs during general anesthesia. Succinylcholine is contraindicated, however, because of the exces-sive release of potassium from denervated muscle and resultant ventricular fibrillation.

The occurrence of other abnormalities affecting anesthetic man-agement depends on the amount of time that has elapsed since the initial injury to the spinal cord. During the first few weeks after injury, urinary and fecal retention is common, which may cause impairment of respiration from elevation of the diaphragm. Disim-paction and bladder decompression or catheterization are therapeu-tic. Pneumonia may also be present. The chronic phase of injury is marked by return of muscle tone, positive Babinski sign, and the recurrence of the hyperreflexia syndromes.

VI. **Hazards and complications**

A. **Respiratory insufficiency.** Quadriplegic and most paraplegic pa-tients suffer from respiratory compromise and kyphoscoliosis. A complete cord lesion causes total paralysis of the intercostal mus-cles. Diaphragmatic innervation remains intact when the lesion is at or below the level of the sixth cervical vertebra. Lesions at the fifth cervical segment are associated with partial compromise of dia-phragmatic innervation. The diaphragm is deprived of its major segmental nerve supply, and its function is grossly impaired when the injury occurs at or above the level of the fourth cervical segment. The prompt placement of an endotracheal tube and controlled ventilation are mandatory for these patients.

The combination of high cervical injury and inadequate ventilation can cause a decrease in vital capacity, expiratory reserve volume, and PaO_2; retention of secretions; increase in $PaCO_2$ and dead space; vasoconstriction; abnormalities in the ventilation-perfusion ratio; respiratory failure; and pulmonary edema. All of these conditions predispose the patient to postoperative pulmonary problems. Assisted or controlled ventilation and monitoring of arterial blood gases are required during operation and in the recovery period.

Postural drainage and chest physiotherapy are important adjuncts after operation. Aspiration, the danger of which is always present and heightened in the immediate postoperative period, should be anticipated and prevented but treated aggressively if it occurs. In addition, neuromuscular activity may be depressed by electrolyte imbalance; unless recognized and corrected, it may lead to serious problems with ventilation in the postoperative period.

B. **Hypotension.** The paraplegic patient should be moved to the operating table and positioned with care to avoid complications from the orthostatic hypotension that accompanies autonomic insufficiency. This basic problem can be exacerbated in these patients by inadequate intravascular volume and insufficient release of norepinephrine.

C. **Pressure necrosis.** The protection of vulnerable skin areas from ischemic pressure, maceration, and abrasion is essential, since 2 hours of continuous pressure on a particular area below the level of the lesion can cause a decubitus ulcer. This time is reduced to 20 minutes when the patient has a high fever. The incidence of pressure sores in quadriplegic patients is double that in paraplegic patients. All pressure points should therefore be carefully padded during operation. In the postoperative period, the patient's position should be changed frequently.

D. **Pathologic fractures.** Gentle transfers of the patient are indicated to avoid pathologic fractures of the femoral shaft and hip joints through areas of osteoporosis or necrosis from secondary osteomyelitis at sites of pressure decubiti (ischium, greater trochanter, sacrum, and heel).

E. **Electrolyte and calcium abnormalities.** In the early phases of spinal cord injury, electrolyte abnormalities may occur. Flaccid paralysis from the failure of nerve conduction to voluntary muscle fibers reduces muscle activity and increases mobilization of calcium. This produces hypercalcemia and hypercalciuria, which start about 10 days after injury. The increase in serum calcium may predispose the patient to ventricular arrhythmias during anesthesia. Calcium levels should therefore be measured preoperatively in patients who have spinal cord injury. Appropriate antiarrhythmic drugs and potassium chloride should be available during operation.

F. **Renal abnormalities.** Patients who have spinal cord injury develop recurrent urinary tract infection, ascending pyelonephritis, amyloidosis, and chronic renal failure. Impaired renal function represents a significant complication, causing loss of protein, elevation of blood urea nitrogen and creatinine, and reduction in total body sodium and potassium. Consequently, electrolyte balance and intravascular volume should be assessed preoperatively.

Anesthetic precautions include avoiding drugs that are metabolized primarily by the kidneys and are potential renal toxins. Extubation should be accomplished after complete reversal of muscle relaxation. Special precaution is indicated after irrigation of body cavities with antibiotic solution such as neomycin.

G. **Temperature regulation.** The spinal cord–injured patient is poikilothermic from the loss of autonomic function. Maintaining normal body temperature is difficult. Careful monitoring as well as temperature control with warming blanket, heated humidified air, increased ambient temperature, and warmed solutions should be instituted, and overheating should be carefully avoided.

References

1. Albin, M. S. Resuscitation of the spinal cord. *Crit. Care Med.* 6:270, 1978.
2. Albin, M. S., White, R. J., Acosta-Rua, G., et al. Study of functional recovery produced by delayed localized cooling after spinal cord injury in primates. *J. Neurosurg.* 29:113, 1968.
3. Burke, D. C., and Murray, D. D. The management of thoracic and thoracolumbar injuries of the spine with neurological involvement. *J. Bone Joint Surg.* [Am.] 58B:72, 1976.
4. Desmond, J. Paraplegia: Problems confronting the anesthesiologist. *Can. Anaesth. Soc. J.* 17:435, 1970.
5. Dohrmann, G. J., Wagner, F. C., Jr., and Bucy, P. C. The microvasculature in transitory traumatic paraplegia: An electron microscopic study in monkey. *J. Neurosurg.* 35:263, 1971.
6. Faden, A. I., Jacobs, T. P., and Holaday, J. W. Endorphin-parasympathetic interaction in spinal shock. *J. Auton. Nerv. Syst.* 2:295, 1980.
7. Faden, A. I., Jacobs, T. P., and Holaday J. W. Opiate antagonist improves neurologic recovery after spinal injury. *Science* 211:493, 1981.
8. Faden, A. I., Jacobs, T. P., Mougey, E., and Holaday, J. W. Endorphins in experimental spinal injury: Therapeutic effect of naloxone. *Ann. Neurol.* 10:326, 1981.

9. Gronert, G. A., and Theye, R. A. Pathophysiology of hyperkalemia induced by succinylcholine. *Anesthesiology* 43:89, 1975.
10. Hardy, R. W., Brodkey, J. S., Richards, D. E., et al. Effect of systemic hypertension on compression block of spinal cord. *Surg. Forum* 23:434, 1972.
11. Hartzog, J. T., Fischer, R. G., and Snow, C. Spinal Cord Trauma: Effect of Hyperbaric Oxygen Therapy. In *Proceedings of the Veterans Administration Spinal Cord Injury Conference* 17:70, 1971.
12. Heiden, J. S., Weiss, M. H., Rosenberg, A. W., et al. Management of cervical spinal cord trauma in Southern California. *J. Neurosurg.* 43:732, 1975.
13. Holaday, J. W., and Faden, A. I. Naloxone acts at central opiate receptors to reverse hypotension, hypothermia and hypoventilation in spinal shock. *Brain Res.* 189:295, 1980.
14. Kajihara, K., Kawanaga, H., de la Torre, J. C., et al. Dimethyl sulfoxide in the treatment of experimental acute spinal cord injury. *Surg. Neurol.* 1:16, 1973.
15. Kendrick, W. W., Scott, J. W., Jousse, A. T., et al. Reflex sweating and hypertension in traumatic transverse myelitis. *Treat. Serv. Bull.* (Ottawa) 8:437, 1953.
16. Kuchner, E. F., and Hansebout, R. R. Combined steroid and hypothermia treatment of experimental spinal cord injury. *Surg. Neurol.* 6:371, 1976.
17. Mackenzie, C., Shin, B., Krishnaprasad, D., and McCormack, F. Cardiac function during anesthesia for acute paraplegics (abstract). Presented at the Society of Neurosurgical Anesthesia and Neurologic Supportive Care Annual Meeting, St. Louis, Oct. 1980.
18. Means, E. D., Anderson, D. K., Nicolosi, G., et al. Microvascular perfusion: Experimental spinal cord injury. *Surg. Neurol.* 9:353, 1978.
19. Naftchi, N. E., Wooten, G. F., Lowman, E. W., et al. Relationship between serum dopamine-β-hydroxylase activity, catecholamine metabolism, and hemodynamic changes during paroxysmal hypertension in quadriplegia. *Circ. Res.* 35:850, 1974.
20. Osterholm, J. L. The pathophysiological response to spinal cord injury: Current status of related research. *J. Neurosurg.* 40:5, 1974.
21. Parker, A. J., Park, R. D., and Stowater, J. L. Reduction of trauma-induced edema of spinal cord in dogs given mannitol. *Am. J. Vet. Res.* 34:1355, 1973.
22. Rivlin, A. S., and Tator, C. H. Effect of duration of acute spinal cord compression in a new acute cord injury model in the rat. *Surg. Neurol.* 10:39, 1978.
23. Sandler, A. N., and Tator, C. H. Effect of acute spinal cord compression injury on regional spinal cord blood flow in primates. *J. Neurosurg.* 45:660, 1976.
24. Schneider, R. C., Crosby, E. C., Russo, R. H., et al. Traumatic spinal cord syndromes and their management. *Clin. Neurosurg.* 20:424, 1973.
25. Smith, R. B., and Grenvik, A. Cardiac arrest following succinylcholine in patients with central nervous system injuries. *Anesthesiology* 33:558, 1970.
26. Sussman, B. J. Fracture dislocation of the cervical spine: A critique of current management in the United States. *Paraplegia* 16:15, 1978.
27. Tator, C. H., and Rowe, D. W. Current concepts in the immediate management of acute spinal cord injuries. *Can. Med. Assoc. J.* 121:1453, 1979.
28. Thompson, P. D., and Melmon, K. L. Clinical assessment of autonomic function. *Anesthesiology* 29:724, 1968.
29. Yashon, D. *Spinal Injury.* New York: Appleton-Century-Crofts, 1978.
30. Young, W., and Flamm, E. S. Effect of high-dose corticosteroid therapy on blood flow, evoked potentials, and extracellular calcium in experimental spinal injury. *J. Neurosurg.* 57:667, 1982.

15. Pediatric Neurosurgery

Mark A. Rockoff

I. Pathophysiology

A. **Cerebrospinal fluid.** Under normal conditions, cerebrospinal fluid (CSF) exists in dynamic equilibrium, with absorption equal to production. The average adult has between 90 and 150 ml of CSF throughout the brain and spinal subarachnoid space. Children have lesser amounts and in neonates, often only a few drops of CSF can be obtained from the spinal canal. CSF is produced predominantly in the choroid plexus, and total CSF replacement occurs about 5 times each day. Production of CSF is affected little by alterations of intracranial pressure (ICP) and is usually unchanged in children who have hydrocephalus. Drugs such as acetazolamide, furosemide, and corticosteroids decrease CSF production. Unusual tumors that produce CSF, such as choroid plexus papillomas, are more likely to occur during childhood.

Absorption of CSF is not as well understood. It appears that the arachnoid villi are important sites for absorption of CSF into the venous system. Absorption increases with elevation of ICP. Intracranial hemorrhage, infections of the central nervous system (CNS), and congenital abnormalities that obstruct CSF flow and/or the arachnoid villi are conditions of childhood that decrease CSF absorption. In the presence of open fontanelles and open cranial sutures, the effects of CSF obstruction that increase ICP may be attenuated by increasing head circumference.

B. **Cerebral blood flow and cerebral blood volume.** In addition to CSF translocation, the brain compensates for increases in ICP by decreasing intracranial blood volume. Although cerebral blood volume occupies only about 10% of the intracranial space, dynamic, blood volume–related changes occur that are often initiated by anesthesia or intensive care procedures. As with other vascular beds, most blood is contained in the low-pressure, high-capacitance venous system. Increases in intracranial volume are met by decreases in cerebral blood volume. Accordingly, in hydrocephalic infants a shift of venous blood from intracranial to extracranial vessels produces distended scalp veins. Ultimately, increases in cerebral blood volume result in elevation of ICP.

Factors that increase cerebral blood flow (CBF) usually increase cerebral blood volume. CBF in infants and children is affected by the same drugs and maneuvers that produce alterations in adults, but there may be quantitative differences in response (Rodgers, 1980). The limits of responsiveness may vary with age. Hypoxia appears to increase CBF, but the CBF may not be affected until PaO_2 falls below 50 mmHg. CBF also appears to be directly related to $PaCO_2$, but the response may be blunted in neonates at values below 30 mmHg. Finally, autoregulation of CBF occurs with gradual changes in blood pressure, but clearly at different absolute values from adults. Mean arterial pressure (MAP) does not normally reach 60 mmHg until the child is approximately 1 year of age. The lower limit of acceptable blood pressure that will ensure adequate CBF is unknown and may change with the child's age (including gestational age). Likewise, excessive blood pressure elevations may exceed the limits of autoregulation at different pressures at different ages.

C. **Cerebral perfusion pressure.** Since CBF is not easily determined, cerebral perfusion pressure (CPP) is often used to estimate cerebral circulation. (CPP is equal to MAP minus ICP.) As with CBF, acceptable limits for young children are not known and may vary with age. It is helpful to be familiar with normal blood pressure values for different ages.

Age	Average systolic blood pressure (mmHg)
30 wk*	45
35 wk*	55
term	65
2 yr	95
12 yr	115

*Refers to gestational age at birth

D. **Intracranial pressure.** Elevation of intracranial pressure (ICP) may not be apparent on clinical examination. Pupillary dilatation, increasing blood pressure, and bradycardia do not always develop in association with intracranial hypertension. However, when they are associated with increased ICP, they are usually late and dangerous signs. Papilledema may not be present in children who die as a result of intracranial hypertension. An abnormal level of consciousness, especially when associated with abnormal motor responses to painful stimuli, is frequently associated with elevated ICP.

Computerized tomography (CT) scanning demonstrates small or obliterated ventricles, hydrocephalus, or mass effect. Increases in ICP occurring soon after head injury in children are not often from intracranial hematomas (as they are in adults), but are more likely to be secondary to diffuse brain swelling caused by excessive CBF.

Techniques used to monitor ICP in adults have been useful in children. Unfortunately, ventricular catheters may be difficult to insert into ventricles compressed by diffuse brain swelling. Subarachnoid bolts are most commonly used to monitor ICP in children, but they are difficult to stabilize in infants less than 1 year old because of the thin calvaria. An epidural transducer secured noninvasively to the anterior fontanelle has recently been used to assess neonatal ICP.

Normal values of ICP in children are generally accepted as less than 15 mmHg. The occurrence of frequent pressure waves in children who have intracranial disorders should be considered hazardous. Before the fontanelles have closed, significant increases in head circumference can occur and ICP remains in the normal range on intermittent measurements. Intracranial hypertension may also exist without bulging fontanelles, especially if the increase in ICP develops slowly.

II. Anesthetic management

A. Preoperative evaluation is the same as for all pediatric patients, with special attention to the following concerns:

1. History

    a. Previous drug reactions, allergies, or asthma (especially if contrast agents may be used for neuroradiologic evaluation)

    b. Associated medical problems (such as seizures, diabetes, croup, or asthma)

    c. Use of medications (antihypertensives, corticosteroids, anticonvulsants, etc.)

    d. Family history of **adverse reaction to anesthetics**

2. Physical examination

    a. Age

    b. Temperature

    c. Heart rate

    d. Blood pressure

    e. Weight (to guide drug and fluid administration and to aid in intraoperative assessment of blood loss and volume replacement)

    f. Respiratory system (pneumonia, asthma, adenoid hypertrophy)

    g. Cardiovascular system (congenital heart disease, especially right-to-left shunts that predispose the patient to arterial embolization)

h. Hydration (may be altered as a result of prolonged vomiting, poor appetite, diabetes insipidus, inappropriate antidiuretic hormone secretion, iatrogenic dehydration secondary to fluid restriction or osmotic agents)

i. Neurologic assessment

(1) Presence of intracranial hypertension

(2) Level of consciousness (ability to cooperate with induction of anesthesia)

(3) Motor weakness (ability to cough and breathe adequately, presence of gag and swallowing mechanisms to protect airway, and muscle dysfunction, which may alter response to muscle relaxants or confuse assessment of their effectiveness)

(4) Pupillary responsiveness and equality (detection of benign congenital anisocoria)

3. **Laboratory data**

   a. **Hematocrit**

   b. **Urinalysis**

   c. **Additional studies** including chest x-ray films, electrocardiogram (ECG), evaluation of clotting parameters, serum (and occasionally urine) electrolytes and osmolality, and arterial or capillary blood gases

   d. **Neuroradiologic studies** (CT scan, angiogram, skull x-ray film)

   e. Clot to blood bank for **type and crossmatch**

4. **Permission for anesthesia** from parents or legal guardian. Good rapport with the patient will facilitate a smooth induction.

5. **NPO orders:** no solid food or milk products for at least six to eight hours before induction.

   a. **Neonate:** offer glucose water two hours before induction; then NPO

   b. **One to six months:** offer glucose water four hours before induction; then NPO

   c. **Six to thirty-six months:** offer clear liquids six hours before induction; then NPO

    d. More than three years: offer clear liquids eight hours before induction; then NPO

B. Premedication (withheld if the patient has a full stomach)

  1. Atropine: not given on ward as its vagolytic effect is usually gone by the time of induction, its drying effect on secretions is annoying and usually unnecessary, and it may be administered during induction if needed.

  2. Narcotics: avoided if intracranial hypertension, CNS depression, or hypotonia is suspected (respiratory depression).

  3. Sedatives: avoided if intracranial hypertension, CNS depression, or hypotonia is suspected (respiratory depression, airway obstruction). Pentobarbital (4–5 mg/kg) or diazepam (0.3–0.5 mg/kg) may be given orally with a sip of water to anxious and alert patients who are 18 months or older.

  4. Corticosteroids: continued in the perioperative period.

  5. Anticonvulsants: continued in the perioperative period.

  6. Rectal drugs: the ability to promise no perioperative intramuscular injection often greatly improves cooperation. An effective drug is methohexital (20–30 mg/kg in a 10% solution of sterile water). Advantages and contraindications are as follows:

    a. Produces sleep within 10 minutes that lasts about 45 minutes

    b. Is particularly useful in patients between 1 and 5 years of age who may be uncooperative

    c. Is often administered to healthy children in their parents' presence, but should only be given by an anesthesiologist in an area where suction equipment and oxygen are available

    d. Does not require a preoperative enema, but someone must hold the buttocks together to prevent the drug from being eliminated

    e. Probably lowers ICP in the same manner as intravenous barbiturates if airway obstruction is prevented

    f. Best avoided in patients who have psychomotor, temporal, or mixed seizure disorders, as it can induce convulsions in the presence of these conditions; rectal pentothal in the same dose is then preferable

    g. Smaller amounts may calm a child sufficiently to allow an intravenous catheter to be placed or a smooth induction with an inhalation anesthetic

h. May be repeated if the first dose fails

i. May be given intramuscularly, 8–10 mg/kg, in a 5% solution of sterile water

C. Monitoring

1. Essential for all children

a. Stethoscope: precordial or esophageal

b. Blood pressure: appropriately sized cuff (should cover about ⅔ of upper arm) with measurement by palpation, oscillation, or Doppler device; direct arterial pressure monitoring may also be indicated

c. ECG

d. Temperature

2. Additional monitoring.
All monitoring devices used for adults can be applied to infants and children when necessary. The small size of the patient may actually be an indication for a more aggressive, if necessarily invasive, approach, since changes occur more rapidly and are often more difficult to detect accurately. Doppler devices, end-tidal carbon dioxide analyzers, neuromuscular blockade monitors, electroencephalograms (EEG), and ICP monitors are used in children as in adults.

3. Technical problems.
The risk of technical problems is less if catheters are inserted after induction.

a. Arterial catheters. 22-Gauge catheters can be placed percutaneously (or by cutdown) in the radial or dorsalis pedis artery, even in infants weighing less than 1000 gm. An umbilical artery can be cannulated in the first days of life, providing an intra-aortic catheter for monitoring, blood sampling, and drug and fluid administration.

b. Central venous catheters may be inserted through the umbilical vein in the first days of life. Commercially available kits use small introducer needle, guide wire, and catheter (down to size 3 French for neonates) for percutaneous venous cannulation (jugular, subclavian, or femoral vein).

c. Urinary catheters. Infant feeding tubes are useful if Foley catheters are too large, although leaking may occur around them. Urine volume is more accurately estimated when collected into large syringes rather than drainage bags.

D. Special problems

1. **Inaccessibility,** frequently encountered during neurosurgical procedures, is more pronounced with pediatric patients. All tubes, catheters, and devices must be securely fastened, preferably with benzoin. Slight displacement of the endotracheal tube (whether from motion of the tube or change in head position) can cause either extubation or bronchial intubation in small children. Disconnection of catheters under the drapes can rapidly result in hypovolemia, hypotension, or air embolism. When possible, a small, well-lit tunnel is created to provide a view of the patient, the airway, and the catheters.

2. **Positioning.** Children are at great risk if all pressure points are not protected during positioning. The consequences of someone's leaning on the patient may be serious. Mechanical devices (such as a metal triangle or Mayo stand) may be secured to the operating table and placed between the surgeon and the patient. Care must be taken to ensure the patient's immobility to avoid stretching of nerves (as when an arm falls over the table) or compression of vital areas (as when the head moves off the headrest and causes pressure on eyes or chin).

   Fortunately, the sitting position is rarely used for children less than two years of age. For the prone position, care must be taken to ensure free abdominal and chest wall motion to avoid both impairment of respiration and increased intra-abdominal pressure. The child is usually supported by padding under the chest and pelvis; pressure on the genitalia is avoided. Inevitably, some equipment must be disconnected while the patient is positioned; constant attention should be directed toward the heart tones audible with the esophageal stethoscope, and periods of monitoring "black-out" should be minimal.

3. **Temperature control.** Hypothermia is a common problem during anesthesia for pediatric neurosurgery. Children have a greater surface area-to-weight ratio, have less insulating fat, and have higher metabolic rates. They therefore produce more heat that can be lost. Central nervous system abnormalities, such as hydrocephalus, may predispose the child to autonomic dysfunction and temperature instability. Pediatric operations are also often performed in rooms that are not designed for pediatric anesthesia.

   Although mild hypothermia decreases brain energy requirements and may be beneficial in paralyzed patients, its deleterious effects become important during the recovery period. Shivering will increase ICP and oxygen consumption. Metabolic acidosis will depress cardiac output, and arrhythmias commonly occur when the body temperature falls below 30°C. If the patient is to remain paralyzed and sedated, then mild hypothermia is permissible. In other cases, efforts must be made to maintain near normal body temperature, since it is difficult to rewarm a patient in the operating room once the temperature has fallen.

Aids in maintaining normothermia in children include the following:

a. Warm the room before induction.

b. Limit the time of body exposure, especially to the cleansing solutions.

c. Provide overhead warmers for infants (servocontrolled to body temperature to avoid overheating) and heating lamps for older children. Placement too close to the skin can cause burns, however.

d. Provide a heated water mattress, especially for children less than 10 kg (about 1 year of age).

e. Place warm blankets over uninvolved areas of the body.

f. Heat inspired gases with a heated humidifier. Avoid airway burns by measuring inspired gas temperature.

g. Warm all intravenous solutions and blood products.

4. **Anesthesia circuits.** All systems applicable to the general practice of pediatric anesthesia can be used for neurosurgical procedures. Mechanical ventilation is desirable for procedures that require careful, stable control of $PaCO_2$. All systems should provide a method of heating and humidifying inspired gases. Unnecessary dead space should be eliminated. For children more than about 3 years of age, the standard semiclosed reabsorber circuit is used. The resistance provided by the one-way valves may be excessive for younger children unless ventilation is controlled. For neonates and small children, a Mapleson or Baines circuit is used, with fresh gas flows of at least twice the minute ventilation to prevent rebreathing (normal neonate minute ventilation is approximately 100 ml/kg).

5. **Fluid and electrolyte replacement.** Various formulas are used to estimate maintenance fluid requirements and deficits

where deficit = hourly requirement × hours NPO + any additional fluid deficit (e.g., from dehydration). One reliable formula for hourly requirement is:

4 ml/kg/hr	0–10 kg
2 ml/kg/hr	10–20 kg
1 ml/kg/hr	>20 kg
Example: A 25-kg child	
4 ml/kg/hr × 1st 10 kg	40 ml/hr
2 ml/kg/hr × 2nd 10 kg (10–20 kg)	20 ml/hr
1 ml/kg/hr × 5 kg (20–25 kg)	5 ml/hr
Total hourly requirement	65 ml/hr

If extensive blood loss is anticipated, the blood is administered gradually, early in the procedure as the losses occur. In cases in which blood loss is not a major concern, one half the deficit is replaced with crystalloid solution over the first hour and the rest as the case progresses. The choice of electrolyte solutions is similar to that for adults, except that infants receive supplementation with glucose (usually Ringer's lactate solution with 5% dextrose) to avoid hypoglycemia. When large quantities of glucose-containing solutions are given, however, hyperglycemia can occur if the serum glucose is not monitored and its administration is not limited. Hypotonic solutions are avoided.

6. **Blood loss and replacement.** Blood loss is difficult to estimate accurately. Much of the blood lost is absorbed on the drapes, and irrigation solutions confuse sponge weights and suction measurement. Nevertheless, it is important to estimate losses. Accuracy can be improved if the surgeon communicates the volume of blood lost as it occurs and if all suctioned blood is collected in calibrated bottles (such as empty 250-ml IV fluid bottles). Knowledge of the amount of intravenous solution required to maintain the child's intravascular volume is also useful. Serial measurement of the hematocrit (hct) will reflect blood loss during replacement with crystalloid solution.

Preoperatively, an adequate amount of crossmatched blood should always be available, and clotting studies should be normal. It is important to be certain that all neonates receive prophylactic vitamin K_1, 1 mg IM, to prevent hemorrhagic disease of the newborn. Preoperative dehydration may cause a false elevation of hematocrit so that blood requirements may actually be increased.

Adequate blood replacement is essential. Whereas an adult must lose approximately 500 ml to suffer a 10% loss of blood volume, the comparable amount in a neonate may be less than 25 ml. The transfusion of blood may be avoided if a postoperative hematocrit of 30 or greater is anticipated, but blood should be administered from the beginning of the operation (on a milliliter-for-milliliter basis) when large losses are expected. Calcium chloride, 10 mg/kg, is useful when hypotension accompanies the rapid administration of blood or plasma that contains citrate as an anticoagulant. Reconstituting packed cells with fresh frozen plasma, 5% albumin, or saline permits rapid administration. An adequately sized intravenous line must be secured preoperatively when much blood loss is anticipated, even if a cutdown is necessary. Great care is necessary to prevent air bubbles from entering the line because unsuspected right-to-left intracardiac shunts may be present (especially in neonates).

The blood volume is approximately 80 ml/kg in children and about 70 ml/kg in adolescents. The acceptable blood loss may be estimated in a number of ways. One useful method is to calculate the red cell mass at the start of the operation (blood volume × hct/100) and the red cell mass with a hematocrit of 30 (blood volume × 30/100). The red cell mass at a hematocrit of 30 is then subtracted from the original red cell mass to obtain the acceptable red cell loss. The acceptable blood loss is approximately 3 times the acceptable red cell loss.

Example
Beginning hct = 40
Weight = 20 kg
1. Estimate blood volume
   20 kg body weight × 70 ml/kg = 1400 ml
2. Estimate red cell mass at the start of the operation
   1400 ml × 40/100 = 560 ml
3. Estimate red cell mass with hct = 30
   1400 ml × 30/100 = 420 ml
4. Estimate acceptable red cell mass loss
   560 ml − 420 ml = 140 ml
5. Estimate acceptable blood loss
   140 ml × 3 = 420 ml

Alternatively, the acceptable blood loss can be estimated by multiplying the percentage of tolerable hematocrit loss (based on a lower limit of 30) by the blood volume (i.e., beginning hct − 30/beginning hct × estimated blood volume).

If the amount of actual blood loss is less than half the acceptable blood loss, replacement is with Ringer's lactate solution. If the loss is greater than this but less than the acceptable blood loss, 5% albumin is used. Losses greater than the calculated acceptable blood loss are replaced with packed red cells diluted with equal amounts of either colloid or crystalloid. In cases of massive blood replacement (greater than the child's blood volume), the administration of fresh frozen plasma (10 ml/kg) and platelets (1 bag/5 kg) may be necessary to correct coagulopathies.

A major part of the blood loss during a craniotomy occurs with the initial surgical incision. Although bleeding from the bone is difficult to control, losses from the scalp can be decreased by the subcutaneous infiltration of lidocaine with epinephrine. Not more than 3 mg/kg of lidocaine should be given at a time. If halothane is used, 1 µg/kg of epinephrine is safe, and 3 times this dose can be used with neuroleptanesthesia (about 0.5 ml/kg of lidocaine 0.5% with 1:200,000 epinephrine). Infiltration of the scalp with lidocaine also provides additional anesthesia for the stimulation caused by the surgical incision.

7. **Drug doses.** All medications should be titrated to effect, although familiarity with average milligram per kilogram requirements is helpful. For emergency situations, doses for children can be estimated as a percentage of the average adult dose.

Dose estimates

Age	Weight (kg)	Fraction of adult dose
Neonate	3	$\frac{1}{10}$
1 yr	10	$\frac{1}{4}$
7 yr	25	$\frac{1}{2}$
12 yr	40	$\frac{3}{4}$

E. Induction

1. **Intravenous induction.** All patients who have major medical problems, whether adults or children, should have an intravenous cannula securely in place before the induction of anesthesia. In children less than 3 years who have high metabolic rates, a critical situation can develop rapidly, and attempts to insert a catheter intravenously under emergency conditions during or after induction can be difficult. Pediatricians routinely place catheters in children of all ages without the child's cooperation; when necessary, anesthesiologists should do the same. The procedure is greatly simplified if local anesthesia is used at the insertion site before placing the catheter. The sicker the child, the easier the procedure.

Once an intravenous catheter is in place, induction can proceed as with adults. If attempts to insert an intravenous line provoke enough crying and struggling to make the procedure extraordinarily difficult, the child probably has adequate intracranial compliance to tolerate an inhalation induction, as described in section **II.E.3.c.** In the presence of intracranial hypertension, spontaneous hyperventilation with oxygen and the use of mannitol, 0.25 to 1 gm/kg, can improve compliance.

2. **Emergency induction.** Intubation is performed in neonates while they are awake. Gastric contents are first emptied with a large suction catheter. Atropine, 0.1 mg, is given beforehand, intramuscularly or intravenously, to prevent a vagal response to laryngoscopy. The effect of awake intubation on ICP in neonates is unknown, but may be less harmful than in older patients because of the immaturity of their nervous systems. At approximately 1 month of age, awake intubation becomes more difficult unless the child is gravely ill or heavily sedated. A rapid sequence induction using a barbiturate, muscle relaxant, and cricoid pressure is preferred for older infants and children after the insertion of an intravenous catheter. A large-bore tube should be used to aspirate gastric contents after intubation is accomplished and before extubation.

3. **Elective surgery**

   a. **Neonates:** awake intubation as described in section **2.**

   b. **Children less than 5 years of age:** Children in this age group usually resist separation from their parents and are frightened by the smell of inhalation anesthetics. Rectal barbiturates (described in section **B.6**) are particularly useful. Once consciousness is blunted, an intravenous catheter can be placed or an inhalation induction performed, as described in section **c.**

   c. **Children more than 5 years of age:** Older children will usually cooperate with an inhalation induction when given this as an alternative to a needle. When the intracranial compliance is reduced, inhalation of halothane to light levels of anesthesia will allow intravenous access to be secured. Early hyperventilation before inhalation agents are introduced appears to blunt the ICP-increasing effects of these cerebral vasodilators in adults, but the effect of this maneuver in children is unknown. It would certainly appear safe, however, to combine the use of muscle relaxants with low concentrations of halothane. The deep level of anesthesia necessary to accomplish intubation using inhalation drugs alone will reduce blood pressure and simultaneously elevate ICP, thereby decreasing CPP.

F. Intubation

1. A small **air leak** should be audible around the endotracheal tube when an airway pressure of approximately 25 cmH$_2$O is applied. If no leak is audible, the tube is probably too large and should be replaced with a smaller one.

2. A rough guide to the choice of **endotracheal size** is as follows:

Age	Size (mm I.D.)
28 weeks' gestation (about 1000 gm)	2.5
28–38 weeks' gestation (1000–3000 gm)	3.0
term neonate	3.5
2 yr	4.5
>2 yr	4.5 + age%

   Example: A 6-year-old child would require a 5.5 tube (4.5 + %)

3. **Cuffed endotracheal tubes** are used only in children who require size 6.0 mm or greater.

4. **Straight laryngoscope blades** are easier to use for children less than 5 years of age.

5. Tubes must be securely fastened with **benzoin,** since slight motion can cause displacement.

6. **Nasal tubes** are easier to secure. If oral tubes are used, they should be placed on the side of the mouth that will be turned upward, so that saliva will not loosen the tape.

7. To prevent gastric dilatation, an **oral airway** should be inserted to allow for the venting of gases that leak around the endotracheal tube. Leaving the orogastric tube used for aspiration of stomach contents in place will also help.

8. **Relaxants**

   a. **Depolarizing drugs:** succinylcholine is frequently used to facilitate intubation because of its rapid onset and brief duration. However, it may induce a hyperkalemic response in patients who have stroke, encephalitis, peripheral nerve injuries, muscular dystrophies, tetanus, spinal cord dysfunction, severe head injuries, burns, or massive trauma. The hyperkalemic response has not been reported to occur with isolated intracranial hypertension, but caution is advised if motor dysfunction is present. Succinylcholine can also initiate malignant hyperthermia in susceptible children. The dose for intubation is 1 to 1.5 mg/kg or 3 to 4 mg/kg IM. It is helpful to pretreat children less than 12 years of age with atropine, 0.01 mg/kg, to prevent the arrhythmias induced in children by the vagomimetic properties of succinylcholine.

b. Nondepolarizing drugs: pancuronium (0.1–0.15 mg/kg) is particularly useful in children, since cardiac output is better maintained when the heart rate is high. Increasing the dose will effect a more rapid onset so that pancuronium may be used when succinylcholine is contraindicated. Curare, 0.5 mg/kg, is usually avoided because of its histamine-releasing properties (unless hypotension is desired and ICP is not elevated). Metacurine, 0.25 mg/kg, has also been used in children.

9. **Lidocaine:** 1.0 to 1.5 mg/kg IV given a few minutes before laryngoscopy and intubation may help blunt the ICP-increasing effects of these procedures in patients who have poor intracranial compliance.

10. **Barbiturates:** thiopental, 4 to 5 mg/kg, or methohexital, 1 to 2 mg/kg, are ultrashort-acting anesthetics that have ICP-lowering properties and may be used for induction. Long-acting barbiturates (pentobarbital and phenobarbital) take longer to equilibrate with the CNS and have more prolonged effects.

G. Anesthetic techniques

1. **Local anesthesia** is not usually applicable to children. Ventricular catheters may occasionally be used to facilitate CSF drainage before induction of anesthesia. Lidocaine should be limited to less than 3 mg/kg during a given case. Local anesthesia may be supplemented with intravenous sedation in adolescents to facilitate brief, usually radiologic, procedures involving little stimulation.

2. **General anesthesia.** Ventilation is controlled in all infants. All the halogenated inhalation anesthetics are cerebral vasodilators, and they should be avoided or used in low concentrations when ICP is elevated until the dura is opened. Halothane is usually chosen, especially since enflurane in combination with hyperventilation may be epileptogenic. Halothane hepatitis has not been reported in children, even after repeated exposure. Isoflurane, at equipotent concentrations, appears to have a smaller vasodilatory effect than halothane on cerebral blood vessels.

   All the intravenous drugs used in adults produce the same effects in children. Numerous cases of sudden and severe increases in ICP have been reported after administration of ketamine, especially in infants and children who have hydro-cephalus. Most other intravenous sedatives reduce CBF and metabolism when ventilation is controlled. A balanced tech-nique using nitrous oxide, oxygen, barbiturates, muscle relax-ants, narcotics, and sedatives can be used for all age groups.

H. Postoperative care. Repeated neurologic examination is the most important factor in assessing postoperative recovery. Deterioration in neurologic function is often a sign of intracranial bleeding. For this reason, it is usually desirable to have the child as fully alert as possible immediately after the operation. Neuromuscular blockade can be pharmacologically reversed with neostigmine (0.06–0.08 mg/kg) and atropine (0.02–0.04 mg/kg). Intracranial pressure can be determined most effectively in unconscious patients by continu-ous monitoring.

Computerized tomographic scans are extremely valuable in evaluating increasing ICP or deteriorating neurologic status to de-termine the presence of surgically correctable causes. Cranial ul-trasound techniques may be useful if the fontanelles are open. Care-ful assessment of fluid and electrolyte status is necessary to avoid imbalances attendant on alterations in secretion of pituitary hor-mone induced by operation. Close observation in an intensive care unit familiar with the care of children is vital to the early detection and treatment, if not prevention, of all postoperative problems.

III. Special procedures. With an understanding of the special problems presented by children, the anesthesiologist can offer the same standard of care to patients of all ages. Each procedure should not be ap-proached as an unusual difficulty, but their special requirements should be taken into account. The following is a brief discussion of the common operations and diagnostic studies that require anesthesia and the relevant considerations.

A. Neurosurgical procedures

1. Craniotomy. Most craniotomies performed in children are for tumors. Brain tumors are the most common solid tumor in childhood and are second only to leukemia as the leading cause of cancer. Contrary to the situation in adults, most pediatric brain tumors are infratentorial. Intracranial hypertension is al-ways a possibility. Additional neurosurgical conditions are aneu-rysms, frequently fatal during childhood, and large arteriove-nous malformations, which may cause congestive heart failure in neonates.

2. Trauma. Accidents are the most frequent cause of death among children. The majority of these fatalities are caused by head injury. Because children may suffer coincident cervical spinal injuries without radiologic evidence of fracture, great care must be taken during tracheal intubation and positioning of the patient. The cribriform plate is easily fractured, and nasal tubes of any sort should be placed with caution (if at all) if the child has midfacial injury or nasal discharge. The prognosis for children suffering severe head injury is much better than it is for adults who have a similar degree of injury.

3. **Craniofacial deformities.** Craniosynostosis, either alone or in combination with facial anomalies (Apert's syndrome and Crouzon's disease), often entail extensive reconstructive procedures involving huge blood loss, and preparations for adequate replacement must be made. Intracranial hypertension may be present if multiple sutures have fused. Drainage of cerebrospinal fluid (CSF) through a lumbar subarachnoid catheter may improve exposure of the surgical field if ICP is not elevated. Controlled hypotension can be used to reduce blood loss when intracranial hypertension is not a problem.

4. **Dysraphism.** Whether dysraphism occurs in the spine (myelodysplasia) or in the head (encephalocele), neurologic deficits are often present. Hydrocephalus usually coexists in children who have neurologic impairment; this is most often due to an associated Arnold-Chiari malformation (a downward displacement of brainstem structures into a deformity of the upper cervical spine). Extremes of head flexion can cause brainstem compression, as it can with tumors of the posterior fossa. Turning the patient on the side may facilitate intubation; if the left side is down, the tongue falls away from the laryngoscope. Neuromuscular blockade must be avoided (or carefully monitored) if the surgeon plans direct stimulation of neural tissue. Other congenital anomalies may coexist in these children.

5. **Hydrocephalus.** Cerebrospinal fluid is shunted from the ventricle to the peritoneum in children who have hydrocephalus. If the distal end is placed in the right atrium, care must be taken to ensure accurate positioning. The child usually has intracranial hypertension; if shunt revision is to be performed, ICP may be reduced preoperatively by withdrawing CSF from the shunt reservoir when only the peritoneal end of the catheter is obstructed. The sudden removal of CSF from the ventricles may result, however, in upward displacement of the brainstem, producing signs similar to brain herniation. Replacement of the fluid (with CSF or saline) can be an effective temporizing measure.

B. **Neuroradiologic procedures** entail special risks. They are usually performed in an environment not designed for pediatric anesthesia and located far from support facilities. When contrast agents are used, the danger of allergic reactions exists. The osmotic load of these agents will induce diuresis so that adequate amounts of fluid should be administered. The anesthesiologist must be certain all necessary equipment is available and functioning.

1. **Computerized tomographic (CT) scan** requires that the patient be immobilized. Intravenous sedation may be necessary for uncooperative patients, but young children are well controlled with rectal barbiturates. Neonates and small babies (5 to 7 kg) can usually be scanned when they sleep immediately after a feeding, but they may require oral or rectal chloral hydrate, 10–20 mg/kg, to guarantee that they remain still.

2. **Arteriography.** The intra-arterial injection of contrast material produces pain and causes children to move. General anesthesia is usually required. Having the patient spontaneously breathe an inhalation anesthetic allows the anesthesiologist to move away from the site of maximum radiation. If intracranial hypertension exists, however, ventilation should be controlled to produce hypocapnia. The resultant vasoconstriction slows the transit time of contrast agents through the brain and improves the resolution of the angiograms.

3. **Pneumoencephalography (PEG)** has been much less common since the advent of CT scanning. If intracranial hypertension is suspected, the study is performed through a ventriculostomy and not by way of the lumbar subarachnoid space. The extreme changes of position during the procedure require that all tubes and lines be firmly anchored and that a patient's distress be promptly detected through close monitoring so he can be returned promptly to the supine position.

   If air is used as the contrast medium, the administration of nitrous oxide (N_2O) as part of the anesthetic will cause expansion of the intracranial gas bubble. This problem may be eliminated by using either O_2 or N_2O as the contrast agent. In comparison with air, the more rapid absorption of N_2O from the ventricles appears to reduce postcontrast headache, but large volumes must be used and the study must be completed quickly before absorption occurs.

   The rapid or excessive injection of any gaseous contrast can precipitate an acute increase in ICP. Slight hyperventilation (to reduce ICP) and light anesthesia and muscle relaxation (to support blood pressure during changes in body position) are indicated. Any injected gas may embolize intravascularly, especially when the patient has a ventriculoatrial shunt.

4. **Myelography and polytomography.** Like pneumoencephalography, these procedures often involve much movement of the patient. All tubes and lines should be secured and any signs of distress must be recognized immediately to initiate therapy. Metrizamide, a water-soluble contrast agent, can produce seizures when introduced intracranially in high concentrations; the patient's head should therefore remain slightly elevated.

5. **Radiation treatment** requires that the anesthesiologist observe the patient from outside the room, usually by television. An ECG and a monitor of respiration (such as an oral airway or a piece of foam rubber taped to the chest) should be readily visible. As with CT scans, rectal barbiturates may be the only anesthetic required, although absolute immobilization for prolonged periods usually entails general anesthesia.

References

1. Allan, D., Kim, H. S., and Cox, J. M. The anaesthetic management of posterior fossa exploration in infants. *Can. Anaesth. Soc. J.* 17:227, 1970.
2. Bruce, D. A., Berman, W. A., and Schut, L. Cerebrospinal fluid pressure monitoring in children: Physiology, pathology and clinical usefulness. *Adv. Pediatr.* 24:233, 1977.
3. Cohen, E. N. (Ed.). Symposium on pediatric anesthesia. *Anesthesiology* 43:141, 1975.
4. Elwyn, R. A., et al. Nitrous oxide encephalography: Five-year experience with 475 pediatric patients. *Anesth. Analg.* (Cleve.) 55:402, 1976.
5. Kallar, S. K., et al. The use of rectal thiopental in children for computerized axial tomography. *Anesth. Rev.* 7:30, 1980.
6. Meridy, H. W., Creighton, R. E., and Humphreys, R. P. Complications during neurosurgery in the prone position in children. *Can. Anaesth. Soc. J.* 21:445, 1974.
7. Raju, T. N. K., Vidyasagar, D., and Papazafiraton, C. Intracranial pressure monitoring in the neonatal ICU. *Crit. Care Med.* 8:575, 1980.
8. Rockoff, M. A. Anesthesia for children with hydrocephalus. *Anesth. Rev.* 6:28, 1979.
9. Rogers, M. C., Nugent, S. K., and Traystman, R. J. Control of cerebral circulation in the neonate and infant. *Crit. Care Med.* 8:570, 1980.
10. Schroeder, H. G., and Williams, N. E. Anesthesia for meningomyelocoele surgery. *Anaesthesia* 21:57, 1966.
11. Shapiro, H. M. Monitoring in Neurosurgical Anesthesia. In L. J. Saidman and N. T. Smith (Eds.), *Monitoring in Anesthesia*. New York: Wiley, 1978. Pp. 171–204.
12. Shillito, J., and Matson, D. D. Craniosynostosis: A review of 519 surgical patients. *Pediatrics* 41:829, 1968.
13. Smith, R. M. *Anesthesia for Infants and Children* (4th ed.). St. Louis: Mosby, 1980.

16. Pediatric Neurogenic Airway and Swallowing Disorders

Lee D. Rowe

This chapter presents a neuroanatomical approach to the evaluation and management of neurogenic airway and swallowing disorders in children. An understanding of pediatric neurogenic abnormalities of the aerodigestive tract also provides guidelines for successful treatment of acquired adult neurogenic airway dysfunction. Anesthetic techniques, perioperative problems, and surgical approaches to supranuclear, nuclear, and infranuclear lesions of the ninth and tenth cranial nerves are analyzed.

I. **Functional anatomy.** Neuronal control of the pharynx and larynx is divided into three elements: supranuclear, nuclear, and infranuclear (Fig. 16-1).

A. **Supranuclear.** Corticobulbar motor fibers originate in area 4 on the rostral side of the sylvian (lateral) fissure, enter the corona radiata, and pass into the internal capsule. Neurons emerge from the cerebral peduncle, forming the pyramidal tracts, and descend through the pons. Decussating and uncrossed fibers terminate in the nucleus ambiguus.

B. **Nuclear**

1. The nucleus ambiguus is the primary source of pharyngeal and laryngeal motor supply. The orientation of adductor and abductor nuclei (which innervate the intrinsic and extrinsic laryngeal muscles) is dorsoventral. **Adductor neurons,** which innervate the lateral cricoarytenoid, cricothyroid (the sole extrinsic laryngeal muscle), interarytenoid, and external thyroarytenoid muscles, are loosely arranged in the dorsal portion of the medulla. **Abductor neurons** innervate the posterior cricoarytenoid muscle (the *only* laryngeal abductor) and form the more compact ventral division.

2. The retrofacial nucleus, rostral to the nucleus ambiguus, is a second source of abductor neurons to the posterior cricoarytenoid muscle and of adductor neurons to the lateral cricoarytenoid muscle.

3. Nuclei controlling deglutition are located within the nucleus ambiguus.

C. **Infranuclear**

1. Efferent axons from laryngeal motor nuclei emerge in the rostral first and second rootlets of the vagus nerve. These neurons cross the posterior cranial fossa and enter the superior (jugular) ganglion at the level of the jugular foramen. Below the jugular foramen, axons are joined by the cranial (bulbar) spinal accessory nerve, which is proximal to the inferior (nodose) ganglion.

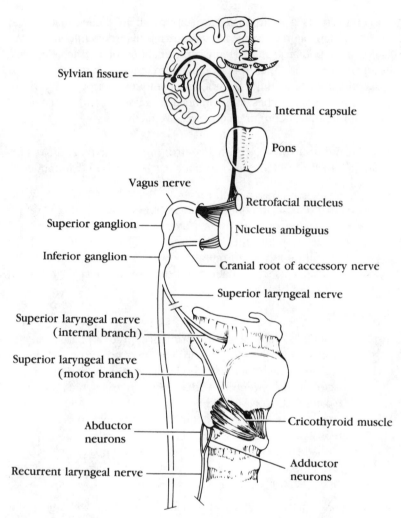

Fig. 16-1. Neuroanatomical pathways of laryngeal function.

This ganglion contains sensory cell bodies of the internal branch of the superior laryngeal nerve, which innervates the entire larynx above the level of the true vocal cords. The external branch of the superior laryngeal nerve carries efferent motor output to the cricothyroid muscle, the chief tensor of the vocal cord.

2. The recurrent laryngeal nerve carries the remaining vagal innervation to the larynx. Abductor and adductor neurons separate into two distinct groups, approximately 1 to 2 cm above their entrance into the larynx. Additional afferent sensory fibers, car-

rying stretch and mucosal receptor information from the true vocal cords and subglottic space, terminate in the nodose ganglion. Secondary neurons ascend to the nucleus solitarius.

3. The pharyngeal plexus, which is separate from the superior laryngeal and recurrent laryngeal nerves, carries motor input to the superior, middle, and inferior pharyngeal constrictor muscles and to striated muscles of the upper esophagus. Pharyngoesophageal sensory output is primarily carried to the nucleus solitarius in the glossopharyngeal and vagus nerves.

II. Physiology

A. Respiration

1. The primitive role of the larynx is to function as a sphincter separating the tracheobronchial tree from ingested material and secretions. Phylogenetically, abductor fibers have appeared only recently and are fewer in number (4:1 ratio of adductor to abductor neurons). With gradual evolutionary conversion to additional respiratory and phonatory roles, the abductor nuclei have received increasing input from the reticular formation neurons and coordinate inspiration through neuronal interconnections with the posterior cricoarytenoid muscle, diaphragm, intercostal muscles, and accessory neck muscles.

2. Respiration requires a complex interaction of the adductor and abductor laryngeal nuclei and reticular formation neurons. During inspiration the vocal cords abduct (Fig. 16-2A). Neuronal output to the posterior cricoarytenoid muscle is increased through the recurrent laryngeal nerve; adductor activity is inhibited. During expiration, slight adduction maintains a physiologic positive end-expiratory pressure.

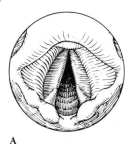
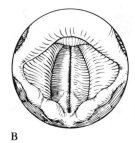

A B

Fig. 16-2. Endoscopic view of the endolarynx. *A.* Inspiration: abduction of the true vocal cords. The posterior cricoarytenoid muscle is the sole abductor of the true vocal cords. *B.* Phonation: midline approximation of the true vocal cords.

3. Phonation requires tensing of the cricothyroid muscle, increased adductor activity, and approximation of the vocal cords in the median position (Fig. 16-2B).

4. Voluntary coughing and reflex clearance of foreign material from the airway are mediated by the nucleus ambiguus.

B. Swallowing

1. Deglutition is initiated by a voluntary oral phase that moves a bolus of food to the base of the tongue and oropharynx. The palate elevates and the lateral wall narrows, stimulating the involuntary pharyngeal phase. Respiration ceases and the larynx rises under the base of the tongue. The constrictor muscle fibers contract sequentially in a rostral-to-caudal direction, and the tonically contracted (15–40 cmH_2O resting pressure) cricopharyngeal muscle relaxes.

2. Food enters the proximal esophagus and is carried by gravity and striated muscle activity in a 100-cm pressure zone to the gastroesophageal junction in 3 to 7 seconds. Normal swallowing function depends, therefore, on adequate mobility of the tongue, sequential relaxation of the cricopharyngeal muscle, and separation of ingested food from the tracheobronchial tree.

III. Etiology and clinical findings

A. Supranuclear lesions

1. Isolated supranuclear anomalies are difficult to recognize in the neonate because lower nuclear pharyngeal and laryngeal reflexes remain intact and speech has not yet been acquired. As a result, supranuclear lesions produce minimal airway, swallowing, or speech dysfunction unless associated with cerebral agenesis, hydrocephalus, or severe encephalitis (Table 16-1).

Table 16-1. Supranuclear lesions

Congenital	Acquired
Hydrocephalus	Hydrocephalus
Cerebral agenesis	Tuberculosis
Kernicterus	Meningoencephalitis
Cerebral palsy	Birth trauma
Charcot-Marie-Tooth syndrome	Cryptococcosis
Toxoplasmosis	
Neurosyphilis	
Intraventricular hemorrhage	
Intra-axial neoplasms	

Table 16-2. Supranuclear lesions: clinical findings

Persistent jaw jerk, snout, Moro, or Babinski reflexes
Delayed speech acquisition
Basal ganglia disorders: rigidity and hyperkinesis
Intact cough and swallowing reflexes

---

    2. Clinical features include persistent abnormal reflexes such as snout, jaw jerk, Moro, and Babinski. Delayed acquisition of speech and disorders of the basal ganglia, including rigidity and hyperkinesia, may be present. Cough and swallowing reflexes are intact. Characteristic signs of spastic dysarthrophonia and slurring of articulation often occur in older children and adolescents (Table 16-2).

B. Nuclear lesions

    1. Nuclear lesions produce striking aerodigestive tract impairment in neonates and infants including dysphagia, aspiration, and upper airway obstruction. Concomitant cranial neuropathies and congenital anomalies are frequently encountered (Table 16-3).

    2. The Arnold-Chiari malformation, a congenital anomaly of the lower brainstem and inferior cerebellum associated with caudal displacement of the medulla, cerebellar tonsils, and fourth ventricle into the upper vertebral canal, is the most common cause of nuclear pharyngolaryngeal dysfunction. Hydrocephalus is severe, and meningomyelocele is almost always present.

    3. Neurogenic airway and swallowing dysfunction probably results from increased intracranial pressure (ICP), which causes intracranial stretching of the vagus, traction on vagal rootlets, and ischemia or hemorrhage from medullary compression. These

Table 16-3. Nuclear lesions

Congenital	Acquired
Brainstem neoplasms	Trauma
Arteriovenous malformations	Polioencephalitis
Dandy-Walker syndrome	Diphtheria
Arnold-Chiari malformation	Rabies
Syringobulbia	Brainstem hemorrhage
Nuclear dysplasia or agenesis	Guillain-Barré syndrome
Riley-Day syndrome	Tetanus
Klippel-Feil syndrome	

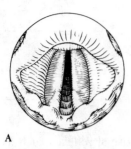 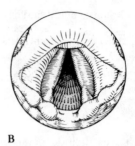

A   B

Fig. 16-3. Endoscopic view of the endolarynx in an infant with bilateral vocal cord paralysis secondary to the Arnold-Chiari malformation. *A.* Inspiration: bilateral abductor vocal cord paralysis with the true vocal cords in the paramedian position. *B.* Phonation: bilateral abductor *and* adductor vocal cord paralysis with both vocal cords in the intermediate position. Failure to achieve closure of the vocal cords during swallowing results in life-threatening aspiration.

conditions frequently develop after removal of the accompanying meningomyelocele or after obstruction of a ventriculoperitoneal shunt previously placed to correct the hydrocephalus. Bilateral impairment of the phylogenetically newer abductor neurons results in paralysis of the vocal cords in the median or paramedian position (Fig. 16-3A). Paradoxically, the cry is normal with high-pitched inspiratory stridor exacerbated by agitation. Persistent adductor neuronal activity probably permits normal phonation (Table 16-4).

Table-16-4. Nuclear lesions: clinical findings

Bilateral vocal cord paralysis	Unilateral vocal cord paralysis
Abductor neurons	Weak or hoarse cry
Normal cry	Minimal stridor or aspiration
Inspiratory stridor	Frequent associated cranial
Minimal aspiration	neuropathies
Vocal cords in paramedian position	Swallowing function: feeding difficulties
Abductor and adductor neurons	
Weak cry	
Minimal inspiratory stridor	
Significant aspiration	
Vocal cords in intermediate position	
Swallowing function	
Feeding difficulties with	
cricopharyngeal achalasia	
Associated cranial neuropathies and	
congenital anomalies	

Table 16-5. Infranuclear lesions

Congenital	Acquired
Congenital heart disease	Trauma
Tracheoesophageal fistula	Botulism
Mediastinal neoplasms	Polyneuritis
Aortic arch anomalies	Demyelinization disorders
	Idiopathic
	Meningitis
	Mediastinitis
	Diphtheria
	Parapharyngeal neoplasms

4. With additional nuclear adductor neuronal involvement, the vocal cords assume a more abducted or intermediate position (Fig. 16-3B). The cry becomes weak and the stridor decreases. However, severe dysphagia and life-threatening aspiration also develop. Children who have the Arnold-Chiari malformation who exhibit these signs should be examined for evidence of increasing ischemia of the brainstem.

5. Bilateral abductor vocal cord paralysis may, in rare circumstances, be inherited as a genetic defect. In addition, dysphagia and aspiration can occur because of either an isolated congenital cricopharyngeal achalasia or pharyngoesophageal dyskinesia. Discoordination of pharyngeal and palatal mobility with failure of cricopharyngeus relaxation results in excessive oropharyngeal secretions, nasal reflux, recurrent aspiration, and bronchopneumonia.

6. Isolated unilateral nuclear vocal cord paralysis is rare but does occur more commonly in association with other brainstem nuclear dysplasia or agenesis. Clinically, the cry is weak or hoarse with minimal stridor and aspiration (see Table 16-4).

C. Infranuclear lesions

1. Congenital infranuclear lesions of the vagus nerve in the neonate are primarily caused by congenital heart disease, mediastinal neoplasms, vascular anomalies, or tracheoesophageal fistulas. Frequently, these disorders are associated with unilateral vocal cord paralysis secondary to recurrent laryngeal nerve involvement (Table 16-5).

2. The cry is weak and one vocal cord is in either the median or the paramedian position (Fig. 16-4A). Aspiration and swallowing

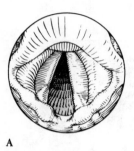 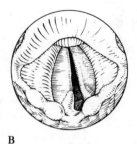

A   B

Fig. 16-4. Right vocal cord paralysis secondary to recurrent laryngeal nerve paralysis. *A.* Inspiration: right vocal cord in paramedian position fails to abduct. *B.* Phonation: the left true vocal cord crosses the midline to approximate the opposite cord
incompletely resulting in a weak, breathy cry. Failure to effect glottic closure completely during swallowing may lead to aspiration.

difficulties may be significant clinical problems, depending on
the degree of compensatory glottic closure by the opposite vocal
cord (Table 16-6; Fig. 16-4B).

3. Acquired infranuclear lesions of the vagus nerve, on the other
hand, frequently involve both vocal cords and affect the recurrent laryngeal nerve, superior laryngeal nerve, and pharyngeal
plexus (see Table 16-5). Infants who have polyneuritis, demy-
elinating disorders, and botulism exhibit a weak or absent cry,
vocal cords in an intermediate position, no stridor, recurrent
aspiration, and difficulty in swallowing. Neonates who sustain
significant cervical trauma during forceps delivery may demonstrate transient unilateral or bilateral vocal cord paralysis. Prolonged intubation of the larynx and trachea may also be associated with recurrent laryngeal nerve injury.

Table 16-6. Infranuclear lesions: clinical findings

Unilateral vocal cord paralysis	Bilateral vocal cord paralysis

Recurrent laryngeal nerve
  Weak cry
  Minimal aspiration
  Normal swallowing
  Vocal cord in paramedian position
Recurrent laryngeal nerve, superior
  laryngeal nerve, pharyngeal plexus
  Weak or absent cry
  Recurrent aspiration
  Vocal cord in intermediate position
  Swallowing function variably im-
    paired
	Recurrent laryngeal nerve, superior
	  laryngeal nerve
	Severe dysphagia
	Aspiration
	Recurrent bronchopneumonia

IV. Diagnosis. Neurogenic laryngeal and swallowing abnormalities are unrecognized in the neonatal period unless associated with significant airway obstruction, aspiration, or other congenital anomalies. Respiratory failure secondary to perinatal anesthetics, hypoxia, or central nervous system damage because of maternal incompatibility or diabetes mellitus must be excluded. In addition, hyaline membrane disease and congenital obstructive lesions of the aerodigestive tract must be ruled out. The congenital lesions include laryngomalacia (the most common cause of congenital laryngeal stridor), subglottic stenosis, and subglottic hemangiomas.

A. In the neonatal period and early infancy, **direct laryngoscopic examination** of the larynx and pharynx provides information concerning vocal cord mobility and the presence or absence of congenital laryngeal and pharyngeal lesions.

B. Careful examination of the cranial nerves and assessment of the quality of respiration provide clues for sites of possible airway obstruction.

1. Stridor represents partial obstruction of the respiratory tract from either external compression of, or partial occlusion within, the air channels. Occurring during inspiration, expiration, or both, the source of the compression may vary from the external nares to the distal bronchioles. The character and intensity of the noise depend on the site and degree of obstruction and the air flow, velocity, and pressure gradient across the point of obstruction. In the evaluation of an infant who has neurogenic airway and swallowing disorders, several signs are useful in localizing the site of obstruction.

a. Normally, inspiration and expiration require approximately equal periods of time. The phase of respiration in which stridor occurs is more likely to be inspiratory in the presence of upper respiratory obstruction.

b. When there is obstruction at the level of the true vocal cords, the stridor is usually high-pitched in character.

c. Stridor during expiration is associated with tracheal and bronchial obstruction. The expiratory phase of respiration is prolonged and the tone of the stridor is lower.

d. Stridor can occur during both inspiration and expiration when there is tracheal obstruction.

2. The quality of the cry remains normal in the majority of infants who have airway obstruction but no laryngeal lesion. A weak or absent cry at birth suggests neurogenic impairment of the vocal cords. Paradoxically, infants who have Arnold-Chiari malformation and bilateral abductor paralysis of the vocal cords may have marked impairment of the airway but a normal cry.

3. With compression of the trachea by either supraglottic tumors or vascular rings, **hyperextension of the neck** is frequently observed. This finding is rare in neurogenic vocal cord disorders, subglottic stenosis, and endotracheal lesions.

4. **Recurrent pneumonitis** is frequently associated with tracheobronchial obstruction, tracheoesophageal fistulas, bilateral abductor *and* adductor neuronal impairment, bilateral recurrent laryngeal and superior laryngeal nerve disorders, and a tracheobronchial foreign body.

C. **Radiographic techniques**

1. **Chest films** during inspiration and expiration are necessary to rule out foreign bodies in the tracheobronchial tree, neoplasms, or cardiac or great vessel anomalies in the mediastinum. Fluoroscopy of the chest during respiration provides additional information when a lucent foreign body of the main bronchus is suspected. Obstructive emphysema will produce a mediastinal shift away from the site of obstruction; atelectasis secondary to complete occlusion of the main bronchus will shift the mediastinum toward the involved side.

2. Nuclear and infranuclear lesions affecting swallowing are most effectively evaluated by rapid **cineradiography** of palatopharyngeal and esophageal motility. Tracheoesophageal fistulas with associated bronchopneumonia and failure to thrive may mimic infranuclear lesions of the vagus nerve and require a **barium swallow** (Fig. 16-5). Occasionally, the diagnosis requires careful endoscopy of the esophagus and tracheobronchial tree under general anesthesia. Cineesophagography is also necessary to rule out isolated cricopharyngeal achalasia.

3. **Plain films of the skull and cervical spine** are obtained in patients in whom congenital nuclear lesions are suspected. The Klippel-Feil syndrome includes a characteristic malformation of the atlanto-occipital joint and vertebrae. Bulging of the lower occipital region is diagnostic of the Dandy-Walker syndrome.

4. Confirmation of the Arnold-Chiari malformation requires **posterior fossa pneumoencephalography or computed tomography** (CT) with metrizamide. CT is also useful in assessing the size of the ventricles before and after insertion of a shunt.

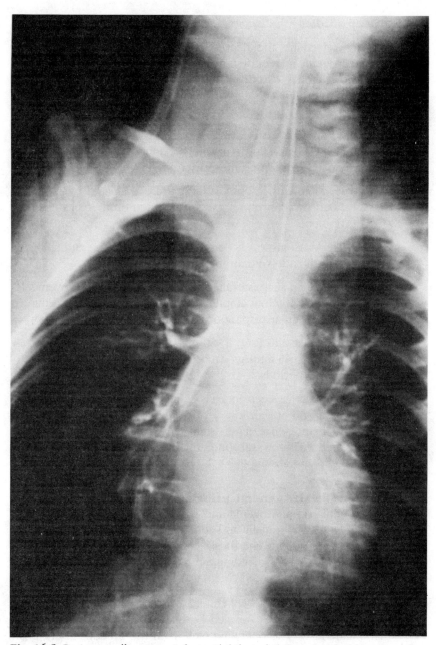

Fig. 16-5. Barium swallow in an infant with bilateral abductor and adductor vocal cord paralysis. A characteristic tracheobronchogram results from nuclear neurogenic dysfunction in an infant with the Arnold-Chiari malformation. There is no filling of the esophagus, and a feeding nasogastric tube can be seen.

D. Sleep studies

1. To determine the degree of sleep-induced exacerbation of neurogenic airway dysfunction, **skin surface oxygen (PsO$_2$) and carbon dioxide (PsCO$_2$) tensions** are continuously monitored during sleep by means of surface electrodes. Associated central, obstructive, or mixed causes of sleep apnea can be identified.

   a. The PsO$_2$ and PsCO$_2$ parallel the arterial O$_2$ and CO$_2$ tensions closely; response times vary from 45 seconds to 2 minutes.

   b. Concomitant respiratory efforts are evaluated by mercury-filled capillary strain gauges mounted on the chest and abdomen.

   c. The nasal airflow is determined by measuring end-tidal carbon dioxide with an infrared CO$_2$ analyzer.

   d. The sleep state is evaluated as active (rapid eye movements, intermittent low amplitude movements of the extremities, and irregular respirations) or quiet (absence of the above).

   e. A decrease in PsO$_2$ to 50 mmHg or less and an increase in PsCO$_2$ to 45 mmHg or more during sleep correlate well with apneic periods.

   f. Obstructive sleep apnea is defined as a complete cessation of nasal and oral airflow during sleep for more than 10 seconds in the presence of persistent chest wall and abdominal movement. With central apnea, thoracic and diaphragmatic excursions are absent.

V. Neuroanesthesia: general principles. Early diagnosis and treatment of pediatric neurogenic and swallowing abnormalities require direct laryngoscopy initially and additional bronchoscopy and esophagoscopy under general anesthesia. Of primary concern is maintaining an adequate airway and avoiding aspiration in patients who have vocal cord paralysis and impaired cough and gag reflexes.

A. Anesthesia is induced with an inhalation anesthetic (halothane or isoflurane) and 100% oxygen by mask while the child breathes spontaneously. The operating table is in the Trendelenburg position.

1. **Suction** is immediately available. Muscle relaxants are not used to preserve pharyngolaryngeal muscle tone and spontaneous respiration, permitting either direct laryngoscopy or intubation. Ventilation may be assisted or controlled to prevent hypoventilation, accumulation of CO$_2$, and ventricular arrhythmias.

2. The surgeon is prepared to perform either bronchoscopy or an **emergency tracheotomy** if the airway becomes obstructed.

3. When the depth of anesthesia is adequate, direct laryngoscopy is performed to evaluate intrinsic laryngeal muscle function during quiet respiration and to rule out congenital laryngeal anomalies such as laryngomalacia or webs. Care is taken not to insert the tip of the laryngoscope into the glottic folds and provoke laryngospasm.

4. **Bronchoscopy** may be accomplished under general anesthesia without the use of an endotracheal tube. After achieving adequate anesthesia by mask, a pediatric ventilating bronchoscope of appropriate size is inserted with the aid of a Jackson pediatric laryngoscope. This plane of anesthesia should be maintained at the conclusion of bronchoscopy to facilitate direct laryngoscopy without danger of laryngospasm.

   It is important to note that during bronchoscopy, the suctioning of secretions and saline introduced into the tracheobronchial tree should be limited to brief periods of time to prevent altered ventilation-perfusion relationships and hypoxia. A mean decrease in arterial O_2 of 12 mmHg has been observed secondary to loss of effective tidal volume during overzealous suctioning and bronchial lavage.

5. When **esophagoscopy** is planned, an endotracheal tube is inserted initially. After completion of endoscopic inspection of the esophagus, the endotracheal tube is removed while the child is still deeply asleep, and the bronchoscope is inserted into the trachea. The function of the vocal cords during quiet respiration may be assessed by direct laryngoscopy after removal of the bronchoscope if a plane of anesthesia sufficient to prevent laryngospasm is maintained.

B. The **endotracheal tube** is removed from infants and children who have neurogenic airway disorders while they are still deeply asleep to prevent laryngospasm, coughing, and straining, which may increase ICP if there is decreased intracranial compliance. Patients are transported and nursed in the lateral decubitus position until fully awake. This places the pharynx in a dependent position and avoids potential aspiration.

VI. **Treatment.** Surgical management of neurogenic disorders of the aerodigestive tract is directed toward alleviation of laryngeal airway obstruction, recurrent aspiration, and dysphagia because these conditions, when coupled with the effect of concomitant hypoxia and poor nutrition on developing brainstem nuclei, may cause periodic apnea,

Table 16-7. Treatment of neurogenic disorders of the aerodigestive tract

Swallowing	Respiration
Upright position	Tracheotomy
Nasogastric tube	Brainstem decompression
Hyperalimentation	Arytenoidectomy
Gavage	Laryngeal reinnervation
Gastrostomy	Ventriculoperitoneal shunt
Cricopharyngeal myotomy	Laryngeal closure
	Teflon injection

sudden infant death syndrome (SIDS), and impaired intellectual development (Table 16-7).

A. Supranuclear lesions (see Table 16-1)

1. Neonates and infants who have congenital supranuclear lesions rarely require surgical intervention unless the lesions are secondary to hydrocephalus or intra-axial neoplasms. Airway and swallowing reflexes remain intact although there is intellectual and functional impairment.

2. Extensive speech therapy, physiotherapy, and feeding assistance may ultimately be necessary for many of these patients.

B. Nuclear lesions (see Table 16-3)

1. Infants who have the **Arnold-Chiari malformation who develop hydrocephalus without vocal cord impairment** are candidates for ventriculoperitoneal shunt. Close observation is necessary because the subsequent development of inspiratory stridor may be an indication of shunt obstruction and increasing ICP, meningitis, or high pressure in the cervical subarachnoid space (with normal ICP). Obstruction of the shunt necessitates immediate revision.

2. Infants who have the **Arnold-Chiari malformation who develop hydrocephalus with bilateral abductor vocal cord paralysis** and airway obstruction require immediate intubation and insertion of a shunt. Airway obstruction and vocal cord immobility resolve within 2 weeks of shunt placement in more than 50% of patients.

   a. Persistent stridor, aspiration, and cyanosis during feeding are indicative of bilateral abductor vocal cord paralysis. Treatment includes decompression of the posterior fossa and cervical canal to the level of the cerebellar tonsils.

b. Infants who exhibit unremitting bilateral abductor vocal cord paralysis will require a permanent tracheotomy to improve respiratory function, prevent airway obstruction and aspiration, and permit increased oral feedings. Tracheotomy may not relieve episodes of central apnea, hypoxia, or cyanosis, so the patient will require apnea monitoring during sleep.

3. **Bilateral abductor paralysis of the vocal cords,** in association with additional adductor neuronal impairment or bilateral superior and recurrent laryngeal nerve paralysis, causes life-threatening aspiration and bronchopneumonia and mandates closure of the larynx.

a. The larynx may be closed by suturing the vocal cords through a laryngofissure approach. A tracheotomy is mandatory.

b. The larynx may be separated from the trachea by closure of the subglottic space and first tracheal ring with creation of a permanent tracheostoma.

4. **Nuclear swallowing dysfunction** is initially treated with semirecumbent positioning, gavage or nasogastric feeding, and frequent nasopharyngeal suctioning.

a. Cricopharyngeal myotomy through a transverse lower left cervical incision is indicated for those children who have isolated cricopharyngeal achalasia but no gastroesophageal reflux.

b. Gastrostomy is reserved for those infants who have severe feeding difficulties and failure to thrive.

c. Parenteral hyperalimentation with carbohydrates, proteins, essential fatty acids, and phospholipids may prevent brain damage from malnutrition.

C. **Infranuclear lesions** (see Table 16-5)

1. **Isolated unilateral paralysis of the left recurrent laryngeal nerve** is the most common type of congenital or acquired infranuclear lesion. When no underlying surgically treatable lesion is identified, these patients are evaluated periodically by direct laryngoscopy. Persistent positioning of the true vocal cord in the paramedian position results in a weak, breathy voice.

This vocal cord malposition is subsequently treated in early adulthood by injection of teflon lateral to the paralyzed vocal cord. The involved cord is mobilized medially and vocal quality is improved by providing an accessible vibratory point for the nonparalyzed cord. This technique is not feasible in neonates or infants because of the extremely small size of the airway, need for general anesthesia, and rapid laryngeal growth. The procedure is done with local anesthesia so the patient can phonate, permitting a judgment as to when an adequate amount of teflon has been injected. In addition to topical 4% lidocaine, bilateral superior laryngeal nerve blocks are performed by injecting two milliliters of 1% lidocaine with a 22-gauge needle 1 cm anterior to the superior corner of the thyroid cartilage in a line drawn midway between the hyoid bone and thyroid cartilage. The ECG is monitored throughout the procedure.

2. **Bilateral paralysis of the recurrent laryngeal nerve** is commonly treated with a tracheotomy and valved Tucker tracheostomy tube. Although used in adults, arytenoidectomy, through either an external or a transoral approach, is not recommended in children because of the aggravation of aspiration and the resultant poor vocal quality.

3. Functional reinnervation of the larynx in adults who have **bilateral abductor paralysis of the vocal cords** has been successful. Neurotization of the posterior cricoarytenoid muscle, the only laryngeal abductor, is achieved through the implantation of a neuromuscular pedicle of the ansa cervicalis nerve and a block of the associated omohyoid muscle. The value of this technique in children is currently unknown, however. Patients who do not have intact posterior cricoarytenoid muscle fibers capable of accepting implanted motor endplates are not candidates for this surgery. Congenitally denervated abductor muscle fibers or fibers traumatically denervated for more than 18 months will probably not be successfully reinnervated. These unique neurogenic airway problems will require a permanent tracheotomy.

References

1. Brown, E. S. Anesthesia in pediatric otolaryngology. *Otolaryngol. Clin. North Am.* 10:113, 1977.
2. Burtner, D. D., and Goodman, M. Anesthetic and operative management of potential upper airway obstruction. *Arch. Otolaryngol.* 104:657, 1978.
3. Fearon, B. Respiratory distress in the newborn. *Otolaryngol. Clin. North Am.* 3:185, 1970.
4. Haddad, G. G., and Mellins, R. B. The role of airway receptors in the control of respiration in infants: A review. *J. Pediatr.* 91:281, 1977.
5. Hart, C. W. Functional and neurological problems of the larynx. *Otolaryngol. Clin. North Am.* 3:609, 1970.
6. Holinger, P. H. Clinical aspects of congenital anomalies of the larynx, trachea, bronchi and esophagus. *J. Laryngol. Otol.* 75:1, 1961.

7. Holinger, L. D., Holinger, P. C., and Holinger, L. D. Etiology of bilateral abductor vocal cord paralysis. *Ann. Otol. Rhinol. Laryngol.* 85:428, 1976.
8. Holinger, P. C., Holinger, L. D., Reicher, T. J., et al. Respiratory obstruction and apnea in infants with bilateral abductor vocal cord paralysis, meningomyelocoele, hydrocephalus, and Arnold-Chiari malformation. *J. Pediatr.* 92:368, 1978.
9. Naeye, R. L. The sudden infant death syndrome. *Arch. Pathol. Lab. Med.,* 101:165, 1977.
10. Rontal, M., and Rontal, E. Lesions of the vagus nerve: Diagnosis, treatment, and rehabilitation. *Laryngoscope* 87:72, 1977.
11. Rowe, L. D., Hansen, T. N., Nielson, D., et al. Continuous measurements of skin surface oxygen and carbon dioxide tensions in obstructive sleep apnea. *Laryngoscope* 90:1797, 1980.
12. Rowe, L. D., and Newfield, P. Airway and swallowing disorders in the Arnold-Chiari malformation. In *Trans. Pac. Coast Otoophthalmol. Soc.* Vol. 61, 1980. Pp. 203–210.
13. Smith, R. M. Pediatric anesthesia in perspective. *Anesth. Analg.* (Cleve.) 57:634, 1978.
14. Snow, J. B., Jr. Clinical evaluation of noisy respiration in infancy. *Lancet* 2:504, 1965.
15. Snow, J. B., and Rogers, K. A. Bilateral abductor paralysis of the vocal cord secondary to Arnold-Chiari malformation and its management. *Laryngoscope* 75:316, 1965.
16. Strohl, K. P., Saunder, N. A., Feldman, N. T., et al. Obstructive sleep apnea in family members. *N. Engl. J. Med.* 299:969, 1978.
17. Venes, J. L. Multiple cranial nerve palsies in an infant with Arnold-Chiari malformation. *Dev. Med. Child Neurol.* 16:817, 1974.
18. Wealthall, S. R., Whittaker, G. E., and Greenwood, N. The relationship of apnea and stridor in spina bifida to other unexplained infant deaths. *Dev. Med. Child Neurol.* 16 (Suppl. 32): 107, 1974.
19. Wolfe, J. A., Rowe, L. D., Pasquariello, P., et al. Tracheotomy for infant botulism. *Ann. Otol. Rhinol. Laryngol.* 88:861, 1979.
20. Wolfsdorf, J. The acute care of respiratory problems in the neonate, infant, and child. *Int. Anesthesiol. Clin.* 13:73, 1975.
21. Work, W. P. Paralysis and paresis of the vocal cords. *Arch. Otolaryngol.* 34:267, 1941.

17. Neuroradiologic Procedures

Bernard Wolfson
William D. Hetrick
Khurshed J. Dastur

Radiology has played an integral part in neurodiagnosis since the introduction of roentgenography in 1895. Although the bony skull and vertebral column provide excellent protection for the enclosed brain and spinal cord, they also make it difficult to obtain information about their contents from simple x-ray films. Contrast material has therefore been injected intravascularly and intrathecally to delineate specific portions of the brain and spinal cord. Dandy injected air into the lateral ventricles in 1918 and into the spinal subarachnoid space in 1919 (pneumoencephalogram). In 1922, Sicard and Forestier injected a radiopaque substance, iodized oil (Lipiodol), into the spinal subarachnoid space (myelogram). Moniz injected radiopaque sodium iodide directly into the carotid artery in 1927, thus performing the first cerebral angiogram. In 1973, the first computed tomographic (CT) brain scanning units were introduced to the United States. This new technique provides information about intracranial contents quickly, efficiently, and noninvasively.

All these techniques are used today. Most of the changes through the years have involved improvements in apparatus, technique, and contrast media to enhance the quality of the radiographs and reduce their general toxic effects.

I. General considerations

A. Evaluation.
The patient requiring a diagnostic procedure should initially undergo a general evaluation. According to the nature of his disease, additional factors must be considered. The presence or absence of increased intracranial pressure (ICP) should be noted. Systemic vascular disease may suggest cerebrovascular disease and, conversely, transient ischemic attacks may suggest generalized as well as cerebral arteriosclerotic disease. Prolonged bed rest after trauma or neurologic disease may cause general debility, which may compound the depressant effect of anesthesia. A hyperkalemic response to succinlycholine has now been noted not only in patients who have burns and acute trauma but also a variety of neurologic diseases including (but not limited to) upper and lower motor neuron lesions, multiple sclerosis, encephalitis, and some muscular dystrophies. Acute head trauma, a common reason for neuroradiologic investigation, may cause unconsciousness, which precludes taking an adequate history. In such instances, the possibility of a full stomach, cervical spine injury, and multiple organ damage must always be considered.

B. Choice of technique.
Although most neurodiagnostic procedures are to some degree invasive and may involve considerable discomfort, none is so traumatic or painful as to make general anesthesia mandatory. These procedures require the patient's total immobility, but in most instances, discomfort can be mitigated and immobility produced by vocal encouragement and sedation. In some cases the patient will not or cannot adequately cooperate, a

situation most commonly found in children who do not comprehend what the procedure involves. An adult may be unable to cooperate because of either fear or disease-related impairment of cerebral function (as in the case of retarded or semicomatose patients). In some instances, general anesthesia with endotracheal intubation, by providing complete airway control and avoiding hypoxia and hypercapnia, may be preferable to the less predictable effects of intravenous sedatives, especially for poor-risk patients.

In most hospitals, radiology suites have not been designed as anesthetizing locations. Anesthetic apparatus must often compete for space with x-ray machines and, in general, conditions are less than optimal. It is essential, however, not to compromise the fundamental requirements of an adequate anesthetic machine and all equipment necessary for administering a general anesthetic and for cardiopulmonary resuscitation. Suction should be available, and monitoring capabilities should be equivalent to the general operating room. Electrocardiographic monitoring is particularly important because, in the presence of controlled ventilation, an arrhythmia may be the earliest sign of pressure on the brainstem. In addition, a defibrillator should be immediately available. This equipment should also be available when sedation is used because of the possibility that general anesthesia may be needed and, more important, because of the potential for complications from the diagnostic procedure.

II. **Computed tomography.** Computed tomography (CT) has become the most widely used neuroradiologic procedure. The quality and detail of the images produced by this noninvasive combination of x-ray and computer instrumentation, coupled with almost total safety, are unparalleled by such conventional techniques as cerebral pneumoencephalography and angiography.

A. **Basic considerations**

1. **Technical facts.** A CT scan provides tomographic images of serial sections through the head. Each image is produced by computer integration of measurements of x-ray absorption obtained by scanning the periphery of the head. The differences in the radiation absorption coefficient between different normal tissues and between normal and abnormal tissues enable the computer to separate these tissues. The image of the brain structures is generated by feeding the relative absorption values (CT numbers) into a cathode ray tube, the brightness of the image being proportional to the absorption value. In addition to being displayed on the cathode ray tube, the image may be obtained on x-ray film, photographed with an instant camera, or transferred to a magnetic disc for permanent storage.

2. **Procedure.** For scanning of the brain, the patient lies on a table with his head inside a rotating gantry (a large square "donut" with a hole in the center, the periphery of which contains the x-ray source, detectors, and associated electronics). In old scanners, the head was encased in a water jacket to eliminate computer artifacts at the scalp level. The water jacket is no longer necessary in new scanners, and the patient's head is simply immobilized with a Velcro belt applied across the forehead. One rotation of the gantry produces one axial slice or "cut." A series of cuts is made; the usual interval is 7 mm but can be larger or smaller, depending on the particular diagnostic information sought. The duration of the procedure reflects the sophistication of the scanner. The first generation scanners took 4½ minutes per cut, whereas the newest scanners take only 2 to 4 seconds per cut. A complete examination of the head usually consists of about 6 cuts. The whole procedure may be repeated after rapid intravenous infusion of contrast medium if contrast enhancement is indicated.

3. **Complications.** Since CT is noninvasive, there are no complications associated with its performance per se. However, examination of the posterior fossa may occasionally require extreme degrees of head flexion, which may either compromise blood flow to the brain or obstruct the airway (including by kinking the endotracheal tube). Many of the CT body scanners can tilt on their axis, eliminating the need for extreme flexion with its associated problems; if available, the body scanners are preferred for examination of the posterior fossa. When contrast medium is injected intravenously, its attendant complications are also possible (see section **VIII**).

4. **Exposure of personnel to radiation.** It has been estimated that anesthesia personnel standing behind a lead screen at the side of a patient undergoing CT scanning will receive a skin dose of 1 to 2 mrad per hour (Aidinis, 1976). This level would make it feasible, if necessary, to participate in a full daily schedule without receiving excessive exposure to radiation.

B. **Management**

1. **Sedation.** Most adults and older children require no medication for a CT scan. Young children may respond well to intramuscular or peroral sedation. Pentobarbital, 6 mg/kg IM in children weighing up to 15 kg and 5 mg/kg IM in children weighing more than 15 kg, may be used. The maximum recommended dose is 200 mg given 20 to 30 minutes before the examination. A mixture containing meperidine hydrochloride (Demerol) 25 mg, chlorpromazine (Thorazine) 6.25 mg, and

promethazine hydrochloride (Phenergan) 6.25 mg in each milliliter has also been suggested. The dose is 1 ml/10–12 kg IM with a maximum dose of 2 ml given 10 to 20 minutes before the procedure. This "cocktail" has been associated with respiratory depression (Mitchell, 1982). Rectal barbiturates (e.g., methohexital, 25 mg/kg) have been used successfully for relatively short procedures (20–25 min). Senile or disoriented adults may be given sedative doses of diazepam (2.5-mg increments IV) and/or small doses of a short-acting narcotic such as fentanyl (0.025-mg increments IV); the usual precautions against respiratory depression must be observed. Special care must be taken when giving sedatives to patients who have head injury or suspected increased ICP. In these cases, it may be preferable to administer general anesthesia with controlled ventilation.

2. **General anesthesia.** General anesthesia may be indicated in situations in which sedation is either hazardous or ineffective (e.g., combativeness or cardiovascular instability). It may also be preferable when there are potential airway problems or when control of ICP is critical. As the patient's head is inaccessible during the CT scan, it is mandatory to place an endotracheal tube, no matter what the reason for using general anesthesia. The scan itself demands only that the patient remain motionless and tolerate the endotracheal tube. Thus, if spontaneous ventilation is acceptable, topical anesthesia (4% lidocaine) to the larynx may be helpful. When ICP is increased, controlled ventilation is essential. When the patient has intracranial hypertension, total flaccidity should be produced before intubation, either with succinylcholine, 1.5 mg/kg, after pretreatment with tubocurarine, 3 mg, or with a nondepolarizing relaxant such as pancuronium, 0.1–0.15 mg/kg. Monitoring of neuromuscular blockade with a peripheral nerve stimulator before intubation is helpful.

   a. **Induction of anesthesia** is performed with thiopental. Anesthesia is maintained with nitrous oxide (N_2O), oxygen, small doses of narcotics, and muscle relaxants. When an inhalation induction is necessary, the lowest concentration permitting insertion of an intravenous cannula should be used; hyperventilation should be instituted as soon as possible. Ketamine increases cerebral blood flow (CBF) and ICP and does not predictably prevent the patient from moving. It is therefore not advocated.

   b. **Control of temperature** is especially important because many of the patients are babies or small children. Scanner rooms are maintained at cool temperatures (approximately

65°F) to avoid artifacts and damage to the circuits (x-ray equipment is heat-sensitive). With early scanners, it was possible to fill the water bag surrounding the head with warm water. Because the water bag is not used with the new machines, the use of standard techniques such as heating lamps and warmed IV solutions may be necessary.

   c. Space is often at a premium in the neurodiagnostic suite. The authors have alleviated this problem in their institution by installing flow meters, gas cylinders, and suction apparatus on a bracket mounted on the wall of the scanner room, thus eliminating the conventional gas machine. A coaxial circuit (Bain Circuit) is used between the bracket and the endotracheal tube, thus keeping the amount of bulky equipment to a minimum.

III. **Pneumoencephalography.** Pneumoencephalography is rarely performed in centers possessing a CT scanner. In some institutions, however, it is still important in the diagnosis of small mass lesions in the sellar and cerebellopontine angle regions. Also, pneumoencephalography is still used where scanners are unavailable. After the introduction of gaseous contrast into the lumbar subarachnoid space, the patient undergoes a number of positional changes to move the gas intracranially, including forward or backward somersault maneuvers. "Minor" complications include headache, nausea, vomiting, tachycardia, bradycardia, extrasystoles, hypotension, and hypertension. Intraprocedural and postprocedural headache and nausea combine to make pneumoencephalography one of the most uncomfortable and unpopular diagnostic procedures to which patients have ever been submitted. Major complications include cardiovascular collapse, air embolus, respiratory irregularities, and herniation of the cerebellar tonsils and brainstem with potential fatality.

   A. Sedation. Despite the discomforts caused by pneumoencephalography, it is most commonly performed using sedation without general anesthesia. This is partly because the serious complications already described are probably more easily diagnosed if the patient is conscious and partly because of the technical problems associated with positional changes and the presence of bulky x-ray apparatus. A useful technique consists of the intermittent administration of a tranquilizer (such as diazepam in 2.5-mg increments) intravenously as a sedative and amnesic in combination with a short-acting narcotic (such as fentanyl in 0.025-mg increments) for the severe headache that usually develops after administration of the gas.

   If hypotension in response to positional change occurs, especially if accompanied by bradycardia, it should be treated aggressively, lest syncope develop. Either ephedrine in 5-mg increments or an infusion of metaraminol, 20 mg/250 ml, is useful because of the short duration of action. Once the gas has been injected, it is not uncommon for hypertension rather than hypotension to occur. Nausea is also common, as is headache. Both nausea and hypertension commonly respond well to droperidol, 2.5 to 7.5 mg IV. The headache is often resistant to modest doses of narcotic, and care must be taken that overenthusiastic medication does not lead to impaired consciousness, hypoventilation, or even apnea.

B. General anesthesia. Nitrous oxide should not be included as part of the general anesthetic when air is used as the gaseous contrast because N_2O is approximately 30 times more soluble in blood than nitrogen. Because of this, the nitrogen component of the air introduced into the ventricles may be replaced by much larger quantities of N_2O, leading to undue distention of the ventricles and increased ICP.

The anesthetic technique should be selected to avoid both over-exaggeration of postural responses and increases in ICP from hypercapnia, anesthetic drugs, and coughing or straining on the endotracheal tube. A technique using thiopental, muscle relaxant, and controlled ventilation, with or without the addition of small doses of narcotic, is usually satisfactory. Intravenous lidocaine has also been suggested as a useful supplement. N_2O need not be included in such a technique.

N_2O may, and indeed must, be used as part of the anesthetic technique when N_2O instead of air is used as the contrast medium. If N_2O is not included, it is absorbed so swiftly from the ventricles that it is almost impossible to obtain adequate films. This technique has the advantage from the patient's point of view of causing less postinvestigation morbidity: because of the rapidity of absorption of N_2O from the ventricles, the headache caused by the presence of gas in the ventricles is reduced. When air has been used as the contrast medium, it remains in the ventricles for a considerable length of time; any subsequent anesthetic administered within a week of the study (and perhaps even longer) should not include N_2O.

Shortly after its introduction into clinical practice, ketamine was suggested as a good drug for pneumoencephalography because of its ability to produce anesthesia while maintaining cardiovascular and respiratory reflexes. Ketamine's effect on ICP, which later became apparent, tempered initial enthusiasm and made it unsuitable for use during pneumoencephalography. Even in the absence of intracranial hypertension, the intracranial compliance may be impaired to such an extent that the patient is unable to tolerate any further increase in ICP.

The effects of the rare but dangerous complications of air embolus and brainstem herniation may be difficult to distinguish from each other and from acute cardiovascular collapse from anesthesia. If the air has not yet been injected intrathecally, then air embolus is not the cause; if a large quantity of CSF has just been drained, herniation is the probable diagnosis. If air has just been injected or if cardiovascular collapse is preceded by sudden hyperventilation, then air embolus may be suspected. The treatment of cardiovascular collapse, whether from air embolus, brainstem herniation, or anesthetic drugs, consists of immediate resumption of the supine position and the initiation of cardiopulmonary resuscitation. Additionally, the left lateral position may be helpful for air embolus. If the diagnosis of brainstem herniation is confirmed, then the reinjection of fluid into the lumbar subarachnoid space in an effort to disimpact the brainstem may be considered.

IV. **Angiography.** Computerized tomography has reduced the use of angiography in neurodiagnosis. Unlike pneumoencephalography, however, angiography is still used fairly frequently to delineate the vasculature of either the brain or the spinal cord. Technical advances in recent years include the use of catheter techniques for selective angiography and of contrast media that are less toxic and cause less discomfort. The introduction of catheters through the femoral and axillary arteries has virtually replaced the direct puncture of the common carotid artery. In addition to eliminating the hazards of puncturing the common carotid artery, the use of catheters allows the selective study of the internal and external carotid systems and the vertebrobasilar system of the posterior circulation. The injection of contrast into the internal carotid artery eliminates facial discomfort in the distribution of the external carotid artery, which was one of the main subjective complaints associated with common carotid injection. Patients may still, however, experience a burning sensation behind the eye or a flash of light.

Accompanying the reduction in discomfort has been a reduction in the number of patients requiring general anesthesia. The anesthesiologist may be asked, however, to administer sedative medications and to monitor the patient's vital signs and neurologic function. It is therefore important to understand the risks and problems associated with angiographic techniques.

A. **Spinal cord angiography.** Angiography of the spinal cord, pioneered by Djindjian in France, virtually always involves selective studies and subtraction techniques. Many of the patients have damage to the cord already. The possibility of further spinal cord damage induced by the injection of contrast is a significant hazard. Although the examination may be prolonged and therefore uncomfortable, it is usually performed without general anesthesia so the patient's neurologic status can be assessed after each injection of contrast medium. Paroxysmal contractions of the lower limbs (which may occur when dye is injected into the anterior spinal artery) respond to the direct injection of diazepam, 5 mg, through the angiography catheter.

B. Complications. Arterial puncture and catheterization may produce arterial spasm, hematoma, or embolization of arteriosclerotic plaques or thrombi forming at the tip of the catheter. Injection into the wall of the vessel may cause either subintimal dissection or occlusion of the vessel. The contrast media, all of which are iodine-containing salts, produce vasodilatation that in turn causes burning discomfort in the area supplied by the vessels injected. The degree of vasodilatation is affected by the osmolality of the contrast medium. Although solutions of low osmolality are becoming available, those currently in common use, such as meglumine iothalamate (Conray), are highly ionized with resultant high osmolality.

Serious neurologic complications from contrast media include dizziness, convulsions, unconsciousness, hemiplegia, blindness, and aphasia. These effects are related to the hyperosmolality of the contrast medium, which may temporarily impair the blood-brain barrier and allow the medium access to brain cells. The damage may also be caused by hypoxic microvascular damage. The concentration of the agent appears to be the critical factor.

Premonitory signs such as slurring of speech or confusion should suggest the need for termination of the procedure. For more serious problems (e.g., hemiplegia, aphasia, or blindness) that do not resolve swiftly after discontinuation of the procedure, a number of therapies have been recommended including the use of steroids and low molecular weight dextran and the elevation of systemic blood pressure by vasopressors to restore blood flow to the areas that have presumably become ischemic.

Allergic reactions to contrast media include itching nose, sneezing, and conjunctival swelling; mild cardiovascular changes such as bradycardia or tachycardia; and marked hypotension and arrhythmias (see section **VIII**). Respiratory problems include bronchospasm, laryngeal edema, and respiratory arrest. Pulmonary edema, congestive heart failure, and even cardiac arrest may occur.

C. Anesthetic management

1. Sedation. Sedation has a number of advantages over general anesthesia for angiography. These advantages may be lost, however, if the patient becomes confused or unconscious from the drugs administered. For this reason the drugs should be selected with care and given in small incremental intravenous doses. The use of a short-acting narcotic such as fentanyl may ameliorate some of the discomfort and provide some mood elevation but care should be taken to avoid respiratory depression. The addition of diazepam in incremental doses may also be valuable but the achievement of hypnosis may be quite unpredictable with this combination. The patient's level of consciousness should therefore be ascertained regularly. The phenothiazines, although effective sedatives, should not be used in these cases because of their ability to lower the convulsive threshold. Droperidol rarely produces unconsciousness in modest doses and, when combined with a narcotic, may be valuable; its ability to produce Parkinson-like central nervous system symptoms should be kept in mind.

2. **General anesthesia.** General anesthesia for angiography is more comfortable for the patient and ensures complete immobility during x-ray exposures. Some European radiologists believe that general anesthesia is essential where subtraction techniques* are used but in the United States, general anesthesia is rarely requested to improve the radiological technique. General anesthesia may be necessary, however, for uncooperative patients and for young children.

In planning the anesthetic technique, some factors should be considered. If hyperventilation is used to produce a moderate reduction in $PaCO_2$ ($PaCO_2$ 30–35 mmHg), a greater concentration of the contrast medium will be produced by constricting cerebral vessels and slowing cerebral circulation. This improvement in the clarity of the film is of particular value in children whose fast cerebral circulation times make it difficult to obtain good angiograms. The new rapid-filming techniques have made hyperventilation a refinement rather than a necessity, however. Hyperventilation has also been shown to improve the quality of angiograms in patients who have brain tumors because it provokes intracerebral steal. In contrast, the cerebral vasodilatation induced by the inhalation drugs may produce the opposite effect. If these drugs are necessary, hyperventilation should be established before their introduction and continued during the study. However, a technique using thiopental, muscle relaxant, N_2O/O_2, and controlled ventilation, with or without additional narcotics, is usually satisfactory.

---

*A radiologic process in which the shadows of the bony skeleton are "subtracted" from the final x-ray picture, leaving the vascular shadows intact. It requires obtaining a series of identical films before and after the injection of dye.

Because of the neurotoxicity of the contrast agents and the potential toxicity of the anesthetic drugs, it is essential that the patient be adequately monitored during general anesthesia. As hypoxia can mimic many of the toxic effects of the anesthetic and contrast drugs, the use of an in-line oxygen analyzer to measure the concentration of inspired oxygen is essential.

There should be open communication between the radiologist and the anesthesiologist, especially with regard to the patient's blood pressure. If the contrast medium is injected during a period of hypotension and if compensatory vasoconstriction is taking place, the proportion of dye delivered to the brain and spinal cord will be greater than anticipated because these vascular beds do not take part in the compensatory process. As the toxicity of these agents is related to their concentration, their toxicity may increase. This effect may be enhanced if a predominantly alpha-adrenergic vasopressor is used to treat the hypotension.

The use of an alpha agonist to treat hypotension before the injection of dye differs from the situation in which toxic symptoms have already appeared and a vasopressor is used in an effort to improve cerebral circulation. In the latter instance, the dye has already been distributed. If hypotension does occur, therefore, it is wise to advise the radiologist and avoid injection during this time. The hypotension is probably best treated initially by withdrawal of anesthetic drugs and administration of fluid. If urgent therapy is required, the use of a predominantly beta-adrenergic drug such as ephedrine may be preferable.

V. Myelography. It is uncommon for the anesthesiologist to be involved in myelography except for studies in children who may not cooperate during the spinal puncture and the required positioning. Since the patient is prone, almost any anesthetic technique that ensures protection of the airway may be used. The introduction of metrizamide (Amipaque), a water-soluble contrast agent, has occasioned greater involvement of the anesthesiologist. Metrizamide has a number of advantages over iophendylate (Pantopaque). It is much less viscous and therefore disperses more widely within the CSF, giving better definition of the conus and the nerve roots. Being water soluble, it is also totally absorbed from the CSF and cleared by the kidneys and therefore does not require removal by way of either the original or a second lumbar puncture. There is also no evidence associating arachnoiditis with the use of metrizamide. Unlike the other water-soluble agents, metrizamide is nonionic and therefore not grossly hypertonic, which reduces its potential neurotoxicity.

Metrizamide's disadvantage is that headache occurs in 21% to 62% of patients and nausea in 13% to 39% of patients. In the majority of cases this presumably represents chemical toxicity rather than spinal headache from lumbar puncture since the 22-gauge needle used in most studies reduces CSF leakage. Most reactions occur 6 hours after the injection of material into the lumbar sac, reflecting a mean time for peak intracranial concentration.

Because metrizamide is readily absorbed from the subarachnoid space, the blood level increases rapidly, which may cause allergic reactions similar to those seen with venography and angiography. Pharmacokinetic studies reveal that metrizamide appears in the blood in approximately 15 minutes; and the concentration peaks at approximately 2 hours. Metrizamide can also cause mental changes including confusion, disorientation, nightmares, hallucinations, hyperacusis, lightheadedness, depression, dysphagia, and anxiety as well as convulsions, presumably from cortical irritation. Seizures are more likely to occur with the concomitant use of drugs that lower the epileptigenic threshold (e.g., phenothiazines, MAO inhibitors, and alcohol), with higher volumes or concentrations of metrizamide, with increased cortical contact time, and in patients who have a seizure disorder. If general anesthesia is required during metrizamide myelography, the use of ketamine should probably be avoided because of its associated EEG changes. Side effects of metrizamide can be prevented by good hydration before and after the study. Maintaining the patient in the semierect position is also important.

VI. **Therapeutic embolization.** The expertise obtained by the radiologist during selective angiography has now been applied to producing selective occlusion of extracranial and intracranial vessels to obliterate feeding arteries of arterial venous malformations, to close carotidcavernous sinus fistulas, or to decrease the vascularity of tumors. Embolization may be either an adjunct to or a substitute for surgery. Occlusion may be produced by particulate emboli (e.g., absorbable gelatin sponge [Gelfoam]), by polymerizing agents (glue), or by detachable balloons.

A. **Complications.** Each technique is associated with problems: vessels may be occluded inadvertently; arterial hemorrhage may occur after injury to the vessel wall by a balloon. In addition, as selective angiography is part of each technique, the possibility of a reaction to the contrast medium is always present.

B. **Management**

1. **Sedation.** It is essential that the diagnosis of neurologic complications be made immediately. The procedures are therefore preferably performed without general anesthesia. Because the

procedures are potentially hazardous and may be prolonged, uncomfortable, and, at some stages, even painful, the involvement of the anesthesiologist is essential to ensure adequate monitoring, cooperation, and comfort. Modest doses of neuroleptic drugs (droperidol, 0.1 mg/kg; fentanyl, 0.002 mg/kg) may be used, either alone or as an adjunct to the use of hypnotic suggestion to produce the necessary conditions. Constant monitoring is essential with particular attention to level of consciousness, motor strength, respiratory and cardiac rhythms, and blood pressure. If signs suggestive of cerebral ischemia appear (e.g., hemiplegia, slurred speech, altered level of consciousness, or aphasia), the procedure should be discontinued immediately. Other measures to promote cerebral blood flow (CBF) include the use of low molecular weight dextran and maintenance of blood pressure in the high normal range, using pressors if necessary, in an effort to maintain cerebral perfusion.

2. **General anesthesia.** General anesthesia is required for infants and children. It is important to prevent movement during the procedure but consciousness should be restored as soon as possible so that a neurologic evaluation may be carried out. The most practical method of achieving these aims involves the use of N_2O/O_2, a muscle relaxant, and controlled ventilation. Whether thiopental or an inhalation drug is used for induction will depend on the availability of suitable veins and the cooperation of the patient. Normocapnia or modest hypocapnia should be maintained; hypocapnia is necessary when inhalation drugs are used. Sudden changes in vital signs should be correlated with the radiologist's activity. The presence of hypertension and bradycardia should raise concern about a possible intracranial hemorrhage.

VII. **Nuclear magnetic resonance.** Nuclear magnetic resonance (NMR) is a new imaging modality that does not use ionizing radiation, depending rather on magnetic fields and radio frequency pulses for the production of its images. It is now available in only a few centers, yet there is little doubt that its use will spread rapidly. Although it produces images similar to those obtained with CT, it has certain advantages over this technique. For example, it can differentiate clearly between white and gray matter in the brain, thus making possible the in vivo diagnosis of multiple sclerosis. It can also display its images in sagittal, coronal, or axial planes with equal ease and, unlike computed tomography, is effective in visualizing disease in the posterior fossa.

There is, as yet, virtually no reported experience of anesthetic management for patients undergoing NMR imaging, but the presence of a powerful magnetic field as an integral part of a unit introduces specific unique problems: anything affected by a magnetic field will either affect or be affected by the unit. For example, television monitors will not function adequately within 20 feet of an NMR unit. Fortunately, the technique is painless and noninvasive; thus the potential role of the anesthesiologist is limited. However, a supportive role either in providing sedation, monitoring, or resuscitation must certainly be envisaged, and it must be assumed that special techniques (perhaps using specialized apparatus and monitoring devices) will be devised. At this time, an anesthesiologist asked to assist with NMR imaging will presumably employ his or her own imagination and resourcefulness to provide adequate monitoring, particularly of respiration, and to allow for immediate resuscitation should the patient's condition deteriorate suddenly.

VIII. **Adverse reactions to contrast media.** Reactions to intravascularly administered contrast media vary from pruritus, mild rashes, and vasomotor phenomena (flushing, burning) on injection to anaphylactic reactions including dyspnea, wheezing, syncope, and cardiovascular collapse. Although these reactions are immediate in onset and mimic IgE-mediated allergic responses, they most likely result from the nonimmunologic release of histamine and other vasoactive mediators from mast cells and basophils (Kelly, 1974). Pulmonary function studies have shown reduction in the peak flow rate and FEV_1 after contrast administration in normal patients. This effect is more pronounced in patients who have a history of allergies. The mildest of these reactions require little, if any, treatment other than reassurance, whereas the most severe of these reactions are truly life-threatening and necessitate immediate treatment.

A. **Basic considerations**

1. **Incidence.** In a prospective study reported by the Committee on Contrast Media of the International Society of Radiology in 1975 (Shehadi, 1975), there was a 2.33% incidence of nonfatal reactions and 4 fatal reactions in 27,628 vascular studies. As many as 500 deaths occur in the United States each year (Lieberman, 1980). Repeat studies in patients who have had a previous untoward response were associated with a threefold increase in reactions as compared to the general population.

2. **Predictive tests.** There are no generally accepted predictive tests. Intradermal testing is unreliable (Witten, 1973) and has been virtually abandoned. The use of small intravenous doses of contrast before the procedure is not a sure method of detection and has been associated with some deaths.

B. Management

1. **Prophylaxis.** Patients who have either allergies or a history of reaction to intravascularly administered contrast media should be evaluated by an allergist and medicated with corticosteroids and antihistamines for 36 to 48 hours before the proposed injection of contrast (Zweiman, 1975). A suggested regimen consists of prednisone, 25 mg q.i.d. and either hydroxyzine, 25 mg, or diphenhydramine (Benadryl), 50 mg q.i.d., starting 2 days before injection of contrast and continued for 24 hours after the investigation (Miller, 1975). In addition, diazepam, 10 mg, is given intramuscularly 30 minutes before the patient comes to the x-ray department; diphenhydramine, 50 mg, is given intravenously immediately before the examination. It is essential to be prepared for all degrees of resuscitation.

2. **Treatment.** Rashes or mild vasomotor reactions require little except reassurance and intravenous diphenhydramine. A severe anaphylactic reaction, including respiratory distress from bronchospasm or laryngeal edema, severe hypotension, or syncope, may be treated with epinephrine 1:1000 subcutaneously or intravenously in doses of 0.3 to 0.5 ml in an adult. Bronchospasm may respond to aminophylline, terbutaline (0.25 mg subcutaneously), or nebulized isoproterenol. Intravenous fluids and pressors will be necessary to treat hypotension. Arrhythmias should be controlled with antiarrhythmic drugs, cardioversion, or both. Corticosteroids may be required in pharmacologic doses. Endotracheal intubation with positive pressure ventilation may be necessary, as well as cardiopulmonary resuscitation if cardiac arrest occurs.

References

1. Aidinis, S. J., Zimmerman, R. A., Shapiro, H. M., et al. Anesthesia for brain computer tomography. *Anesthesiology* 44:420, 1976.
2. Campkin, T. V. General anaesthesia for neuroradiology. *Br. J. Anaesth.* 48:783, 1976.
3. Ferrer-Brechner, T., and Winter, J. Anesthetic considerations for cerebral computer tomography. *Anesth. Analg.* 56:344, 1977.
4. Kelly, J. F., and Patterson, R. Anaphylaxis—Course, mechanisms and treatment. *J.A.M.A.* 227:1431, 1974.
5. Lieberman, P., Siegle, R. L., and Taylor, W. W. Anaphylactoid reactions to iodinated contrast material. *J. Allergy Clin. Immunol.* 62:174, 1980.
6. Miller, W. L., Doppman, J. L., and Kaplan, A. P. Renal arteriography following systemic reaction to contrast material. *J. Allergy Clin. Immunol.* 56:291, 1975.
7a. Mitchell, A. A., Louik, C., Lacouture, P., et al. Risks to children from computed tomographic scan premedication. *J.A.M.A.* 247:2385, 1982.
7. Shehadi, W. H. Adverse reactions to intravascularly administered contrast

media; A comprehensive study based on a prospective survey. *Am. J. Roentgenol. Radium Ther. Nucl. Med.* 124:145, 1975.

8. Witten, D., Hirsch, F. D., and Hartman, G. W. Acute reactions to urographic contrast medium. Incidence, clinical characteristics, and relationship to history of hypersensitivity states. *Am. J. Roentgenol.* 119:832, 1973.

9. Wolfson, B., and Hetrick, W. D. Anesthesia for Neuroradiologic Procedures. In J. E. Cottrell and H. Turndorf (Eds.), *Anesthesia and Neurosurgery*. St. Louis: Mosby, 1980. Pp. 138–149.

10. Zweiman, B., Mishkin, M. M., and Hildreth, E. A. An approach to the performance of contrast studies in contrast material-reactive persons. *Ann. Intern. Med.* 83:159, 1975.

Index

Index

Abortion, spontaneous, 236
Abscess, cerebral
  in pregnancy, 227
  syndrome of inappropriate antidiuretic
    hormone secretion after, 168
Acceleration-deceleration injury, 283, 284,
    291, 314. *See also* Automobile ac-
    cidents
Acetazolamide, 11–12, 353
Acetoacetate, and cerebral metabolism in
    starvation, 10
Acid-base disturbances, 103–106. *See also*
    Acidosis; Alkalosis
Acidosis
  in central neurogenic hyperventilation, 110
  cerebrospinal fluid lactic, 302
  and oxyhemoglobin dissociation curve,
    101
  primary metabolic, 105–106
  primary respiratory, 103–105
  renal compensation in, 105
  vasopressor drugs for, 165
Acoustic neuroma, 50
Acromegaly, 263, 265, 272, 273
Adenoid hypertrophy, in pediatric patient,
    355
Adenosine diphosphate (ADP), and inor-
    ganic phosphate, 10–11
Adenosine triphosphate (ATP) depletion, re-
    tarded by hypothermia, 90
Adenosine triphosphate (ATP) equation, in
    cerebral production of phosphate
    compounds, 10–11
Adrenalin. *See* Epinephrine
Adrenergic agonists, 125–126. *See also*
    specific drugs
  alpha-
    and angiography, 400
    avoidance of in pregnancy, 236
    and fetal hypoxia, 234
    and surgery for head trauma, 330
    and vasoconstrictors, 125–126
  beta-, 132–133, 137
  and sympathomimetic amines, 126
Adrenergic antagonists. *See also specific*
    drugs
  alpha-
    droperidol. *See* Droperidol
    phenoxybenzamine, 344
  beta-
    and control of arrhythmia, 137
    and control of hypertension, 138
Adrenergic receptors
  beta-2, 133
  in cerebral arteries, 128
  in cerebral circulation, 122
  and positive inotropic drugs, 134–135
  presynaptic and postsynaptic, 126
  stimulation by catecholamines, 126

Adrenocorticotropic hormone (ACTH), 263,
    264, 267, 269, 270–271, 310
Adriamycin, and free-radical formation, 64
Adult respiratory distress syndrome (ARDS),
    71
  and blunt chest trauma, 107
  and continuous positive airway pressure,
    109
  and fat embolism syndrome, 113
  vs. neurogenic pulmonary edema, 109, 167
  pathophysiology of, 109
  and pulmonary capillary wedge pressure,
    109
  and shock, 303–305
Aerodigestive disorders. *See* Pediatric neuro-
    genic aerodigestive disorders
Aging, and free-radical activity, 64
Air-contrast study, and posterior fossa proce-
    dures, 247. *See also* Pneumoenceph-
    alography
Air embolism
  as angiography complication, 398
  after head trauma, 327
  and pneumoencephalography, 397
  and posterior fossa procedures, 252–254,
    256, 257
  in transsphenoidal procedures, 277–278
Airway pressure, positive, 109, 116–117. *See
    also* Ventilation
Alcohol
  in aspiration pneumonitis, 111
  and gastrointestinal tract bleeding, 312
  instillation, in spinal cord injury, 342
  and metrizamide interaction, 401
Alcoholics, subdural hematomas in, 284
Aldosterone, 310
Alkalosis
  and oxyhemoglobin dissociation curve, 101
  primary metabolic, 106
  primary respiratory, 105–106
Allergic reactions to contrast medium, 369,
    393, 398, 401, 403–404
Allergies in pediatric patient, 355
Alveolar concentration, minimum, 36
Amblyopia, tobacco, as contraindication to ni-
    troprusside, 199
Amenorrhea, 272, 308
ε-Aminocaproic acid (Amicar), 178, 230
Aminophylline, 131
  for cerebral arterial spasm, 141, 179
  in contrast media reaction, 404
  and fluid management of cerebral vaso-
    spasm, 166
Amipaque. *See* Metrizamide
Amitriptyline, potential interactions with,
    148
Amnesia, 283
Amyloidosis in spinal cord injury patients,
    350

Droperidol—*Continued*
and cerebral hemodynamics, 23–24
and cerebral metabolism, 317
and evoked potential monitoring, 47–48
and head trauma, 324
pharmacologic characteristics of, 130
in posterior fossa procedures, 256, 258
during surgery for head trauma, 331
and therapeutic embolization, 402
Drowning, near-, barbiturates for, 62, 74, 76, 83–84
Drug overdose, and controlled ventilation, 116
Drugs. *See also specific drugs and drug types*
anticancer, and free-radical formation, 64
anticholinesterase, avoidance in pregnancy 236
and blood-brain barrier, 121–122. *See also* Blood-brain barrier
teratogenic, 227, 234, 235–236
Dysplasia, nuclear, 377
Dysraphism, 368

ECG. *See* Electrocardiography
Edema
and barbiturates, 65, 68, 71
brain, and intraoperative fluid management, 162
cardiogenic pulmonary, 111
cerebral, 66–68, 162, 165, 213
and head trauma, 286, 287, 291, 316
in hypertension, 143, 145, 146
cytotoxic, 66–68
and failure of sodium-potassium pump, 66
interstitial pulmonary, 257
and ischemia, 66–68
neurogenic pulmonary, 110–111, 166–167
vs. adult respiratory distress syndrome, 109
and head trauma, 305–306
and no reflow into capillaries, 66–67
spinal, 339
vasogenic, 66
Edrophonium, after transsphenoidal procedures, 276
EEG. *See* Electroencephalography
Elastic stockings, 183
Electro-Cap, 32
Electrocardiography (ECG)
and barbiturates, 88
in carotid endarterectomy, 218, 219
continuous, for neurosurgical patient, 117
after head trauma, 306–307, 326
before intracranial aneurysm surgery, 189
and neuroradiologic procedures, 392
in posterior fossa procedures, 249, 258
and spinal shock, 340
in subarachnoid hemorrhage, 187–188
after surgery for intracranial aneurysm, 203

Electrodes. *See also* Electrophysiologic monitoring
in evoked potential monitoring, 46
gold cup, 31
Silastic, 31
subdermal platinum, for somatosensory evoked potentials, 53
wick, 31, 55
Electroencephalography (EEG)
abnormal patterns, 36–37
biocalibration, 34
during carotid endarterectomy, 30–31, 36, 40, 218, 219
and cerebral blood flow, 3, 125
cf. Cerebral Function Monitor, 219
and cardiac output, 125
and cerebral perfusion pressure, 4, 29
and enflurane, effect on seizure patterns, 20
and generator cells, 33
and head trauma, 297, 329
and intracranial aneurysms
before induction of anesthesia, 190
and intraoperative rupture, 185
isoelectric, thiopental after head injury, 77
normal patterns, 35–36
and oxygenation, compromised, 29
and pharmacologic management, 56
and physiologic management, 57
and preoperative assessment, 55
signal processing and display, 37–43
alarm generation, 43
automated pattern recognition, 43
Cerebral Function Monitor, 39–40
compressed spectral array, 37–39
Fast Fourier Transform, 37
hardware, 39
Neurometrics Monitor, 42–43
single-channel, 30, 31
traditional recording, 33–34
waves, beta, delta, and theta, 35–36
Electrolytes. *See also* Fluid management of the neurosurgical patient; *specific electrolytes*
composition of body fluid, 156, 158–159
after head trauma, 297, 310
imbalance, 161
intracellular vs. extracellular, 155, 156
and intracranial aneurysm, 187
loss, 158
in pediatric neurosurgical patient, 360–361
in posterior fossa procedures, 257, 259
potassium, 159
sodium, 158
in spinal cord injury, 349–350
after surgery for intracranial aneurysm, 183
zinc, 159
Electrophysiologic monitoring. *See also specific types*
and cerebral perfusion pressure, 29